Clinical Review of Vascular Trauma

Anahita Dua • Sapan S. Desai
John B. Holcomb • Andrew R. Burgess
Julie Ann Freischlag

Editors

Clinical Review of Vascular Trauma

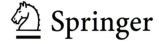

Springer

Editors
Anahita Dua, MD
Department of Surgery
Medical College of Wisconsin
Milwaukee, WI
USA

Center for Translational Injury Research
Houston, TX
USA

Sapan S. Desai, MD, PhD, MBA
Department of Surgery
Duke University
Durham, NC
USA

Department of Cardiothoracic
and Vascular Surgery
University of Texas Medical School
Houston, TX
USA

John B. Holcomb, MD
Division of Acute Care Surgery
Department of Surgery, Center for
Translational Injury Research (CeTIR)
Houston, TX
USA

Department of Surgery
University of Texas
Houston, TX
USA

Andrew R. Burgess, MD
Department of Orthopedic Surgery
University of Texas
Houston, TX
USA

Julie Ann Freischlag, MD
John Hopkins Medical Institutions
Baltimore, MD
USA

ISBN 978-3-642-39099-9   ISBN 978-3-642-39100-2   (eBook)
DOI 10.1007/978-3-642-39100-2
Springer Heidelberg New York Dordrecht London

Library of Congress Control Number: 2013950485

Dedicated to all of our trauma patients – past, present, and future

Foreword

The American Heritage Dictionary of the English Language defines evolution as a gradual process in which something changes into a significantly different, especially more complex or more sophisticated, form. The same dictionary defines revolution in several ways. For this foreword, I would use an assuredly momentous change in any situation. I believe these two definitions apply to the last 10 years in vascular injuries. What has caused this evolution/revolution? Clearly, there are many issues. To a great extent, it is the vendors who provide endovascular stents in the rapid evolution from the original stents for the thoracic aorta to almost any vessel in the human body. An equally important concept was when surgeons stepped forward and learned the techniques of interventional radiologists. Another evolutionary concept was the hybrid operating room where surgery could be carried out as well as placement of endovascular prosthetics. This is an extremely important concept because we are just now developing management protocols in patients with vascular injuries. There are some significant problems. When does the surgeon make a decision to locate the injury with open surgery, tomography, or arterial visualization with injected contrast agents into the vascular system? Alternatively, if an injury can be demonstrated, it may be simpler to control the bleeding blood vessel (artery or vein) by balloon technology. Protocols and treatment algorithms will help as more experience is gained over the next few years. It will be particularly important to define our limitations particularly in some vascular areas. The use of stents may not be the best for intracranial acute vascular injuries.

This book *Clinical Review of Vascular Trauma* is one of the first of many to take on the challenge of defining the problems today, and in their first part they address vascular surgery essentials. This part outlines general vascular principles such as the use of vascular diagnostics, scoring systems, and the hematologic perspectives that includes a discussion on anticoagulation, vascular trauma resuscitation, and hemostatic monitoring. The subject of anticoagulation is extremely important. From my perception, anticoagulation contributes more to morbidity than any one other single entity. Other chapters in vascular surgery essentials include an overview of vascular trauma, a chapter on the mangled extremity, and another chapter by Burgess on fasciotomy. These are important due to recent activities in the Middle East as well as the bombing in Boston. The chapter on surgical critical care is particularly important because I believe the vascular surgeon must be involved in critical care decisions. Very few interventional radiologists care about surgical critical care and delegate it to other specialties. There must be surgical input!

The rest of the book is dedicated to the various regions of the anatomy, and the second part is on cerebral vascular and upper extremity injuries. This part is particularly important because of the limitations of some of the bony canals and the skull base.

The third part is on the chest which is the area where endovascular surgery had its beginnings. The fourth part is on abdominal vascular injuries and focuses on the abdominal aorta and the branches. I think there is particular merit in having a separate subsection of the IVC and other major veins. During my surgical career I have gained a major respect for large veins. I have successfully repaired avulsion of the left hepatic vein in two patients and avulsion of the right hepatic vein in two patients with one survivor.

The pelvis is the fifth part and this can be very important to the patient with grade IV and V pelvic fractures.

The sixth part covers the lower extremity and this particular anatomical region is evolving rapidly. I am also pleased to see a special consideration of military injuries, pediatric and vascular trauma, neurologic injuries, and the use of shunts particularly in far forward military situations. This concept could be used in rural areas, particularly farm country where vascular injuries are common but the surgeons are not there to care for them. Why not teach the same concepts of shunts to the rural general surgeon?

I believe that modern vascular trauma surgery is an exciting and worthwhile venture. Hopefully, we will be able to develop treatment protocols based on experience that would tell us whether to open a chest or abdomen to gain control or we can do it with balloons above or below the injury or directly in the injured artery or vein.

Portland, OR, USA   Donald Trunkey, MD

Preface

Caring for people who are afflicted by trauma is an honor and a privilege. These people who come into our trauma bays are exactly that, people; hence in trauma, there is no such thing as a "vascular" patient, an "orthopedic" patient, or a "plastics" patient. There is but the patient.

As surgeons we certainly strive to provide excellent, holistic care for our patients but sometimes the silo nature of our healthcare systems hinders instead of helps. Specialist services have taken over for the general surgeon in many areas with a noble aim: to provide expert care by dedicated surgeons. However, this double-edged sword can simultaneously prevent us from engaging as we should with other disciplines, and it is this issue of communication that can lead to devastating consequences for our patients. This book was inspired by a patient who sustained a gunshot wound to the abdomen resulting in a bowel and iliac injury. After trauma surgery stabilized the patient, vascular surgery was consulted to fix the iliac artery injury. They opted to use vein graft which got infected and disintegrated 7 days later, leading to frank hemorrhage and near death for our patient. As per the "vascular" literature, the choice of conduit was correct: a contaminated field meant vein graft to reduce the infection risk. However, recent "trauma" literature from the Iraq and Afghanistan wars advocated for the use of prosthetic graft in a contaminated field to avoid the complication we faced with our patient. The correct approach here would have been for both the vascular and trauma teams to have been aware of each other's literature so an informed, best-practice decision could have been made for our patient. This text is an attempt to bring together evidence from multiple fields that are involved in the care of trauma patients with vascular pathology.

This book is broken down by vessel injury so it may serve as a reference for any orthopedic, vascular, trauma, acute care, plastics, or cardiothoracic surgeon during that 2 AM trauma call. Every part has been meticulously reviewed by surgeons from various disciplines so that chapters provide a consensus between the disciplines. Our senior editors include a professor of trauma and acute care surgery (Dr. Holcomb), a professor of vascular surgery (Dr. Freischlag), and a professor of orthopedic surgery (Dr. Burgess) along with a vascular fellow (Dr. Desai) and myself (Dr. Dua) a general surgery resident. We are an example of the team that would come to the trauma bay to take care of a vascular trauma patient, and all viewpoints are an essential part of this book as they should be an essential part of patient care.

This text includes dedicated chapters on the mangled extremity and fasciotomy, written by Dr. Burgess, an orthopedic surgeon. In our medical system,
mangled extremities are managed by the trauma or vascular surgery team.
Today, barely any house staff have any orthopedic rotations or basic clinical
experience in the diagnosis of high-energy musculoskeletal injury, especially
when combined with significant vascular injury. Therefore, a text of this
nature brings the orthopedic viewpoint to the forefront so it can be a consideration during a trauma call by all members of the surgery teams involved.

The overall mission of this book is to optimize the care of trauma patients
using a multidisciplinary approach.

Houston, TX, USA   Anahita Dua, MD

Contents

Contributors

Ahmed Al-Adhami, MBChB (Hons), MSc Department of Cardiothoracic Surgery, Golden Jubilee National Hospital, Glasgow, UK

Abdul Aziz, MBChB Department of Trauma and Orthopaedic Surgery, Queens Medical Centre, Nottingham, UK

Ali Azizzadeh, MD Department of Cardiothoracic and Vascular Surgery, University of Texas Medical School, Houston, TX, USA

Memorial Hermann Heart and Vascular Institute, Texas Medical Center, Houston, TX, USA

Gabriel J. Bietz, MD Division of Vascular and Endovascular Surgery, Department of Surgery, University of Kentucky, Lexington, KY, USA

Walter Biffl, MD Department of Surgery, Denver Health Medical Center, University of Colorado School of Medicine, Denver, CO, USA

Joseph L. Bobadilla, MD Division of Vascular and Endovascular Surgery, Department of Surgery, University of Kentucky, Lexington, KY, USA

Karen J. Brasel, MD, MPH Division of Trauma and Critical Care, Department of Surgery, Medical College of Wisconsin, Milwaukee, WI, USA

Kellie Brown, MD Division of Vascular Surgery, Department of Surgery, Medical College of Wisconsin, Milwaukee, WI, USA

Andrew R. Burgess, MD Department of Orthopedic Surgery, University of Texas, Houston, TX, USA

Ruth L. Bush, MD, MPH Department of Surgery, Texas A&M Health Science Center College of Medicine, Round Rock, TX, USA

John Byrne, MCh, FRCSI (Gen) Department of Surgery, Albany Vascular Group, Albany Medical College, Albany, NY, USA

Division of Vascular Surgery, Albany Medical Center Hospital, Albany, NY, USA

Kristofer M. Charlton-Ouw, MD Department of Cardiothoracic and Vascular Surgery, University of Texas Medical School at Houston, Houston, TX, USA

Raul Coimbra, MD, PhD Division of Trauma, Surgical Critical Care and Burns, Department of Surgery, University of California San Diego Health Sciences, San Diego, CA, USA

Todd W. Costantini, MD Division of Trauma, Surgical Critical Care and Burns, Department of Surgery, University of California San Diego Health Sciences, San Diego, CA, USA

R. Clement Darling III, MD Department of Surgery, Albany Vascular Group, Albany Medical College, Albany, NY, USA

Division of Vascular Surgery, Albany Medical Center Hospital, Albany, NY, USA

Sapan S. Desai, MD, PhD, MBA Department of Surgery, Duke University Medical Center, Durham, NC, USA

Department of Cardiothoracic and Vascular Surgery, University of Texas Medical School, Houston, TX, USA

Anahita Dua, MD Department of Surgery, Medical College of Wisconsin, Milwaukee, WI, USA

Center for Translational Injury Research, Houston, TX, USA

John F. Eidt, MD, FACS Division of Vascular Surgery, Greenville Health System, University Medical Center, Greenville, SC, USA

Charles J. Fox, MD Department of Surgery, Denver Health Medical Center, University of Colorado School of Medicine, Denver, CO, USA

Julie A. Freischlag, MD Department of Surgery, The Johns Hopkins Hospital, Baltimore, MD, USA

Mario G. Gasparri, MD Division of Cardiothoracic Surgery, Department of Surgery, Medical College of Wisconsin, Milwaukee, WI, USA

Ronald I. Gross, MD Division of Trauma and Emergency Surgery, Department of Surgery, Tufts University School of Medicine, Boston, MA, USA

Division of Trauma, Acute Care Surgery and Surgical Critical Care, Baystate Medical Center, Springfield, MA, USA

Neal C. Hadro, MD Department of Surgery, Tufts University School of Medicine, Baystate Vascular Services, Boston, MA, USA

Division of Vascular Surgery, Baystate Medical Center, Springfield, MA, USA

Linda Harris, MD Division of Vascular Surgery, Department of Surgery, State University of New York (SUNY), Buffalo, NY, USA

Nathan P. Heinzerling, MD Division of Pediatric Surgery, Children's Hospital of Wisconsin, Milwaukee, WI, USA

Department of Surgery, Medical College of Wisconsin, Milwaukee, WI, USA

Jennifer A. Heller, MD Division of Vascular Surgery, Department of Surgery, The Johns Hopkins Hospital, Baltimore, MD, USA

John B. Hijjawi, MD Departments of Plastic Surgery and General Surgery, Medical College of Wisconsin, Milwaukee, WI, USA

John B. Holcomb, MD Division of Acute Care Surgery, Department of Surgery, Center for Translational Injury Research (CeTIR), Houston, TX, USA

Department of Surgery, University of Texas, Houston, TX, USA

Robert Houston IV, MD Department of Surgery, San Antonio Military Medical Center, Houston, TX, USA

Pär I. Johansson, MD, DMSc, MPA Section for Transfusion Medicine, Capital Region Blood Bank, Rigshospitalet University of Copenhagen, Copenhagen, Denmark

Department of Surgery, Center for Translational Injury Research (CeTIR), University of Texas Medical School – Houston, Houston, TX, USA

William F. Johnston, MD Department of Surgery, University of Virginia, Charlottesville, VA, USA

Jeremy S. Juern, MD Department of Trauma and Critical Care, Medical College of Wisconsin, Milwaukee, WI, USA

Melina R. Kibbe, MD Division of Vascular Surgery, Northwestern University Feinberg School of Medicine, Chicago, IL, USA

Daniel H. Kim, MD Department of Neurosurgery, University of Texas Medical School at Houston, Houston, TX, USA

David R. King, MD Division of Trauma, Emergency Surgery and Surgical Critical Care, Department of Surgery, Massachusetts General Hospital, Boston, MA, USA

M. Margaret Knudson, MD Department of Surgery, University of California San Francisco, San Francisco, CA, USA

Department of Surgery, San Francisco General Hospital and Trauma Center, San Francisco, CA, USA

Leslie M. Kobayashi, MD Division of Trauma, Surgical Critical Care and Burns, Department of Surgery, University of California San Diego Health Sciences, San Diego, CA, USA

John F. Kragh Jr., MD Department of Surgery, US Army Institute of Surgical Research, Fort Sam Houston, TX, USA

Laura A. Kreiner, MD Department of Surgery, University of Texas Medical School at Houston, Houston, TX, USA

SreyRam Kuy, MD, MHS Department of Surgery, Division of Vascular Surgery, Medical College of Wisconsin, Milwaukee, WI, USA

Mark A. Mattos, MD Division of Vascular Surgery, Department of Surgery, Wayne State University, Detroit, MI, USA

Jason McMaster, MD Obstetrics and Gynecology Resident, Medical College of Wisconsin, Milwaukee, WI, USA

Martin A.S. Meyer, BSc Section for Transfusion Medicine, Capital Region Blood Bank, Rigshospitalet, Copenhagen University Hospital, Copenhagen, Denmark

Department of Surgery, Center for Translational Injury Research, The University of Texas Health Science Center, Houston, TX, USA

David J. Milia Division of Trauma and Critical Care, Department of Surgery, Medical College of Wisconsin, Milwaukee, WI, USA

Erica L. Mitchell, MD Division of Vascular Surgery, Oregon Health and Science University, Portland, OR, USA

Victor A. Moon, MD Department of Surgery, Hofstra North Shore – LIJ School of Medicine, Hempstead, NY, USA

Laura J. Moore, MD, FACS Division of Acute Care Surgery, Department of Surgery, Shock Trauma Intensive Care Unit – Memorial Hermann Hospital, The University of Texas Health Science Center at Houston, Houston, TX, USA

Jessica O'Connell, MD Division of Vascular Surgery, Ronald Reagan UCLA Medical Center, Los Angeles, CA, USA

Bhavin Patel, MD Department of Medicine, Medical College of Wisconsinm, Milwaukee, WI, USA

Rushad D. Patell, MD Department of Medicine, Medical College Baroda and SSG Hospital, Vadodara, Gujarat, India

Jasmeet S. Paul, MD Division of Trauma and Critical Care, Department of Surgery, Medical College of Wisconsin, Milwaukee, WI, USA

K. Shad Pharaon, MD Division of Trauma, Critical Care and Acute Care Surgery, Oregon Health and Science University, Portland, OR, USA

Nicolas H. Pope Department of Surgery, University of Virginia, Charlottesville, VA, USA

Todd E. Rasmussen, MD Department of Surgery, USA Institute of Surgical Research, Joint Base San Antonio, Fort San Houston, TX, USA

Jesper B. Ravn, MD Department of Cardiothoracic Surgery, Rigshospitalet, Copenhagen University Hospital, Copenhagen, Denmark

Amy B. Reed, MD Vascular Surgery, Heart and Vascular Institute, Penn State Hershey Medical Center, Hershey, PA, USA

Justin L. Regner, MD Trauma, Critical Care and Acute Care Surgery, Scott and White Memorial Hospital, Texas A&M University, Temple, TX, USA

Peter Rhee, MD, MPH Surgical Critical Care, Burns and Emergency Surgery, University of Arizona, Tucson, AZ, USA

Peter J. Rossi, MD Division of Vascular Surgery, Department of Surgery, Medical College of Wisconsin, Milwaukee, WI, USA

Harleen K. Sandhu, MD Department of Cardiothoracic and Vascular Surgery, School of Public Health, University of Texas Health Science Center at Houston, Houston, TX, USA

Thomas T. Sato, MD Division of Pediatric Surgery, Children's Hospital of Wisconsin, Milwaukee, WI, USA

Department of Surgery, Medical College of Wisconsin, Milwaukee, WI, USA

Martin A. Schreiber, MD Department of Surgery, Oregon Health and Science University, Portland, OR, USA

Sherene Shalhub, MD, MPH Division of Vascular Surgery, University of Washington, Seattle, WA, USA

Mark L. Shapiro, MD, FACS Department of Trauma, Duke University Medical Center, Durham, NC, USA

Nicholas M. Southard, DO Division of Vascular Surgery, Department of Surgery, Medical College of Wisconsin, Milwaukee, WI, USA

Jessica R. Stark, MD Department of Neurosurgery, University of Texas Medical School at Houston, Houston, TX, USA

Benjamin W. Starnes, MD Division of Vascular Surgery, University of Washington, Seattle, WA, USA

William B. Tisol, MD Division of Cardiothoracic Surgery, Department of Surgery, Medical College of Wisconsin, Milwaukee, WI, USA

Donald D. Trunkey, MD Section of Trauma and Critical Care, Department of Surgery, Oregon Health and Science University, Portland, OR, USA

Gilbert R. Upchurch Jr., MD Division of Vascular and Endovascular Surgery, Department of Surgery, Molecular Physiology and Biological Physics, University of Virginia, Charlottesville, VA, USA

John A. Weigelt, MD Division of Trauma and Critical Care, Department of Surgery, Medical College of Wisconsin, Milwaukee, WI, USA

John W. York, MD Division of Vascular Surgery, Greenville Health System, University Medical System, Greenville, SC, USA

Abbreviations

AAST	American Association for the Surgery of Trauma
ABC	Airway, breathing, and circulation
ABI	Ankle-brachial index
ACS	American College of Surgeons
ADP	Adenosine diphosphate
AIS	Abbreviated injury score
AP	Anterior-posterior
APTT	Activated partial thromboplastin time
ASA	Aspirin
AT	Anterior tibial
ATLS	Advanced trauma life support
AV	Arteriovenous
AVF	Arteriovenous fistula
BAAI	Blunt abdominal aortic injury
BAI	Blunt aortic injury
BCI	Blunt cardiac injury
BCVI	Blunt cerebrovascular injury
BPM	Beats per minute
BRAI	Blunt renal artery injury
BTAI	Blunt thoracic aortic injury
CABG	Coronary artery bypass graft
CAD	Coronary artery disease
CAG	Coronary angiography
CCA	Common carotid artery
CCD	Charge-coupled device
CFA	Common femoral artery
CFD	Color flow duplex
CKD	Chronic kidney disease
CNS	Central nervous system
COT	Committee on Trauma
CPN	Common peroneal nerve
CPU	Central processing unit
CT	Computed tomography
CTA	Computed tomographic angiography
DBP	Diastolic blood pressure
DIC	Disseminated intravascular coagulation
DP	Dorsalis pedis

DSA	Digital subtraction angiography
DUS	Duplex ultrasonography
DVT	Deep vein thrombosis
EAST	Eastern Association for the Surgery of Trauma
ECA	External carotid artery
ECMO	Extracorporeal membrane oxygenation
ECRB	Extensor carpi radialis brevis
ECRL	Extensor carpi radialis longus
ED	Emergency department
ePTFE	Expanded polytetrafluoroethylene
FAST	Focused assessment with sonography in trauma
FDA	Food and Drug Administration
FFP	Fresh frozen plasma
FWB	Fresh whole blood
FXIII	Factor XIII
GCS	Glasgow coma score
GDA	Gastroduodenal artery
GONR	Graphene oxide nanoribbon
GSW	Gunshot wound
GWOT	Global war on terror
HES	Hydroxyethyl starch
HOCM	High-osmolar contrast media
HR	Heart rate
HU	Hounsfield unit
IAOB	Intra-aortic occlusion balloon
IAVI	Intra-abdominal venous injury
ICA	Internal carotid artery
ICU	Intensive care unit
IFU	Instructions for use
IMA	Inferior mesenteric artery
IMV	Inferior mesenteric vein
INR	International normalized ratio
IOCM	Iso-osmolar contrast media
ISS	Injury severity score
IV	Intravenous
IVC	Inferior vena cava
IVU	Intravenous urography
KE	Kinetic energy
KUB	Kidney, ureters, and bladder
LMWH	Low-molecular-weight heparin
LSA	Left subclavian artery
LTA	Light transmission aggregometry
Ly	Clot lysis
M	Mass
MA	Maximum amplitude
MAI	Minimal aortic injury
MDCT	Multidetector row computed tomography
MESS	Mangled extremity severity score

MRA	Magnetic resonance angiography
MRI	Magnetic resonance imaging
MT	Massive transfusion
MTP	Massive transfusion protocol
MVC	Motor vehicle collision
NaCl	Sodium chloride
NAP	Nerve action potential
NBCA	N-butyl cyanoacrylate
NPO	Nil per os
NTDB	National Trauma Data Bank
OIS	Organ injury scale
PCI	Percutaneous coronary intervention
PFA	Profunda femoral artery
PLT	Platelet
POSSUM	Physiological and operative severity score for the enumeration of mortality and morbidity
PRBC	Packed red blood cells
PRN	As needed
PT	Posterior tibial
PT	Prothrombin time
PTFE	Polytetrafluoroethylene
PV	Portal vein
PVA	Polyvinyl alcohol
R	Reaction time
RBC	Red blood cell
RNA	Ribonucleic acid
ROTEM	Rotational thromboelastometry
RR	Respiratory rate
RT	Resuscitative thoracotomy
RTS	Revised trauma score
SBP	Systolic blood pressure
SFA	Superficial femoral artery
SMA	Superior mesenteric artery
SMV	Superior mesenteric vein
T	Temperature
TAG	Thoracic aortic graft
TAVI	Transfemoral aortic valve implantation
TEE	Transesophageal echocardiography
TEG	Thromboelastography
TEP	Trauma exsanguination protocol
TEVAR	Thoracic endovascular aneurysm repair
TF	Tissue factor
TIA	Transient ischemic attack
tPA	Tissue plasminogen activator
TPN	Total parenteral nutrition
TPT	Tibioperoneal trunk
TRA	Tibiopedal retrograde access
TRISS	Trauma and injury severity score

TTE	Transthoracic echocardiography
US	Ultrasonography
V	Velocity
VAC	Vacuum-assisted closure
VAI	Vertebral artery injury
VATS	Video-assisted thoracoscopic surgery
VHA	Viscoelastic hemostatic assay
VTE	Venous thromboembolism
vWF	von Willebrand factor
WTA	Western Trauma Association

Introduction

At an urban trauma center, a 15-year-old victim of violence arrives in the emergency department with a GSW through his knee. His distal femur is shattered and his popliteal artery and vein are transected. In the operating room, the orthopedic surgeons bring his leg out to length and stabilize the fracture with an external fixator, while the trauma surgeons harvest the saphenous vein from the opposite leg for the interposition graft. Meanwhile, in the mountains of Afghanistan, a Marine on foot patrol suffers a dismount injury as the result of an IED. His buddy applies a tourniquet to his injured extremity, and he is brought to a Role 4 far forward post where a general surgeon from a community hospital who serves in the Army reserve inserts a shunt into his superficial femoral artery and prepares the warrior for transfer to a combat support hospital where an Air Force vascular surgeon will perform the definitive repair of the vascular injury. And somewhere in the middle of the United States, a young woman survives a major motor vehicle crash but arrives in hemorrhagic shock bleeding from her pelvic fracture. An interventional radiologist successfully performs an embolization of her internal iliac artery and then assists the vascular surgeon with placement of the endovascular stent that bridges across her lacerated thoracic aorta.

As can be appreciated from the above scenarios, the field of vascular surgery does not belong to any one discipline. Indeed, the recently published, multicenter study authored by Shackford et al. (J Trauma Acute Care Surg, 2013;74:716) illustrates that trauma/general surgeons and vascular surgeons have equivalent outcomes following repair of peripheral vascular injuries as long as the principles of both vascular surgery and trauma surgery are adhered to. Recognizing the multidisciplinary nature of the subject, the editors of this textbook have included authors from a wide variety of fields, a feature that makes this textbook both unique in its contributions and useful as a reference for physicians who encounter vascular injuries, regardless of their training and irrespective of the setting.

The book is divided into seven parts. The first part contains a useful review of the advantages and limitations of various imaging techniques in the diagnosis of vascular injuries by Byrne and Darling. They emphasize three relatively recent valuable advances in this area: the omnipresent computed tomographic angiography (CTA), FAST ultrasound exams, and the "hybrid" operating room that facilitates diagnosis, open, and endovascular techniques, all of which can be accomplished without moving the patient out of the room. The chapter on hematologic perspectives by Johansson should be required reading for all physicians dealing with vascular trauma. He emphasizes the importance of an organized transfusion therapy including packages of red blood cells, plasma, and platelets guided by viscoelastic hemostatic assays (VHA) provided by TEG or ROTEM. The potential benefit of antifibrinolytic agents such as TXA following severe injury and shock is a relatively recent discovery and one that requires further investigation. Another proposed topic ripe for prospective research is the development of a scoring system that is capable of predicting mortality based on the severity of the vascular injury. Also unique to this vascular textbook is a chapter on ICU care containing detailed guidelines for monitoring for compartment syndrome in neurologically impaired patients, control of blood pressure in patients with blunt thoracic aortic injuries undergoing delayed repair, the medical treatment of blunt cerebral vascular injuries, and recommendations on venous thromboembolic prophylaxis in critically injured patients.

The next five parts include in-depth descriptions on the management of vascular injuries by anatomic area: cerebrovascular and upper extremity, thoracic, abdominal, pelvic, and lower extremity. Brasel and her coauthor reemphasize the importance of the hybrid operating room for the treatment of the notoriously difficult bleeding vertebral artery injury. Hadro and Gross highlight the major innovations from military and civilian experience that have improved upper extremity limb salvage including arterial repair over ligation, enhanced resuscitation and transport programs, targeted antibiotic therapy, imaging techniques, microvascular repair, an understanding of the importance of concomitant vein repair, timely fasciotomy, endovascular techniques, and VAC wound care therapy. Although uncommonly encountered, the review of radial and ulnar arterial injuries is valuable and suggests that hand surgeons should be considered part of the "vascular trauma team." The overview of chest trauma includes a contemporary review of the indications for and technique of performing emergency department thoracotomy, an appropriate study for all physicians involved in vascular trauma. Pharaon and Schreiber provide an excellent description of the technique of endovascular repair of the subclavian artery and once again emphasize the value of a hybrid operating room for such procedures. The complications of TEVAR therapy for thoracic aortic injuries, nicely summarized in the chapter by Al-Adhami, should be familiar to all vascular surgeons, trauma and acute care surgeons, as well as interventional radiologists. Another unique feature in this book is the chapter on the diagnosis and treatment of thoracic duct injuries, adding VATS to the treatment algorithm.

In the part on abdominal vascular injuries, Starnes reviews newer techniques in the management of blunt aortic injuries including the use of chest tubes as temporary shunts and placement of a transfemoral intra-aortic occlusion balloon (IAOB) for temporary control preoperatively and categorizes the types of injuries that could be managed nonoperatively and which ones would be amenable to endovascular approaches. Placement of an IAOB can be lifesaving and should be mastered by all surgeons who provide emergency coverage. Coimbra and coauthors provide a nice review of abdominal vascular anatomy and the various approaches to injuries of these vessels. In the chapter on iliac artery injuries, we are again reminded that outcomes are improved when the trauma, vascular, and interventional services work in close collaboration. The part on lower extremity vascular trauma emphasizes the importance of performing, recording, and repeating the Doppler-derived ABI following both blunt and penetrating lower extremity trauma and importantly both before and after an associated fracture reduction. Additionally, pre-repair placement of orthopedic hardware requires communication between the orthopedic surgeon and the trauma/vascular surgeon to facilitate exposure of the accompanying vascular injury. Fox, in his chapter on femoral and popliteal artery trauma, opines that the new acute care surgeon should be competent in endovascular techniques, given the continued emergence of this area in the field of vascular trauma. He also suggests that in the face of extensive soft tissue injury in the leg, a longer tunneled interposition graft placed outside of the field of injury may avoid contamination and late graft rupture. The review of renovascular injuries provided in this textbook is appropriate for all involved in trauma care, including urologists.

The last part of this textbook includes chapters on a variety of relatively unique subjects in vascular injury. Heinzerling and Sato outline the nuances to be considered in treating pediatric patients, including the importance of vigilance for potential vascular injury in the presence of supracondylar fractures of the humerus, the association between pedestrian crashes and thoracic aortic injuries in children, and the potential for limb length discrepancy following vascular trauma in very young patients. The important contributions of military medics deployed in the current military conflicts are nicely reviewed by Fox, including the advantages of a two-team surgical approach. Rasmussen provides the reader with a detailed description of the use of vascular shunts, including tips on how to avoid complications and maximize success of this important limb-saving and occasionally lifesaving technique. As important as vascular repair is to limb salvage, nerve injuries, well summarized in this part, must also be addressed in order to maximize functional outcomes.

In summary, this textbook has relevance to an all-inclusive vascular trauma "team" that includes surgeons from many disciplines (trauma, vascular, thoracic, orthopedic, plastics, pediatric, urologic, and military) as well as the integrated nonsurgical fields of emergency medicine and radiology. Following carefully designed practice management guidelines that are patient centered and disease specific, as promoted in this book, assures the highest possibility of a favorable outcome following even the most complex vascular injury.

San Francisco, CA, USA   M. Margaret Knudson, MD

Part I

Vascular Surgery Essentials

Mark A. Mattos, Charles J. Fox, Jennifer A. Heller,
and Jessica O'Connell

Overview of Vascular Trauma

1

Gabriel J. Bietz and Joseph L. Bobadilla

Contents

G.J. Bietz, MD • J.L. Bobadilla, MD (✉)
Division of Vascular and Endovascular Surgery,
Department of Surgery, University of Kentucky,
Lexington, KY, USA
e-mail: jbo244@uky.edu

1.1 Introduction

Classically, vascular injury mechanisms are divided into penetrating or blunt. Following blunt trauma, tissue injury is produced by local compression, rapid deceleration, and the resulting shear forces. In penetrating trauma, the injury is produced by crushing and separation of tissues along the path of the penetrating object along with the resulting concussive shockwave. Understanding the biomechanics of specific injuries is important in determining the potential for vascular injury and the subsequent hemodynamic consequences of these injuries. Injury severity is proportional to the amount of kinetic energy (KE) transferred to the tissues, which is a function of the mass (M) and velocity (V); $KE = (M \times V^2)/2$. This relationship is valid for both blunt and penetrating injury mechanisms. Small changes in velocity alter the kinetic energy transfer more significantly than do changes in mass. This is critical when evaluating high- and low-velocity gunshot wounds and their corresponding injury potential.

This chapter focuses on vascular trauma and the decision processes associated with the workup and treatment of these injuries, both open and endovascular. Vascular injuries resulting from blunt, penetrating, and iatrogenic sources are considered in the following pages. Injuries are grouped in a "head-to-toe"-type organization, similar to that encountered during a trauma survey. The major sections include:

A. Dua et al. (eds.), *Clinical Review of Vascular Trauma*,
DOI 10.1007/978-3-642-39100-2_1, © Springer-Verlag Berlin Heidelberg 2014

1. Head and Neck Vascular Injuries
2. Thoracic Vascular Injuries
3. Abdominal and Pelvic Vascular Injuries
4. Peripheral (Extremity) Vascular Injuries

We present a general overview to the evaluation and workup of each of these regions, followed by a vessel-specific review of the current treatment options and recommendations.

1.2 Head and Neck Injuries

Cervical vascular injuries are notoriously difficult to evaluate and manage as a result of the complex anatomy and confined narrow anatomical space of the neck. The initial evaluation of these injuries can often be obscured by associated injuries in the head, neck, and chest. In addition, signs of cerebral ischemia or focal neurologic deficit may not be obviously present on initial evaluation due to patient condition, sedation, or the need for mechanical ventilation. Advances in noninvasive imaging (primarily computed tomography) have revolutionized the

evaluation of stable patients with cervical vascular injuries. Injuries to the distal internal carotid, proximal common carotid, subclavian, and vertebral arteries are now amenable to endovascular adjuncts to arrest hemorrhage, stabilize dissections, or exclude pseudoaneurysms. Following penetrating cervical trauma, cervical blood vessels are the most commonly injured structures in the neck, accounting for a 7–27 % stroke rate and a 7–50 % mortality rate [1]. Eighty percent of deaths in this population are stroke related.

1.2.1 Penetrating Injury

The neck has classically been divided into three zones that dictate the diagnostic evaluation and treatment: zone I, below the cricoid cartilage; zone II, between the cricoid cartilage and the angle of the mandible; and zone III, above the angle of the mandible (Fig. 1.1). Zone II is the most commonly injured (47 %), followed by zone III (19 %) and zone I (18 %) [2]. The hard and soft signs of vascular injury are present

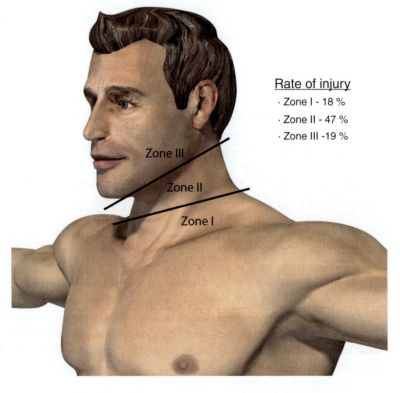

Fig. 1.1 The three zones of the neck. *Zone I* is located below the cricoid cartilage. *Zone II* is located between the cricoid cartilage and the angle of the mandible. *Zone III* is located above the angle of the mandible. Injury to zone I occurs in about 18 % of patients with neck trauma, zone II injuries occur in 47 %, and zone III injuries occur in 19 %

Rate of injury
· Zone I - 18 %
· Zone II - 47 %
· Zone III -19 %

Zone III

Zone II

Zone I

Table 1.1 Hard and soft signs of vascular injury

Hard signs	Soft signs
Shock/refractory hypotension	Non-pulsatile bleeding
Pulsatile bleeding	Stable hematoma
Audible bruit	Nerve injury
Enlarging hematoma	Unequal blood pressures/pulse exam
Loss of pulse with neurologic deficit	Proximity of injury tract

Hard signs of vascular injury are predictive of significant vascular injury in 97 % of patients. Isolated soft signs predict significant vascular injury in less than 5 % of patients; therefore, patients with only soft signs of vascular injury should undergo further work-up prior to an operative intervention

Table 1.2 Blunt cerebrovascular injury grading scale

Grade	Angiographic findings	Stroke risk (%)	Mortality (%)
I	Luminal irregularity, dissection, or intramural hematoma with <25 % luminal narrowing	3	11
II	Luminal irregularity, dissection, or intramural hematoma with ≥25 % luminal narrowing	11	11
III	Pseudoaneurysm	33	11
IV	Vessel occlusion	44	22
V	Vessel transaction	100	100

Adapted from Biffl et al. [8]
Angiographic criterion for the blunt cerebrovascular injury scale. Associated stoke and death rates are included as reference

in Table 1.1. Ninety-seven percent of patients with hard signs have an associated vascular injury, as opposed to only 3 % of those with soft signs [2]. Because of this, patients with hard signs of a vascular injury should proceed directly to the operative suite for exploration and repair, provided that other injuries do not preclude this. All patients should at least have plain radiographs of the chest to diagnose occult hemopneumothorax. Historically, exploration of cervical injuries based solely on platysma muscle penetration carries an unacceptably high negative exploration rate of 50–90 % [3].

1.2.2   Blunt Injury

The overall incidence of blunt cerebrovascular injury (BCVI) has been universally reported as less than 1 % of all admissions for blunt trauma, but this relatively small population of patients has stroke rates ranging from 25 to 58 % and mortality rates of 31–59 % [4–6]. The incidence of BCVI is 0.19–0.67 % for unscreened populations and 0.6–1.07 % for screened populations [7]. The recognition and treatment of BCVI has evolved dramatically over the past two decades. As imaging technology has improved with respect to both image quality and acquisition times, CT has become a fundamental diagnostic tool in blunt trauma evaluation. A current grading scale for blunt cervical vessel injury is presented in Table 1.2.

1.2.3   Evaluation

Computed tomography is the workhorse of trauma evaluation and should be the initial diagnostic step in patients with penetrating neck injuries but no hard signs of vascular injury. Computed tomographic angiography (CTA) has a 90 % sensitivity and 100 % specificity for vascular injuries that require treatment [9, 10]. Occult injuries (intimal flaps, dissections, pseudoaneurysms) identified during the evaluation for penetrating cervical injury should be considered for management similar to those caused by blunt trauma. Table 1.3 summarizes the evaluation criterion from three major investigator groups that should trigger CTA in the evaluation of blunt cervical vessel injuries. CTA evaluation should always include the head and neck, and if zone I injuries are suspected, the aortic arch should also be included. This can be completed with a single contrast bolus in a well-timed exam.

1.2.4   Carotid Artery Injuries

1.2.4.1   Treatment of Blunt Injuries I–IV
The mainstay of treatment for BCVI grades I–IV is antithrombotic therapy, traditionally with heparin infusion followed by warfarin therapy [5]. Because of the concern for full anticoagulation of the recent trauma patient, others have investigated

Table 1.3 Screening criteria for blunt cerebrovascular injury

Denver criteria[a]	Memphis criteria[b]	Modified Biffl criteria[c]
Arterial hemorrhage	Neurologic exam not explained by imaging	GCS <6
Expanding hematoma	Horner's syndrome	
Cervical bruit	Neck soft tissue injury (seat-belt sign, hanging, or hematoma)	
Neurologic exam inconsistent with head CT findings		
New stroke on follow-up imaging		
New focal neurologic deficit		
Le Fort II or III fracture pattern	Le Fort II or III fractures	Le Fort II or III fractures
Basilar skull fracture with involvement of carotid canal	Basilar skull fracture with carotid canal involvement	Petrous fracture
Diffuse axonal injury with GCS <6	Cervical spine fracture	Diffuse axonal injury
Cervical spine fracture		
Near-hanging with anoxic brain injury		

Adapted from Biffl et al. [6], Miller et al. [11], Biffl et al. [12]
Multigroup criterion triggering BCVI screening based on specific clinical and radiographic criterion
CT computed tomography, *GCS* Glasgow Coma Scale score
[a]Adapted from Biffl et al. [6]
[b]Adapted from Miller et al. [11]
[c]Adapted from Biffl et al. [12]

the use of antiplatelet therapy alone [11, 13, 14]. Some have found lower stroke rates with heparin compared to antiplatelet therapy [6]. Unfortunately, there are no prospective head-to-head trials of heparin versus antiplatelet therapy; therefore, a prudent protocol includes heparin therapy and transition to warfarin if an absolute contraindication to systemic anticoagulation does not exist. If full anticoagulation is not able to be completed, antiplatelet therapy should be initiated. These lesions all require follow-up imaging with either CTA or catheter-based angiography anywhere from 1 to 3 months post-injury. Edwards et al. found that at 3 months, one can expect 72 % of grade I injuries to be completely healed [15]. Grade II injuries are fairly evenly distributed: 33 % are improved, 33 % are stable, and 33 % progress [15]. Grade III injuries tend to either remain unchanged or enlarge but rarely resolve [15]. These lesions typically have a low risk of rupture but can be a source of distal embolic events or thrombosis, and as such, continued anticoagulation is recommended [16, 17].

1.2.4.2 Treatment of Penetrating Injuries and Grade V Blunt Injuries

The management of grade V blunt injuries (complete transection) and penetrating injuries is a much more complex decision tree. In essence, they may be treated as synonymous injuries. Penetrating injuries in zone II should be operatively explored and repaired surgically. This can be accomplished via a cervical incision. The external jugular and facial veins may be ligated with little concern. Injuries to the internal jugular vein may be primarily repaired but can be ligated in emergency conditions if necessary. Whenever surgical intervention is undertaken, at least one leg must be prepped to allow for vein harvesting for patch or interposition conduit harvesting. Saphenous vein patch can be used to repair partial injuries and should be harvested from the groin rather than the ankle. Alternatively, some have used bovine pericardium if no vein is present, but this carries increased risk of infection in a contaminated field. Injuries due to iatrogenic cannulation or from stab wounds can often be repaired primarily; ballistic injuries most often require segmental resection and interposition grafting. The saphenous vein offers a good size match for the internal carotid in these cases and in some cases for the distal common carotid. If size mismatch is an issue, some have proposed the use of the superficial femoral artery with interposition polytetrafluoroethylene (PTFE) grafting in the superficial femoral artery (SFA) harvest location [4]. This allows for autologous reconstruction in the contaminated field and prosthetic reconstruction in the clean harvest bed. The patient should always be fully heparinized prior to any clamping of the carotid system; temporary shunts can be used at the discretion of the operative surgeon. Simple ligation of the carotid artery has significant consequences and results in nearly 45 % mortality [1]. Because of this, it should be reserved only for those injuries at the base of the skull that are not amenable to reconstruction or when complete transection with thrombosis is already present without resulting neurologic incident.

Penetrating carotid artery injuries in zone I and III present a much more complex problem. Proximal and distal control can be a significant issue or require much more morbidity with jaw dislocation, mandibulotomy, median sternotomy, or trapdoor incisions. Because of this, endovascular techniques have increased in popularity for control of these injuries. These techniques have the added benefit of being able to be completed under local anesthesia, allowing for continuous neurologic monitoring. Multiple groups have shown low-risk profiles with the use of covered stents for the treatment of hemodynamically significant dissection, pseudoaneurysms, partial transections, and other injuries to the carotid vessels in these zones [18–25].

1.2.5 Vertebral Artery Injuries

Vertebral artery injuries (VAIs) are quite rare, with average incidence of 0.20–0.77 % among all trauma admissions [5, 6]. Other than the first segment of the vertebral artery, V1, the remaining portions of this vessel are difficult to access from open surgical approaches due to the significant bony protection. The vertebral artery is most often injured from cervical spine transverse process fractures, subluxations, or penetrating injuries to the back of the neck [26]. Catheter-based selective angiography remains the gold standard, but as with carotid injury, CTA has gained popularity due to its ease of access and rapid initiation. CTA has been shown to have a sensitivity and specificity of 40–60 % and 90–97 %, respectively [27].

1.2.5.1 Treatment of Blunt Injuries

As with blunt carotid injuries, the mainstay of blunt vertebral injuries is systemic anticoagulation, unless complete transection with extravasation is noted. Studies from the past decade have shown a reduced neurologic incident rate from 20 to 35 % with no anticoagulation to 0–14 % with heparin therapy [7, 28]. Again, as with carotid blunt injury, if systemic anticoagulation cannot be administered, antiplatelet therapy should be given.

1.2.5.2 Treatment of Penetrating Injuries and Blunt Transection Injuries

Because of the difficult surgical access to the vertebral vessel, endovascular techniques have become a first approach to the treatment of penetrating and blunt transection injuries. Selective angiography and crossing of the lesion can allow for proximal and distal coil embolization in most patients. Even in cases of complete transection, crossing of this lesion can be successful, allowing endovascular treatment. Up to 50 % of the time, selective angiography will reveal that the vessel has already thrombosed, and thus no further therapy is needed [29]. There have been rare reports of covered stent graft placement in the vertebral system, but this is not routinely performed [7].

If endovascular techniques are not available or do not succeed in controlling the bleeding, open operative ligation can be completed with an expected stroke rate of 3–5 % [30]. The most straightforward approach involves isolation of the V1 segment of the vertebral artery and ligation at this point, with packing of the wound to assist in retrograde and collateral back bleeding. This portion of the vertebral artery can be obtained through the same exposure as the carotid artery. The sternocleidomastoid muscle attachments to the sternum and clavicle are taken down, the scalene fat pad is mobilized, and the anterior scalene muscle is divided with care not to injure the phrenic nerve. At this point, the subclavian artery and origin of the vertebral artery can be dissected and ligated to control bleeding.

1.3   Thoracic Vascular Injuries

Thoracic vascular injuries carry with them a high degree of lethality. By best estimates, thoracic aortic injuries result in 50–80 % in-the-field mortality. Those patients that do survive to hospital evaluation require rapid and accurate diagnosis and intervention. In most urban environments, upwards of 90 % of these injuries are a result of penetrating mechanisms [31]. In contrast, in more isolated and rural setting, the majority are due to blunt aortic transections from deceleration injuries. Regardless, the initial evaluation should consist of chest radiographs, and in the hemodynamically stable patient, CTA plays a key role in the radiographic survey. Unstable patients with great vessel or thoracic aortic injury often undergo emergency room thoracotomy. Once the chest has been opened, aortic clamping with further resuscitation and transport to the operating theater for definitive repair may be undertaken. This section will focus on the aortic arch, its branches, and the descending thoracic aorta. Both penetrating and blunt injuries will be discussed. The rising use of endovascular techniques for the management of these injuries will be of specific discussion.

1.3.1   Ascending Aorta and Transverse Arch

Injury to the ascending aorta and transverse arch is most often associated with penetrating mechanisms but can be seen with severe blunt force injury. There is exceedingly high in-the-field mortality with these most proximal aortic injuries. Clinical and radiographic signs include cardiac tamponade, widened mediastinum, and apical capping. These injuries should be approached with an open technique via a median sternotomy utilizing cardiopulmonary bypass (Fig. 1.2). Depending on the extent of the injury, primary repair or interposition grafting may be necessitated. Posthospital survival rate depends greatly on clinical presentation, comorbid conditions, and other associated injuries [32, 33].

1.3.2   Innominate Artery

Innominate artery injuries can result from blunt, penetrating, and iatrogenic sources. The most common iatrogenic mechanism is with central line misadventures. Classically, open repair via a median sternotomy with a right cervical extension was the

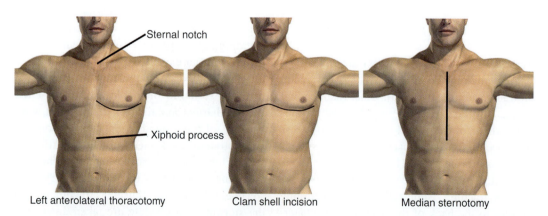

Fig. 1.2 Three major incisions used for access to mediastinal structures. The left anterolateral thoracotomy permits rapid access to mediastinal and left chest contents and is particularly useful for cross clamping the aorta after major trauma with hemorrhage. The clamshell incision permits rapid access to the entire chest and can be used by extending the initial incision made for a left anterolateral thoracotomy if a major right chest trauma is suspected. Finally, a median sternotomy permits access to the mediastinum. A right or left cervical extension can be utilized for access to the subclavian and carotid vessels

approach of choice to repair of these injuries. Primary repair or short segment interposition grafts can be utilized to repair these injuries. Because of the potential morbidity of these procedures, endovascular techniques have gained popularity in recent years. There have been multiple reports of cover stent graft implantation for the management of these injuries [34–37]. As a result of this growing body of literature, consideration for covered stent graft implantation should be given. Because of the immediate proximity to the cerebrovascular circulation, systemic anticoagulation during cannulation and deployment should be complete, and post-implant treatment with antiplatelet agents should be strongly considered.

1.3.3   Proximal Left Carotid Artery

Surgical exposure for intervention on the proximal left common carotid artery is a mirror exposure of that of the innominate artery. Median

sternotomy with left cervical extension is utilized (Fig. 1.2). While primary repair can be completed in some cases, interposition grafting is the preferred method of repair in an open intervention. As with the other arch vessels, management has shifted to endovascular techniques in recent years. The implantation of covered stent grafts has gained significant popularity [38–41]. As with innominate artery stent implantation, full heparinization during the procedure is essential, and post-implantation antiplatelet therapy is strongly advised. Additionally, the use of distal embolic protection is strongly advised when carotid artery interventions are undertaken [42].

1.3.4   Left Subclavian Artery Injuries

Surgical exposure of the left subclavian artery can be difficult and may require both a supraclavicular and anterolateral thoracotomy (Fig. 1.3). Some have connected these with a median

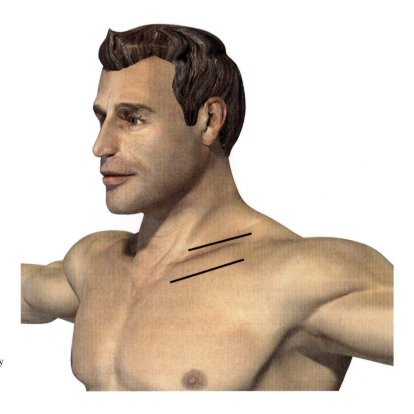

Fig. 1.3 Subclavian exposure. A supraclavicular and infraclavicular incision can be used for access to the subclavian artery. A median sternotomy may be necessary to achieve proximal control, particularly in trauma

sternotomy for full exposure, but this incision is wrought with complications and can be difficult to complete if not experienced in this technique. Clavicle resection may also be needed to gain complete control of these injuries. Because of the complex surgical exposure, interest in endovascular approaches has gained significant momentum. As with other arch vessels, the use of covered stent grafts has shown promising results with injuries in this location [43–46]. These injuries may be approached from either the ipsilateral brachial or either femoral access points depending on the associated bony extremity injuries.

1.3.5 Descending Thoracic Aorta

Most penetrating injuries of the descending aorta result in in-the-field mortality or significant hemodynamic instability prompting emergent thoracotomy. Once identified, these injuries can be repaired with traditional open techniques, including primary repair or interposition graft. With improved prehospital care and automotive safety, survival to hospital presentation with blunt aortic injury is increasingly more common. As a result, this section will deal mostly with the diagnosis and treatment associated with blunt aortic injury (BAI) and traumatic aortic disruption. The exact incidence is not truly known, but the EAST Practice Guideline of 2,000 estimated that BAI accounted for roughly 8,000 deaths annually in the United States [47]. There are multiple theories on how BAI develops, including acute intraluminal pressure spikes, stretch and shear strain, and bony compression, but a description of these in detail is beyond the scope of this chapter. Regardless of the mechanism, BAI typically results in disruption near the aortopulmonary ligament at the embryologic remnant of the ductus arteriosus. Widened mediastinum on chest radiograph is the classic finding, but rib 1–3 fracture, sternal fracture, clavicle or scapular fractures, or apical capping should all raise the index of suspicion. If hemodynamically stable, CTA is essential in case planning, especially for endovascular approaches. If endovascular repair is chosen, CTA through the pelvis is ideal to assess the iliofemoral system for large-bore introducer

cannulation needed to deploy thoracic endografts. Once a BAI has been confirmed, strict blood pressure and heart rate control should be undertaken until the diagnostic work-up is completed and repair has occurred. Fabian et al. have shown that strict impulse control (blood pressure and heart rate) results in decreased morbidity [48, 49]. In summary, they recommend a goal systolic blood pressure <100 mmHg, a goal mean arterial pressure <80 mmHg, and a goal heart rate of <100 BPM [48, 49]. This can be accomplished with esmolol infusion or PRN labetalol with or without the aid of nitroglycerine infusion to assist in vasodilation. Once impulse control has been established and provided that hemodynamic stability persists, the patient can receive the remainder of the trauma evaluation. Other immediately life-threatening injuries can be dealt with first, and if no other emergent operative indications exist, repair of the BAI can be undertaken.

Historically, these injuries have been treated with open left lateral thoracotomy with or without cardiopulmonary bypass and hypothermic circulator arrest (Fig. 1.2). Interposition grafting is almost universally needed, and primary repair is general not advisable. A complete description of the operative exposure and repair is beyond the scope of this chapter; however, as with any thoracic aortic surgery, subsequent paraplegia from spinal ischemia is a feared consequence [50–52]. With aggressive and protocolized approaches to spinal cord protection, this often fatal complication can be prevented in many patients [53–57]. As with the other vessels described in this section, endovascular techniques are a rising component in the management of BAI. The use of thoracic endovascular aneurysm repair (TEVAR) devices for the management of BAI is becoming increasingly common [58–62]. Additionally, others have reported the use of abdominal aortic extension cuff in the thoracic aorta for the treatment of BAI [60]. As with any off-label use, the merits of this technique must be weighed against the benefits and risks of a non-FDA-approved application of such devices. There has been some concern about the long-term implication of device implantation in a typically young trauma patient population. Additionally, concern has been raised about the ability to maintain long-term follow-up in this patient population [63]. Despite these concerns, TEVAR for BAI has been recommended as the treatment of choice by many [60, 62]. The current generation of TEVAR devices is approved for vessel diameters of 16 mm and larger; because of this, the use in very young and pediatric populations is generally not advised due to the absolute vessel size and long-term consequences of future growth. In these extenuating circumstances, open repair is advised.

1.4 Abdominal and Pelvic Vascular Injuries

Vascular injuries within the abdominal and pelvic cavities can be difficult to manage as a result of concomitant injury to both hollow and solid organs. Traditionally, many intra-abdominal vascular injuries have been addressed in an open fashion as there is often an indication for exploration due to these other associated injuries. However, there does exist a subset of abdominopelvic vascular injuries that can be addressed via endovascular approaches. Abdominal vascular injuries account for 30 % of all vascular trauma, and about 90 % are caused by penetrating trauma [64]. In patients undergoing exploratory laparotomy, it is estimated that the incidence of concomitant vascular injury is 14 % for gunshot wounds, 10 % for stab wounds, and 3 % for blunt injuries [65, 66]. Most patients with abdominopelvic vascular injuries present with hard signs of vascular injury or hemodynamic instability due to the large potential space for bleeding and other associated injuries that typically accompany. Because of this, most of these injuries are directly discovered at the time of exploratory laparotomy, and little work-up is typically undertaken. With smaller, more distal branch vessel injury, patients may undergo abdominopelvic CT, allowing for a more thorough evaluation.

1.4.1 Abdominal Aorta Injuries

Abdominal aortic injuries are almost uniformly penetrating in nature. Blunt injury to the abdominal

aorta accounts for 0.04 % of trauma admissions [67]. Gross contamination is common in patients with penetrating trauma, as 93 % of patients have other associated intra-abdominal injuries including the small bowel (45 %), colon (30 %), and liver (28 %) [68]. The use of prosthetic graft has always been an area of controversy. We recommend the use of autogenous tissue for reconstruction whenever possible for these situations. Enteric spillage should rapidly be controlled and the peritoneal cavity irrigated in all cases however. Prosthetic grafts may be necessary for large or complex repairs, and bowel content spillage is not considered an absolute contraindication by some [69].

There have been case reports of the management of abdominal aortic injuries using endovascular techniques, but the current generation of devices is limited in their utility for injuries in this location. Pseudoaneurysms, aortocaval fistulae, and infrarenal aortic dissections have all been treated successfully with stent grafts [67, 70–72]. The limiting factor preventing more widespread application of endovascular techniques in repair of the abdominal aorta is branch graft technology. Until fenestrated and branch graft technology becomes more available, the use of endovascular grafts will have a definitive role in selected cases of infrarenal aortic injury.

1.4.2 Celiac Artery Injuries

Celiac artery injuries are often accompanied by other vascular injuries and most often the result of penetrating injuries. Ligation is generally well tolerated for celiac and celiac branch vessel injury. The portal vein and gastroduodenal artery are often adequate blood supply for liver parenchyma should the common hepatic artery require ligation; however, late bile duct strictures can be encountered if distal hepatic branches are ligated. Because of the rich collateral network in this location, catheter-directed embolization is also a viable technique. Additionally, there have been a few reports of endovascular covered stent grafts, though tortuosity is a complicating factor. Celiac artery injuries are considered a marker of more severe trauma, and published mortality rates range from 38 to 75 % [73]. Many of these mortalities are related to other associated injuries and not directly attributable to the celiac disruption.

1.4.3 Superior Mesenteric Artery (SMA) Injuries

For traumatic injury purposes, the SMA can be divided into two segments, marked by the takeoff of the middle colic artery. Proximal to this, ligation results in significant bowel ischemia from the ligament of Treitz to and including the right hemicolon. Distal to this, ligation can result in partial bowel ischemia, and segmental resection may be needed. In the unstable patient, as an alternative to ligation, damage control with a temporary shunt should be considered [74]. Definitive reconstruction can be performed once the patient is stable at the second laparotomy. Saphenous vein, femoral vein, and PTFE graft may all be used as conduit. Again, the use of autologous tissue is strongly encouraged because of the risks of bowel content spillage and subsequent graft infection. Proximal SMA partial transections can be managed with primary repair in 40 % of cases [75]. Additionally, there have been scattered reports of these injuries being treated with covered stent grafts [76–80]. This is a viable option in the critically ill patient, but long-term patency data is not yet available. Furthermore, these techniques are best utilized in the proximal segment of the SMA and should be avoided distal to the middle colic vessel to prevent covering important side branch vessels and inducing further bowel ischemia. All hematomas near the SMA should be explored in penetrating trauma. In blunt trauma, with a stable hematoma and viable nonischemic bowel, it is recommended to not explore the site. Instead, postoperative SMA evaluation via color-flow Doppler imaging, CT angiography, or angiography is recommended.

1.4.4 Renal Artery and Renal Parenchymal Injuries

Renal artery injuries are rare and account for about 0.05 % of all blunt trauma admissions [81].

The injuries typically present are intimal flaps, partial transections, pseudoaneurysms, traumatic AV fistulas, and acute occlusions. Treatment of traumatic renovascular injuries depends on the warm ischemia time, general condition of the patient, mechanism of injury, and condition of the contralateral kidney. Endovascular treatment should be considered the first-line therapeutic option for patients in stable condition with intimal tears, acute occlusions, false aneurysms, and arteriovenous fistulae. Because of the relatively large diameter, straight anatomical course, and parallel proximal and distal landing zones, endovascular interventions have shown great success in the treatment of renovascular injuries [82–84].

Expanding perinephric hematomas secondary to penetrating trauma should be explored, and most of these are found at the time of laparotomy for other associated injuries. A stable perinephric hematoma, away from the hilum may be considered an exception to this rule [85]. Blunt renovascular injuries are often found after a significant time delay. After 3–6 h of warm ischemia time, renal function is severely impaired. At this point, revascularization is of little use. In this circumstance, roughly 30–40 % of patients will ultimately develop renovascular hypertension [86–88].

1.4.5 Inferior Mesenteric Artery (IMA) Injuries

IMA injuries are rare and most often related to penetrating trauma. They account for less than 1 % of all abdominal vascular traumas [64]. Ligation is generally well tolerated and resultant colorectal ischemia is rare.

1.4.6 Iliac Artery Injuries

Isolated traumatic iliac vessel injuries carry a significant morbidity and mortality and are most often the result of penetrating trauma. In hospitals, mortality has been reported anywhere from 25 to 50 % depending on other associated injuries, the most significant being associated iliac vein injury [89–91]. In addition, iliac arterial injury has been reported numerous times after misadventures in lumbar spine surgery. Finally, with the increasing need for large-diameter transfemoral access for TEVAR and transfemoral aortic valve implantation (TAVI) cases, iatrogenic external iliac artery injury has increased.

Endovascular techniques are now often considered the first-line therapy to address iliac artery injury, particularly after blunt force trauma. Endovascular stents have been shown to be very effective in addressing pseudoaneurysms, arteriovenous fistulae, or major intimal tears with or without thrombosis [92–96]. Furthermore, active bleeding from internal iliac artery braches, often caused by pelvic fractures, is amenable to endovascular coil embolization. During laparotomy, pelvic hematomas due to blunt trauma should only be explored if they are expanding rapidly. Hematomas secondary to penetrating trauma should be explored. If there is an absent or diminished femoral pulse, in-line bypass should be considered. Vein or PTFE patch may be used, depending of amount of wound contamination. A balloon-tipped catheter should be passed proximally and distally to remove any residual thrombus. Simple ligation of the common or external iliac arteries is associated with a high incidence of limb loss. Patients in critical condition that can only tolerate damage control surgery may have the flow restored to the limb by using a temporary shunt. Definitive vessel reconstruction may be performed as a second-stage operation once the patient is hemodynamically stable.

Exposure of the external iliac can be accomplished by a separate retroperitoneal incision or by extending the classic groin cutdown incision upwards and laterally through the inguinal ligament. Classic repair with either saphenous vein or PTFE interposition remains a viable option; however, covered stent graft insertion has gained recent popularity [94, 97, 98]. Depending on the circumstances, location, and type of injury, ipsilateral or contralateral access can be gained. Guidewire access across the injury is necessary, and after this is achieved, a covered graft can be deployed. Covering of the ipsilateral hypogastric artery can be tolerated if the contralateral hypogastric vessel is patent without significant

stenosis but should be avoided if possible. Midterm results of such endovascular treatments are promising, but long-term data is not readily available.

1.4.7 Venous Injuries

The inferior vena cava (IVC) is the most commonly injured abdominal venous structure and accounts for about 25 % of abdominal venous injuries [99]. Blunt trauma is responsible for only about 10 % of IVC injuries with 90 % due to penetrating mechanisms [100, 101]. Eighteen percent of patients with penetrating IVC injuries have an associated aortic injury [100, 101]. Many injuries to the IVC, especially those involving the infrarenal IVC, present with stable hematomas. Hematomas due to penetrating trauma should be routinely explored, with the exception of stable retro-hepatic hematomas. Exploration and vessel control in this location is extremely difficult, resulting in uncontrollable hemorrhage and death. Mortality ranges between 20 and 57 % for IVC injured victims who survive to the hospital [100].

Portal vein (PV) and superior mesenteric vein (SMV) injuries are rare and account for roughly 1–2 % of trauma patients. These injuries should be repaired if this can be accomplished with simple suture repair. Complex reconstructions including interposition grafting are generally not advisable. Reconstruction of the portal vein with a saphenous vein graft or internal jugular vein graft is a viable option but should be considered only in those patients who have had complete transection of the hepatic arteries [102]. Individuals with portal vein ligation and a patent hepatic artery have survival ranges from 55 to 85 % [103]. Contrary, ligation of both the portal vein and hepatic arteries is not compatible with life, and fulminant hepatic failure quickly ensues. Portal vein or SMV ligation results in bowel wall edema. A temporary abdominal closer device is recommended, and a second-stage laparotomy is recommended to evaluate for bowel necrosis.

Renal vein injuries can be managed by primary repair or ligation. Left renal vein ligation near the IVC is acceptable because of collateral venous drainage through the left gonadal vein, left adrenal vein, and lumbar veins. Right renal vein ligation should always be followed by nephrectomy.

Iliac venous injuries can be technically more challenging than arterial injuries because of the difficult exposure and overlying structures. Iliac artery transection to access the underlying vein should only be considered in extreme cases [104]. Often generous mobilization and retraction of the artery provides adequate exposure of the vein for repair. Ligation is generally preferable to a repair that results in a severe stenosis. The risk of pulmonary embolism is low after iliac vein ligation, and the complications are generally minimal. Transient edema is noted in most patients, but this most often responds to compression therapy. Occasionally, massive edema of the leg can develop. Rarely, compartment syndrome has been described, but this is usually in patients with combined arterial and venous injuries. In this instance, the early use of decompressive fasciotomy is recommended.

1.5 Peripheral (Extremity) Vascular Injuries

Peripheral vascular injuries account for upwards of 80 % of all cases of vascular trauma, with most of these injuries involving the arteries and veins of the lower extremities. High-velocity weapons (70–80 %) account for most of these injuries, followed by stab wounds (10–15 %) and blunt trauma (5–10 %). In a series of penetrating injuries, arterial injuries were caused by gunshot wounds in 64 %, knife wounds in 24 %, and shotgun blasts in 12 % [105]. The morbidity of blunt vascular injuries can be magnified by associated fractures, dislocations, and crush injuries to the adjacent muscles and nerves. Occult vascular injuries are usually composed of intimal flaps, segmental narrowing, and hemodynamically insignificant arteriovenous fistulae or pseudoaneurysms. There is growing evidence that most of these injuries heal spontaneously or stabilize without further compromising the distal circulation and perfusion [106, 107]. These findings have been confirmed by independent studies in

animals [108, 109] and humans [108, 110]. Subclinical vascular injuries with intact distal perfusion may be observed with serial monitoring, antiplatelet therapy or systemic anticoagulation, and repeat noninvasive imaging. Subclinical vascular defects have been defined as those exhibiting the following characteristics:

- Low-velocity injury
- Minimal (<5 mm) arterial wall disruption for intimal defects and pseudoaneurysms
- Adherent or downstream protrusion of intimal flaps
- Intact distal circulation
- No active hemorrhage

Interval vascular imaging is essential when expectant management is chosen, but resolution can be seen in 85–90 % of these lesions with no operative intervention [106, 111].

Potential serious complications of untreated clinically evident peripheral vascular trauma include uncontrolled hemorrhage, thrombosis, ruptured pseudoaneurysm, hemodynamically significant arteriovenous fistula, and compartment syndrome. Table 1.1 outlines the hard and soft signs of vascular injury, and the predictive nature of these signs holds true with regard to peripheral vascular injury as well. Most patients who present with hard signs of vascular injury will require operative intervention. Patients with soft signs, who are hemodynamically stable, can undergo noninvasive evaluation. The routine use of contrast angiography (both invasive and noninvasive) is not advisable, resulting in historically high negative yield (up to 90 % with no injury identified). Because of this, the routine use of ankle-brachial indices (ABI) as a screening tool has developed [112, 113]. The presence of an ankle index of less than 0.9 was found to be 95 % sensitive and 97 % specific [112, 113]. The threshold of an ABI <0.9 assumes no history of preexisting vascular arterial insufficiency. Others have modified this observation to include an ABI 10 % lower than the contralateral extremity. Multiple studies have confirmed the safety of selective, rather than routine, contrast angiography [114–116]. If an ABI differential is found, contrast studies may then be advised. A classic paper tested the interobserver agreement between

CTA and invasive angiography and found a kappa statistic of 0.9 [117].

1.5.1 Axillary and Brachial Arteries

Axillary artery injuries are very similar to subclavian injuries. High axillary injuries may be difficult to expose and gain proximal control for open operative repair. Both supraclavicular and infraclavicular incision may be necessary to achieve adequate control of the vessel for open repair. In addition to this, the proximity to the brachial plexus must also be considered [38, 43–45, 118, 119]. Because of this, the use of stent graft has gained recent enthusiasm.

Brachial artery injuries are most often the result of penetrating injury, either ballistic or iatrogenic. Open operative exposure and repair remains the gold standard. Occasionally, primary repair can be accomplished, but many times, short segment saphenous vein interposition grafting is needed. Care must be taken to avoid too long a conduit that will kink once the elbow is bent. Careful planning and observation in both the extended and flexed elbow positions is necessary before completing the distal anastomosis.

1.5.2 Radial and Ulnar Arteries

Single vessel injury of the forearm can be simply ligated, provided that the opposing vessel is intact to the hand and a palmer arch is present. Bedside handheld Doppler evaluation of the palmer arch and digital vessels can be undertaken to confirm viability prior to ligation of the injured vessel. If in-line flow is not present or an incomplete palmer arch is present, primary repair of the injured vessel should be completed. Endovascular approaches and stent graft have no appreciable role in the management of forearm vessel injuries.

1.5.3 Femoral and Popliteal Arteries

Open surgical repair of the femoral vessels at the level of the groin should be undertaken as routine. Primary repair or short saphenous interposition

grafts can be used to reconstruct these vessels. Both the superficial femoral artery (SFA) and profunda femoris vessels should be reconstructed, hemodynamic status allowing. The deep profunda vessel is essential in long-term limb viability and is a vital collateral for patients that develop late SFA atherosclerotic disease; because of this, it should be revascularized unless extreme circumstances prohibit [120]. The mid and distal segments of the SFA should also be repaired operatively. Short segment saphenous interposition grafts serve well in this location, but if the vein is not available, PTFE can be utilized with slightly decreased long-term patency. The use of covered stent grafts has been described, but long-term patency data is not available, and given the relatively low morbidity of short segment venous interposition grafting, it is not widely advisable except under significant extenuating circumstances [97, 121–123].

The popliteal artery provides some clinical controversy. It can be a challenging injury to manage. Historically, amputation rates were as high as 20 % with injuries in this location [124, 125]. Both penetrating and blunt injuries can affect this vessel. Classic traction injury from posterior knee dislocation can result in injuries ranging anywhere from a small hemodynamically insignificant intimal flaps to critical ischemia and complete transection. In most clinically apparent injuries, open repair is indicated, either by primary repair (stab wounds) or short segmental saphenous vein bypass (blunt injury, gunshot wounds). There have been anecdotal reports of covered stent graft repair for trauma and iatrogenic injury, but the long-term durability and patency have not been firmly established in these applications [97, 121–123]. Because of this, most would recommend open operative repair except under significant extenuating circumstances.

1.5.4 Tibial-Peroneal Arteries

As with the upper extremity, injury to one terminal vessel in the lower limb can be dealt with by simple ligation [126]. Injury at the level of the tibioperoneal trunk should prompt open surgical reconstruction [126]. Injury to all three tibial arteries should prompt open operative repair of at least two arteries to avoid a potential risk for future amputation [126, 127]. Currently endovascular techniques have not played a major role in the management of tibial arteries injuries.

References

1. Du Toit DF, Van Schalkwyk GD, Wadee SA, Warren BL. Neurologic outcome after penetrating extracranial arterial trauma. J Vasc Surg. 2003;38:257–62.
2. Demetriades D, Theodorou D, Cornwell E, Berne TV, Asensio J, Belzberg H, Velmahos G, Weaver F, Yellin A. Evaluation of penetrating injuries of the neck: prospective study of 223 patients. World J Surg. 1997;21:41–7; discussion 47–8.
3. Meyer JP, Barrett JA, Schuler JJ, Flanigan DP. Mandatory vs selective exploration for penetrating neck trauma. A prospective assessment. Arch Surg. 1987;122:592–7.
4. Jacobs JR, Arden RL, Marks SC, Kline R, Berguer R. Carotid artery reconstruction using superficial femoral arterial grafts. Laryngoscope. 1994;104:689–93.
5. Fabian TC, Patton Jr JH, Croce MA, Minard G, Kudsk KA, Pritchard FE. Blunt carotid injury. Importance of early diagnosis and anticoagulant therapy. Ann Surg. 1996;223:513–22; discussion 522–5.
6. Biffl WL, Moore EE, Ryu RK, Offner PJ, Novak Z, Coldwell DM, Franciose RJ, Burch JM. The unrecognized epidemic of blunt carotid arterial injuries: early diagnosis improves neurologic outcome. Ann Surg. 1998;228:462–70.
7. Miller PR, Fabian TC, Bee TK, Timmons S, Chamsuddin A, Finkle R, Croce MA. Blunt cerebrovascular injuries: diagnosis and treatment. J Trauma. 2001;51:279–85; discussion 285–6.
8. Biffl WL, Moore EE, Offner PJ, Brega KE, Franciose RJ, Burch JM. Blunt carotid arterial injuries: implications of a new grading scale. J Trauma. 1999; 47:845–53.
9. Munera F, Soto JA, Nunez D. Penetrating injuries of the neck and the increasing role of CTA. Emerg Radiol. 2004;10:303–9.
10. Nunez Jr DB, Torres-Leon M, Munera F. Vascular injuries of the neck and thoracic inlet: helical CT-angiographic correlation. Radiographics. 2004;24:1087–98; discussion 1099–100.
11. Miller PR, Fabian TC, Croce MA, Cagiannos C, Williams JS, Vang M, Qaisi WG, Felker RE, Timmons SD. Prospective screening for blunt cerebrovascular injuries: analysis of diagnostic modalities and outcomes. Ann Surg. 2002;236:386–93; discussion 393–5.
12. Biffl WL, Moore EE, Offner PJ, Brega KE, Franciose RJ, Elliott JP, Burch JM. Optimizing screening for blunt cerebrovascular injuries. Am J Surg. 1999; 178:517–22.
13. Wahl WL, Brandt MM, Thompson BG, Taheri PA, Greenfield LJ. Antiplatelet therapy: an alternative to heparin for blunt carotid injury. J Trauma. 2002;52:896–901.
14. Cothren CC, Moore EE, Biffl WL, Ciesla DJ, Ray Jr CE, Johnson JL, Moore JB, Burch JM. Anticoagulation is the gold standard therapy for blunt carotid injuries to reduce stroke rate. Arch Surg. 2004;139:540–5. discussion 545-6.
15. Edwards NM, Fabian TC, Claridge JA, Timmons SD, Fischer PE, Croce MA. Antithrombotic therapy and endovascular stents are effective treatment for blunt carotid injuries: results from longterm followup. J Am Coll Surg. 2007;204:1007–13; discussion 1014–5.
16. Duke BJ, Ryu RK, Coldwell DM, Brega KE. Treatment of blunt injury to the carotid artery by using endovascular stents: an early experience. J Neurosurg. 1997;87:825–9.
17. Pretre R, Kursteiner K, Reverdin A, Faidutti B. Blunt carotid artery injury: devastating consequences of undetected pseudoaneurysm. J Trauma. 1995;39:1012–4.
18. Coldwell DM, Novak Z, Ryu RK, Brega KE, Biffl WL, Offner PJ, Franciose RJ, Burch JM, Moore EE. Treatment of posttraumatic internal carotid arterial pseudoaneurysms with endovascular stents. J Trauma. 2000;48:470–2.
19. Ellis PK, Kennedy PT, Barros D'Sa AA. Successful exclusion of a high internal carotid pseudoaneurysm using the Wallgraft endoprosthesis. Cardiovasc Intervent Radiol. 2002;25:68–9.
20. Mcneil JD, Chiou AC, Gunlock MG, Grayson DE, Soares G, Hagino RT. Successful endovascular therapy of a penetrating zone III internal carotid injury. J Vasc Surg. 2002;36:187–90.
21. Duane TM, Parker F, Stokes GK, Parent FN, Britt LD. Endovascular carotid stenting after trauma. J Trauma. 2002;52:149–53.
22. Cohen JE, Ben-Hur T, Rajz G, Umansky F, Gomori JM. Endovascular stent-assisted angioplasty in the management of traumatic internal carotid artery dissections. Stroke. 2005;36:e45–7.
23. Bejjani GK, Monsein LH, Laird JR, Satler LF, Starnes BW, Aulisi EF. Treatment of symptomatic cervical carotid dissections with endovascular stents. Neurosurgery. 1999;44:755–60; discussion 760–1.
24. Liu AY, Paulsen RD, Marcellus ML, Steinberg GK, Marks MP. Long-term outcomes after carotid stent placement treatment of carotid artery dissection. Neurosurgery. 1999;45:1368–73; discussion 1373–4.
25. Cothren CC, Moore EE, Ray Jr CE, Ciesla DJ, Johnson JL, Moore JB, Burch JM. Carotid artery stents for blunt cerebrovascular injury: risks exceed benefits. Arch Surg. 2005;140:480–5; discussion 485–6.
26. Reid JD, Weigelt JA. Forty-three cases of vertebral artery trauma. J Trauma. 1988;28:1007–12.

27. Bub LD, Hollingworth W, Jarvik JG, Hallam DK. Screening for blunt cerebrovascular injury: evaluating the accuracy of multidetector computed tomographic angiography. J Trauma. 2005;59:691–7.

28. Biffl WL, Moore EE, Elliott JP, Ray C, Offner PJ, Franciose RJ, Brega KE, Burch JM. The devastating potential of blunt vertebral arterial injuries. Ann Surg. 2000;231:672–81.

29. Mwipatayi BP, Jeffery P, Beningfield SJ, Motale P, Tunnicliffe J, Navsaria PH. Management of extracranial vertebral artery injuries. Eur J Vasc Endovasc Surg. 2004;27:157–62.

30. Thomas GI, Anderson KN, Hain RF, Merendino KA. The significance of anomalous vertebral-basilar artery communications in operations on the heart and great vessels: an illustrative case with review of the literature. Surgery. 1959;46:747–57.

31. Mattox KL, Feliciano DV, Burch J, Beall Jr AC, Jordan Jr GL, De Bakey ME. Five thousand seven hundred sixty cardiovascular injuries in 4459 patients. Epidemiologic evolution 1958 to 1987. Ann Surg. 1989;209:698–705.

32. Symbas PJ, Horsley WS, Symbas PN. Rupture of the ascending aorta caused by blunt trauma. Ann Thorac Surg. 1998;66:113–7.

33. Serna DL, Miller JS, Chen EP. Aortic reconstruction after complex injury of the mid-transverse arch. Ann Thorac Surg. 2006;81:1112–4.

34. Shalhub S, Starnes BW, Hatsukami TS, Karmy-Jones R, Tran NT. Repair of blunt thoracic outlet arterial injuries: an evolution from open to endovascular approach. J Trauma. 2011;71:E114–21.

35. De Troia A, Tecchio T, Azzarone M, Biasi L, Piazza P, Franco Salcuni P. Endovascular treatment of an innominate artery iatrogenic pseudoaneurysm following subclavian vein catheterization. Vasc Endovascular Surg. 2011;45:78–82.

36. Gifford SM, Deel JT, Dent DL, Seenu Reddy V, Rasmussen TE. Endovascular repair of innominate artery injury secondary to air rifle pellet: a case report and review of the literature. Vasc Endovascular Surg. 2009;43:301–5.

37. Ahmed I, Katsanos K, Ahmad F, Dourado R, Lyons O, Reidy J. Endovascular treatment of a brachiocephalic artery pseudoaneurysm secondary to biopsy at mediastinoscopy. Cardiovasc Intervent Radiol. 2009;32:792–5.

38. Joo JY, Ahn JY, Chung YS, Chung SS, Kim SH, Yoon PH, Kim OJ. Therapeutic endovascular treatments for traumatic carotid artery injuries. J Trauma. 2005;58:1159–66.

39. Parodi JC, Schonholz C, Ferreira LM, Bergan J. Endovascular stent-graft treatment of traumatic arterial lesions. Ann Vasc Surg. 1999;13:121–9.

40. Diaz-Daza O, Arraiza FJ, Barkley JM, Whigham CJ. Endovascular therapy of traumatic vascular lesions of the head and neck. Cardiovasc Intervent Radiol. 2003;26:213–21.

41. Gomez CR, May AK, Terry JB, Tulyapronchote R. Endovascular therapy of traumatic injuries of the extracranial cerebral arteries. Crit Care Clin. 1999;15:789–809.

42. Matsumura JS, Gray W, Chaturvedi S, Yamanouchi D, Peng L, Verta P. Results of carotid artery stenting with distal embolic protection with improved systems: protected carotid artery stenting in patients at high risk for carotid endarterectomy (PROTECT) trial. J Vasc Surg. 2012;55:968–76.E5.

43. Castelli P, Caronno R, Piffaretti G, Tozzi M, Lagana D, Carrafiello G, Cuffari S. Endovascular repair of traumatic injuries of the subclavian and axillary arteries. Injury. 2005;36:778–82.

44. Assenza M, Centonze L, Valesini L, Campana G, Corona M, Modini C. Traumatic subclavian arterial rupture: a case report and review of literature. World J Emerg Surg. 2012;7:18.

45. Raval M, Lee CJ, Phade S, Riaz A, Eskandari M, Rodriguez H. Covered stent use after subclavian artery and vein injuries in the setting of vascular Ehlers-Danlos. J Vasc Surg. 2012;55:542–4.

46. Dubose JJ, Rajani R, Gilani R, Arthurs ZA, Morrison JJ, Clouse WD, Rasmussen TE, Endovascular Skills for, T. & Resuscitative Surgery Working, G. Endovascular management of axillo-subclavian arterial injury: a review of published experience. Injury. 2012;43:1785–92.

47. Nagy K, Fabian T, Rodman G, Fulda G, Rodriguez A, Mirvis S. Guidelines for the diagnosis and management of blunt aortic injury: an EAST practice management guidelines work group. J Trauma. 2000;48:1128–43.

48. Fabian TC, Davis KA, Gavant ML, Croce MA, Melton SM, Patton Jr JH, Haan CK, Weiman DS, Pate JW. Prospective study of blunt aortic injury: helical CT is diagnostic and antihypertensive therapy reduces rupture. Ann Surg. 1998;227:666–76; discussion 676–7.

49. Pate JW, Gavant ML, Weiman DS, Fabian TC. Traumatic rupture of the aortic isthmus: program of selective management. World J Surg. 1999;23: 59–63.

50. von Oppell UO, Dunne TT, De Groot MK, Zilla P. Traumatic aortic rupture: twenty-year metaanalysis of mortality and risk of paraplegia. Ann Thorac Surg. 1994;58:585–93.

51. Adams HD, van Geertruyden HH. Neurologic complications of aortic surgery. Ann Surg. 1956;144:574–610.

52. Gharagozloo F, Larson J, Dausmann MJ, Neville Jr RF, Gomes MN. Spinal cord protection during surgical procedures on the descending thoracic and thoracoabdominal aorta: review of current techniques. Chest. 1996;109:799–809.

53. Acher CW, Wynn M. A modern theory of paraplegia in the treatment of aneurysms of the thoracoabdominal aorta: An analysis of technique specific observed/expected ratios for paralysis. J Vasc Surg. 2009;49:1117–24; discussion 1124.

54. Acher CW, Wynn MM, Mell MW, Tefera G, Hoch JR. A quantitative assessment of the impact of intercostal

artery reimplantation on paralysis risk in thoracoabdominal aortic aneurysm repair. Ann Surg. 2008; 248:529–40.

55. Tefera G, Acher CW, Wynn MM. Clamp and sew techniques in thoracoabdominal aortic surgery using naloxone and CSF drainage. Semin Vasc Surg. 2000;13:325–30.

56. Acher C, Wynn M. Outcomes in open repair of the thoracic and thoracoabdominal aorta. J Vasc Surg. 2010;52:3S–9.

57. Mell MW, Wynn MM, Reeder SB, Tefera G, Hoch JR, Acher CW. A new intercostal artery management strategy for thoracoabdominal aortic aneurysm repair. J Surg Res. 2009;154:99–104.

58. Amabile P, Collart F, Gariboldi V, Rollet G, Bartoli JM, Piquet P. Surgical versus endovascular treatment of traumatic thoracic aortic rupture. J Vasc Surg. 2004;40:873–9.

59. Steuer J, Wanhainen A, Thelin S, Nyman R, Eriksson MO, Bjorck M. Outcome of endovascular treatment of traumatic aortic transection. J Vasc Surg. 2012;56:973–8.

60. Celis RI, Park SC, Shukla AJ, Zenati MS, Chaer RA, Rhee RY, Makaroun MS, Cho JS. Evolution of treatment for traumatic thoracic aortic injuries. J Vasc Surg. 2012;56:74–80.

61. Lioupis C, Mackenzie KS, Corriveau MM, Obrand DI, Abraham CZ, Steinmetz OK. Midterm results following endovascular repair of blunt thoracic aortic injuries. Vasc Endovascular Surg. 2012;46: 109–16.

62. Azizzadeh A, Charlton-Ouw KM, Chen Z, Rahbar MH, Estrera AL, Amer H, Coogan SM, Safi HJ. An outcome analysis of endovascular versus open repair of blunt traumatic aortic injuries. J Vasc Surg. 2013;57(1):108–14.

63. Karmy-Jones R, Ferrigno L, Teso D, Long 3rd WB, Shackford S. Endovascular repair compared with operative repair of traumatic rupture of the thoracic aorta: a nonsystematic review and a plea for trauma-specific reporting guidelines. J Trauma. 2011;71: 1059–72.

64. Asensio JA, Chahwan S, Hanpeter D, Demetriades D, Forno W, Gambaro E, Murray J, Velmahos G, Marengo J, Shoemaker WC, Berne TV. Operative management and outcome of 302 abdominal vascular injuries. Am J Surg. 2000;180:528–33; discussion 533–4.

65. Cox EF. Blunt abdominal trauma. A 5-year analysis of 870 patients requiring celiotomy. Ann Surg. 1984;199:467–74.

66. Demetriades D, Velmahos G, Cornwell 3rd E, Berne TV, Cober S, Bhasin PS, Belzberg H, Asensio J. Selective nonoperative management of gunshot wounds of the anterior abdomen. Arch Surg. 1997;132:178–83.

67. Voellinger DC, Saddakni S, Melton SM, Wirthlin DJ, Jordan WD, Whitley D. Endovascular repair of a traumatic infrarenal aortic transection: a case report and review. Vasc Surg. 2001;35:385–9.

68. Demetriades D, Theodorou D, Murray J, Asensio JA, Cornwell 3rd EE, Velmahos G, Belzberg H, Berne TV. Mortality and prognostic factors in penetrating injuries of the aorta. J Trauma. 1996;40:761–3.

69. Accola KD, Feliciano DV, Mattox KL, Bitondo CG, Burch JM, Beall Jr AC, Jordan Jr GL. Management of injuries to the suprarenal aorta. Am J Surg. 1987;154:613–8.

70. Picard E, Marty-Ane CH, Vernhet H, Sessa C, Lesnik A, Senac JP, Mary H. Endovascular management of traumatic infrarenal abdominal aortic dissection. Ann Vasc Surg. 1998;12:515–21.

71. Vernhet H, Marty-Ane CH, Lesnik A, Chircop R, Serres-Cousine O, Picard E, Mary H, Senac JP. Dissection of the abdominal aorta in blunt trauma: management by percutaneous stent placement. Cardiovasc Intervent Radiol. 1997;20:473–6.

72. Kainuma S, Kuratani T, Kin K, Sawa Y. Endovascular aortic repair for spontaneous rupture of a non-aneurysmal infrarenal aorta. Interact Cardiovasc Thorac Surg. 2011;13:526–8.

73. Asensio JA, Forno W, Roldan G, Petrone P, Rojo E, Ceballos J, Wang C, Costaglioli B, Romero J, Tillou A, Carmody I, Shoemaker WC, Berne TV. Visceral vascular injuries. Surg Clin North Am. 2002;82: 1–20, xix.

74. Reilly PM, Rotondo MF, Carpenter JP, Sherr SA, Schwab CW. Temporary vascular continuity during damage control: intraluminal shunting for proximal superior mesenteric artery injury. J Trauma. 1995; 39:757–60.

75. Lucas AE, Richardson JD, Flint LM, Polk Jr HC. Traumatic injury of the proximal superior mesenteric artery. Ann Surg. 1981;193:30–4.

76. Narayanan G, Mohin G, Barbery K, Lamus D, Nanavati K, Yrizarry JM. Endovascular management of superior mesenteric artery pseudoaneurysm and fistula. Cardiovasc Intervent Radiol. 2008;31:1239–43.

77. Miller MT, Comerota AJ, Disalle R, Kaufman A, Pigott JP. Endoluminal embolization and revascularization for complicated mesenteric pseudoaneurysms: a report of two cases and a literature review. J Vasc Surg. 2007;45:381–6.

78. Bikk A, Rosenthal D, Kohlman M, Lai KM, Wellons ED. Traumatic superior mesenteric arteriovenous fistula and aortic pseudoaneurysm 20 years after repair. Vascular. 2005;13:350–4.

79. Krishan S, Mcpherson S, Pine J, Hayden J. Current management of mesenteric extrahepatic arterioportal fistulas: report of a case treated with a gastroduodenal artery stent graft and literature review. Vasc Endovascular Surg. 2010;44:139–45.

80. Price E, Zukotynski K, Chan R. Endovascular repair of traumatic mesocaval fistula. J Vasc Interv Radiol. 2008;19:1659–61.

81. Sangthong B, Demetriades D, Martin M, Salim A, Brown C, Inaba K, Rhee P, Chan L. Management and hospital outcomes of blunt renal artery injuries: analysis of 517 patients from the National Trauma Data Bank. J Am Coll Surg. 2006;203:612–7.

82. Villas PA, Cohen G, Putnam 3rd SG, Goldberg A, Ball D. Wallstent placement in a renal artery after blunt abdominal trauma. J Trauma. 1999;46:1137–9.

83. Sprouse 2nd LR, Hamilton Jr IN. The endovascular treatment of a renal arteriovenous fistula: Placement of a covered stent. J Vasc Surg. 2002;36:1066–8.

84. Lee JT, White RA. Endovascular management of blunt traumatic renal artery dissection. J Endovasc Ther. 2002;9:354–8.

85. Velmahos GC, Demetriades D, Cornwell 3rd EE, Belzberg H, Murray J, Asensio J, Berne TV. Selective management of renal gunshot wounds. Br J Surg. 1998;85:1121–4.

86. Clark DE, Georgitis JW, Ray FS. Renal arterial injuries caused by blunt trauma. Surgery. 1981;90: 87–96.

87. Lock JS, Carraway RP, Hudson Jr HC, Laws HL. Proper management of renal artery injury from blunt trauma. South Med J. 1985;78:406–10.

88. Haas CA, Spirnak JP. Traumatic renal artery occlusion: a review of the literature. Tech Urol. 1998; 4:1–11.

89. Burch JM, Richardson RJ, Martin RR, Mattox KL. Penetrating iliac vascular injuries: recent experience with 233 consecutive patients. J Trauma. 1990; 30:1450–9.

90. Carrillo EH, Spain DA, Wilson MA, Miller FB, Richardson JD. Alternatives in the management of penetrating injuries to the iliac vessels. J Trauma. 1998;44:1024–9. discussion 1029–30.

91. Asensio JA, Petrone P, Roldan G, Kuncir E, Rowe VL, Chan L, Shoemaker W, Berne TV. Analysis of 185 iliac vessel injuries: risk factors and predictors of outcome. Arch Surg. 2003;138:1187–93. discussion 1193–4.

92. Balogh Z, Voros E, Suveges G, Simonka JA. Stent graft treatment of an external iliac artery injury associated with pelvic fracture. A case report. J Bone Joint Surg Am. 2003;85-A:919–22.

93. Lyden SP, Srivastava SD, Waldman DL, Green RM. Common iliac artery dissection after blunt trauma: case report of endovascular repair and literature review. J Trauma. 2001;50:339–42.

94. Nam TK, Park SW, Shim HJ, Hwang SN. Endovascular treatment for common iliac artery injury complicating lumbar disc surgery: limited usefulness of temporary balloon occlusion. J Korean Neurosurg Soc. 2009;46:261–4.

95. Skippage P, Raja J, Mcfarland R, Belli AM. Endovascular repair of iliac artery injury complicating lumbar disc surgery. Eur Spine J. 2008;17 Suppl 2:S228–31.

96. Sato K, Orihashi K, Hamanaka Y, Hirai S, Mitsui N, Chatani N. Treatment of iliac artery rupture during percutaneous transluminal angioplasty: a report of three cases. Hiroshima J Med Sci. 2011;60:83–6.

97. Goltz JP, Basturk P, Hoppe H, Triller J, Kickuth R. Emergency and elective implantation of covered stent systems in iatrogenic arterial injuries. Rofo. 2011;183:618–30.

98. Loh SA, Maldonaldo TS, Rockman CB, Lamparello PJ, Adelman MA, Kalhorn SP, Frempong-Boadu A, Veith FJ, Cayne NS. Endovascular solutions to arterial injury due to posterior spine surgery. J Vasc Surg. 2012;55:1477–81.

99. Demetriades D, Murray J, Asensio J. Iliac vessel injuries. In: Rich N, Mattox K, Hirshberg A, editors. Vascular trauma. Philadelphia: Elsevier/Saunders; 2004.

100. Kuehne J, Frankhouse J, Modrall G, Golshani S, Aziz I, Demetriades D, Yellin AE. Determinants of survival after inferior vena cava trauma. Am Surg. 1999;65:976–81.

101. Buckman RF, Pathak AS, Badellino MM, Bradley KM. Injuries of the inferior vena cava. Surg Clin North Am. 2001;81:1431–47.

102. Buckman RF, Pathak AS, Badellino MM, Bradley KM. Portal vein injuries. Surg Clin North Am. 2001;81:1449–62.

103. Pachter HL, Drager S, Godfrey N, Lefleur R. Traumatic injuries of the portal vein. The role of acute ligation. Ann Surg. 1979;189:383–5.

104. Lee JT, Bongard FS. Iliac vessel injuries. Surg Clin North Am. 2002;82:21–48, xix.

105. Pasch AR, Bishara RA, Lim LT, Meyer JP, Schuler JJ, Flanigan DP. Optimal limb salvage in penetrating civilian vascular trauma. J Vasc Surg. 1986;3:189–95.

106. Stain SC, Yellin AE, Weaver FA, Pentecost MJ. Selective management of nonocclusive arterial injuries. Arch Surg. 1989;124:1136–40; discussion 1140–1.

107. Frykberg ER, Vines FS, Alexander RH. The natural history of clinically occult arterial injuries: a prospective evaluation. J Trauma. 1989;29:577–83.

108. Neville Jr RF, Hobson 2nd RW, Watanabe B, Yasuhara H, Padberg Jr FT, Duran W, Franco CD. A prospective evaluation of arterial intimal injuries in an experimental model. J Trauma. 1991;31:669–74; discussion 674–5.

109. Panetta TF, Sales CM, Marin ML, Schwartz ML, Jones AM, Berdejo GL, Wengerter KR, Veith FJ. Natural history, duplex characteristics, and histopathologic correlation of arterial injuries in a canine model. J Vasc Surg. 1992;16:867–74; discussion 874–6.

110. Dennis JW, Frykberg ER, Veldenz HC, Huffman S, Menawat SS. Validation of nonoperative management of occult vascular injuries and accuracy of physical examination alone in penetrating extremity trauma: 5- to 10-year follow-up. J Trauma. 1998;44: 243–52; discussion 242–3.

111. Frykberg ER. Advances in the diagnosis and treatment of extremity vascular trauma. Surg Clin North Am. 1995;75:207–23.

112. Lynch K, Johansen K. Can Doppler pressure measurement replace "exclusion" arteriography in the diagnosis of occult extremity arterial trauma? Ann Surg. 1991;214:737–41.

113. Johansen K, Lynch K, Paun M, Copass M. Non-invasive vascular tests reliably exclude occult arterial trauma in injured extremities. J Trauma. 1991;31:515–9; discussion 519–22.

114. Dennis JW, Jagger C, Butcher JL, Menawat SS, Neel M, Frykberg ER. Reassessing the role of arteriograms in the management of posterior knee dislocations. J Trauma. 1993;35:692–5; discussion 695–7.

115. Abou-Sayed H, Berger DL. Blunt lower-extremity trauma and popliteal artery injuries: revisiting the case for selective arteriography. Arch Surg. 2002; 137:585–9.

116. Conrad MF, Patton Jr JH, Parikshak M, Kralovich KA. Evaluation of vascular injury in penetrating extremity trauma: angiographers stay home. Am Surg. 2002;68:269–74.

117. Soto JA, Munera F, Cardoso N, Guarin O, Medina S. Diagnostic performance of helical Ct angiography in trauma to large arteries of the extremities. J Comput Assist Tomogr. 1999;23:188–96.

118. Dubose JJ, Rajani R, Gilani R, Arthurs ZA, Morrison JJ, Clouse WD, Rasmussen TE, Endovascular Skills for Trauma and Resuscitative Surgery Working Group. Endovascular management of axillo-subclavian arterial injury: a review of published experience. Injury. 2012;43:1785–92.

119. Xenos ES, Freeman M, Stevens S, Cassada D, Pacanowski J, Goldman M. Covered stents for injuries of subclavian and axillary arteries. J Vasc Surg. 2003;38:451–4.

120. Gorman JF. Combat arterial trauma. Analysis of 106 limb-threatening injuries. Arch Surg. 1969;98:160–4.

121. Kovacs F, Pollock JG, Denunzio M. Endovascular stent graft repair of iatrogenic popliteal artery injuries – a report of 2 cases. Vasc Endovascular Surg. 2012;46:269–72.

122. Zimmerman P, D'Audiffret A, Pillai L. Endovascular repair of blunt extremity arterial injury: case report. Vasc Endovascular Surg. 2009;43:211–4.

123. Trellopoulos G, Georgiadis GS, Aslanidou EA, Nikolopoulos ES, Pitta X, Papachristodoulou A, Lazarides MK. Endovascular management of peripheral arterial trauma in patients presenting in hemorrhagic shock. J Cardiovasc Surg (Torino). 2012;53:495–506.

124. Wagner WH, Yellin AE, Weaver FA, Stain SC, Siegel AE. Acute treatment of penetrating popliteal artery trauma: the importance of soft tissue injury. Ann Vasc Surg. 1994;8:557–65.

125. Wagner WH, Calkins ER, Weaver FA, Goodwin JA, Myles RA, Yellin AE. Blunt popliteal artery trauma: one hundred consecutive injuries. J Vasc Surg. 1988;7:736–43.

126. Shah DM, Corson JD, Karmody AM, Fortune JB, Leather RP. Optimal management of tibial arterial trauma. J Trauma. 1988;28:228–34.

127. Whitman GR, Mccroskey BL, Moore EE, Pearce WH, Moore FA. Traumatic popliteal and trifurcation vascular injuries: determinants of functional limb salvage. Am J Surg. 1987;154:681–4.

Anticoagulation, Resuscitation, and Hemostasis

2

Pär I. Johansson

Contents

P.I. Johansson, MD, DMSc, MPA
Section for Transfusion Medicine,
Capital Region Blood Bank, Rigshospitalet University
of Copenhagen, Copenhagen, Denmark

Department of Surgery,
Center for Translational Injury Research (CeTIR),
University of Texas Medical School – Houston,
Houston, TX, USA
e-mail: per.johansson@regionh.dk

2.1 Introduction

Hemorrhage requiring massive transfusion remains a major cause of potentially preventable deaths. Trauma and massive transfusion are associated with coagulopathy secondary to tissue injury, hypoperfusion, dilution, and consumption of clotting factors and platelets, and coagulopathy, together with hypothermia and acidosis, forms a "lethal" triad [1]. In the last decade, the *concept of damage control surgery* has evolved, prioritizing early control of the cause of bleeding by temporary, non-definitive means. Similarly, the concept of *damage control resuscitation*, i.e., limiting fluid resuscitation and applying the concept of permissive hypotension with the goal of achieving a palpable radialis pulse in patients, has been advocated, whereas in patients with head injury, a systolic blood pressure above 110 mmHg is recommended [2–4]. Also, providing a large amount of blood products to critically injured patients in an immediate and sustained manner as part of an early massive transfusion protocol, reducing the amount of crystalloid administered, has been introduced [3, 5]. The rationale behind this resuscitation concept is to transfuse red blood cells, plasma, and platelets (PLT) in the same proportion as found in circulating whole blood, thus leading toward a unit-for-unit ratio to prevent and treat coagulopathy due to massive hemorrhage. This chapter addresses the clinical problems associated with vascular hemorrhage and massive transfusion in trauma.

2.2 Coagulopathy in Vascular Trauma

2.2.1 Dilution

The dilution of coagulation factors and platelets is an important cause of coagulopathy in trauma patients [6]. The Advanced Trauma Life Support (ATLS) guideline recommends aggressive crystalloid resuscitation, but the dilutional effects of such administration on coagulation competence are well described [7], and this strategy provokes acidosis, formation of interstitial edema with tissue swelling, impairment of the microcirculation, and hence compromised oxygenation [8, 9]. Furthermore, recent studies indicate that increased volume of crystalloids administered is associated with greater incidence of multiple organ failure, abdominal compartment syndrome [10], and mortality [11].

Furthermore, synthetic colloid resuscitation fluids influence coagulation competence more profoundly than crystalloids. Hydroxyethyl starch (HES) causes efflux of plasma proteins from blood to the interstitial space, reduction in plasma concentration of coagulation factor VIII and von Willebrand factor (vWF), inhibition of platelet function, and reduced interaction of activated FXIII with fibrin polymers [12]. A recent meta-analysis of 24 studies evaluating the safety of HES 130/0.4 administration in surgical, emergency, and intensive care patients demonstrated that HES administration promotes a dose-dependent coagulopathy [13]. Also, administration of blood products such as RBC, FFP, and PLT may cause significant dilution since these blood products are stored in anticoagulation solutions reducing coagulation factor concentration

to approximately 60 % and platelet count to approximately $80 \times 10^9/l$ when a hematocrit of 30 % is warranted [14].

2.2.2 Hypothermia

Hypothermia is associated with risk of uncontrolled bleeding and death in trauma patients. Hypothermia-induced coagulopathy is attributed to platelet dysfunction, reduced coagulation factor activity (significant below 33 °C) [15], and induction of fibrinolysis [16], and these effects are reversible with normalization of body temperature.

2.2.3 Acidosis

In trauma patients acidosis is induced by hypoperfusion and excess administration of ionic chloride, i.e., NaCl, during resuscitation [17]. Acidosis impairs almost all essential parts of the coagulation process: At pH <7.4, platelets change their structure and shape [18]. The activity of coagulation factor complexes on the cell surface is reduced, and the resulting impaired thrombin generation is a major cause of coagulopathic bleeding, secondary to reduced clot strength and stability. Furthermore, acidosis leads to increased degradation of fibrinogen [19] which further aggravates the coagulopathy.

2.2.4 Trauma

An early "endogenous" coagulopathy in trauma patients not attributed to dilution and hypothermia with shock and hypoperfusion as the key drivers of acute traumatic coagulopathy through activation of the anticoagulant and fibrinolytic pathways has been identified [20–22]. We recently reported that the early coagulopathy observed in trauma patients, which reflects the state of the fluid phase including its cellular elements, i.e., circulating whole blood, is a consequence of the degree of the tissue injury and the thereby generated sympathoadrenal activity and critically related to the degree of endothelial damage, with a progressively more procoagulant endothelium (solid phase) inducing a gradient of increasing anticoagulation toward the fluid phase (circulating blood) [23]. Though it seems counterintuitive that increasing injury severity is associated with progressive hypocoagulability and hyperfibrinolysis, this may from an evolutionary perspective exert a survival advantage by preserving blood flow through the progressively more damaged and procoagulant microvasculature [23]. In alignment with this, we found that in trauma patients upon hospital admission, a high level of syndecan-1, a marker of endothelial glycocalyx degradation, was associated with high sympathoadrenal activity and increased mortality, even after adjusting for injury severity score [24]. Also, only in patients with high syndecan-1 levels was increasing injury severity associated with increased tissue and endothelial damage, protein C depletion, hyperfibrinolysis, and inflammation [24].

2.2.5 Consumptive Coagulopathy

Tissue injury secondary to trauma induces immediate activation of the coagulation system through upregulation of tissue factor (TF) expression and extensive thrombin generation. Tissue injury in association with extensive endothelial injury, massive soft tissue damage, and fat embolization from long-bone fractures may be associated with the consumption of coagulation factors and platelets and hence development of coagulopathy. Disseminated intravascular coagulation (DIC) is the most extreme form of consumptive coagulopathy and is characterized by systemic activation of pathways leading to and regulating coagulation, which can result in the generation of fibrin clots that may cause organ failure with concomitant consumption of platelets and coagulation factors that may result in clinical bleeding [25, 26]. We recently reported, however, that disseminated intravascular coagulation (DIC) was not a part of the early coagulopathy secondary to trauma [27] though this may develop later in the course of resuscitation [28].

2.2.6 Hyperfibrinolysis

Increased fibrinolysis is observed in patients with profound endothelial activation and damage secondary to trauma, surgery, and ischemia-reperfusion injury where tissue-type plasminogen activator (tPA) is released from the Weibel-Palade bodies of the endothelial cells. In trauma, increased fibrinolysis has been reported in the most severely injured patients, and this correlates with poor outcome [29, 30]. The presence of increased fibrinolysis with increasing injury severity may reflect an evolutionary mechanism aiming at preventing fatal intravascular coagulation secondary to systemic hypercoagulation induced by the trauma [23].

2.3 Anticoagulation

Vitamin K antagonists are used by patients with atrial fibrillation or artificial cardiac valves, and warfarin has been reported to be associated with about 21,000 visits for bleeding complications per year in the USA alone [31, 32]. The use of the International Normalized Ratio (INR, a plasmatic coagulation analysis) to monitor the degree of anticoagulation by warfarin may in part explain this problem. The lack of adequate hemostatic monitoring is also evident with regard to the newer pharmaceutical agents used for secondary prevention and postoperative thromboprophylaxis such as the direct thrombin inhibitor dabigatran [33] and the direct FXa inhibitors apixaban [34] and rivaroxaban [35]. Currently, it is recommended that treatment with these agents does not require hemostatic monitoring [36]. Despite this, however, reports of severe bleedings in patients taking these medications are being reported, including trauma, and since no antidote exists, treatment of these patients is a major challenge [37–39].

Apart from coagulopathy due to iatrogenic heparinization, critically ill patients, including trauma patients, may become endogenously heparinized due to degradation of the endothelial glycocalyx [26, 40], the antiadhesive and anticoagulant carbohydrate-rich surface layer that covers and protects the endothelial cells and contains significant amounts of heparin-like substances [41, 42].

2.4   Platelet Inhibitors

An important cause of excessive bleeding in trauma patients is platelet inhibitors, which an increasing proportion of the population today uses as secondary prevention. Currently, the most important are the platelet ADP receptor inhibitors clopidogrel and the even more potent prasugrel that irreversibly inhibits platelet activation through the platelet ADP receptor and confers more potent platelet inhibition than acetylsalicylic acid.

Importantly, the enhanced antiplatelet activity and greater efficacy seen with prasugrel when compared to clopidogrel in clinical trials have been accompanied by increased bleeding risk, and the FDA advisory committee issued guidance to physicians about the increased risk in low-weight or elderly patients [43].

2.5   Monitoring Hemostasis

2.5.1   Whole Blood Viscoelastic Assays

Introduction of the cell-based model of hemostasis emphasizes the role of platelets for intact thrombin generation and highlights the importance of the dynamics of thrombin generation influencing the quality and stability of the thrombus formed [44]. Consequently, hemostatic assays performed on plasma such as activated partial thromboplastin time (APTT) and prothrombin time (PT) are of limited value [45], and they do not correlate with clinically relevant coagulopathies [46, 47]. Instead, employing a whole blood assay, such as viscoelastic hemostatic assays (VHA) like TEG/ROTEM that records the viscoelastic changes during clot formation and subsequent lysis, is preferable. The TEG reports (Fig. 2.1) the reaction time (R), angle (α), maximum amplitude (MA), maximal clot strength, and clot lysis (Ly) [48, 49]. Typical TEG profiles observed in trauma patients are normocoagulable, hypercoagulable, hypocoagulable, and hyperfibrinolytic profiles (Fig. 2.2), and in actively bleeding patients these should be treated according to an algorithm.

Reduced clot stability correlates with clinical bleeding conditions as demonstrated by Plotkin et al. [50] who, in patients with a penetrating trauma, reported TEG to be an accurate indicator of the blood product requirements. Furthermore, TEG is the gold standard for identifying hypercoagulability [51] and hyperfibrinolysis [29, 30, 52], the latter a significant cause of bleeding in patients with major trauma [29, 30, 52]. The use of VHA in trauma is now recommended by recent guidelines [53] and textbooks [54] and its use in the military field is extensive, and many level 1 trauma centers consider the use of VHA to monitor and guide hemostatic therapy as routine; a recent study of 1.974 trauma patients report that rapid TEG can replace the conventional coagulation tests in trauma patients [55].

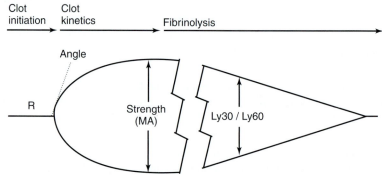

Fig. 2.1 Thromboelastograph (TEG) parameters

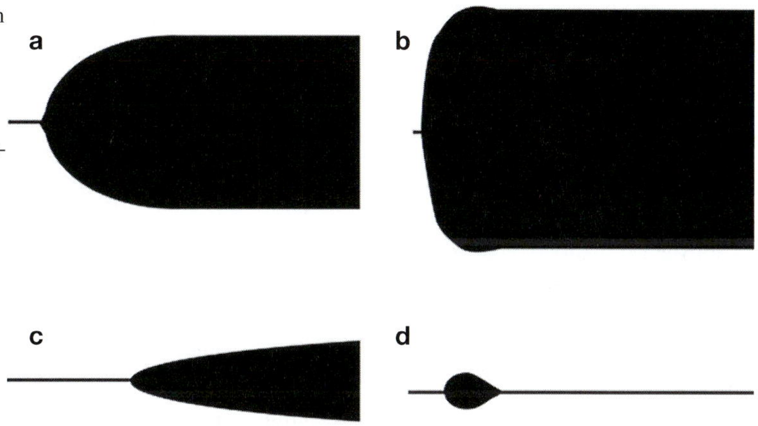

Fig. 2.2 Schematic presentation of various TEG tracings in trauma: (**a**) normal, (**b**) hypercoagulability, (**c**) hypocoagulability (thrombocytopenia/thrombocytopathy), and (**d**) primary hyperfibrinolysis

2.5.2 Whole Blood Platelet Function Analyzers

Different assays evaluating the degree of platelet inhibition secondary to platelet inhibitors exist. Light transmission aggregometry (LTA), previously considered the "gold standard" for investigation of platelet aggregation [56], unfortunately relies on artificially manufactured platelet-rich plasma suspensions, which do not reflect in vivo conditions, and consequently platelet function assays performed on whole blood are today favored. Examples of whole blood platelet function assays are PFA100 (Siemens, Tarrytown, USA), VerifyNow (Accumetrics, San Diego, USA), Multiplate (Verum Diagnostica GmbH, Munich, Germany), and TEG PlateletMapping (Haemonetics Corp, Chicago, USA), which all have been reported to be able to identify clinically relevant platelet inhibition secondary to pharmacological platelet inhibitors.

2.6 Administration of Blood Products

2.6.1 Red Blood Cells

In response to hemorrhage, lowered hematocrit contributes to coagulopathy since erythrocytes promote marginalization of platelets so the platelet concentrations along the endothelium remain almost seven times that of the average blood concentration [57]. In addition, erythrocytes support thrombin generation through exposure of procoagulant membrane phospholipids [58], and they activate platelets by liberating ADP [59] emphasizing that in vivo thrombus formation is a multicellular event [44, 60]. Yet, the optimal hematocrit for platelet-vessel wall interactions remains unknown but it may be as high as 35 % [61].

2.6.2 Fresh Frozen Plasma

It remains controversial when and in what dose plasma should be transfused to massively bleeding trauma patients [62], and the optimal ratio of FFP to RBCs remains to be established although collectively the data indicate that a FFP/RBC ratio greater than 1:2 is associated with improved survival compared to one lower than 1:2 [63, 64]. This is further supported by a review and meta-analysis from 2010 reporting that in patients undergoing massive transfusion, high FFP to RBC ratios were associated with a significant reduction in the risk of death (odds ratio (OR) 0.38 (95 % CI 0.24–0.60)) and multiorgan failure (OR 0.40 (95 % CI 0.26–0.60)) [65] and a meta-analysis from 2012 reports of reduced mortality in trauma patients treated with the highest FFP or PLT to RBC ratios [66].

2.6.3 Platelets

Platelets are also pivotal for hemostasis [44, 66], and several retrospective studies report an association between thrombocytopenia and postoperative bleeding and mortality [67, 68]. Holcomb et al. [63] found that the highest survival was established in patients who received both a high PLT/RBC and a high FFP/RBC ratio. Inaba et al. recently reported from a retrospective study of massively transfused patients that as the apheresis platelet to RBC ratio increased, a stepwise improvement in survival was seen and a high apheresis PLT/RBC ratio was independently associated with improved survival [69]. This is in alignment with Brown et al. who reported that admission platelet count was inversely correlated with 24-h mortality and transfusion of RBCs and that a normal platelet count may be insufficient after severe trauma, suggesting these patients may benefit from a higher platelet transfusion threshold [70]. In a recent meta-analysis, a high PLT/RBC ratio in massively bleeding trauma patients was reported to reduce mortality [66].

2.6.4 Massive Transfusion Protocols and Ratios

A recent meta-analysis of retrospective observational studies evaluating the effect of FFP/RBC and/or PLT/RBC ratios and survival in massively bleeding trauma patients recently reported a significant survival benefit in patients receiving high FFP/RBC and PLT/RBC ratios [66]. A potential confounder of these results is survivorship bias relating to that those surviving long enough will receive FFP and PLT whereas those dying early will not, as reported by Snyder et al. [71]. Survivorship bias, however, does not explain the improved survival in studies concerning the introduction of transfusion packages where both FFP and PLT are immediately available, i.e., where pre-thawed FFP are available. Cotton et al. [72] implemented a trauma exsanguination protocol (TEP) involving 10 RBC, 4 FFP, and 2 apheresis PLT for trauma patients and used it to evaluate 211 trauma patients of who 94 received TEP and 117 were historic controls. The TEP patients received more RBC (16 vs. 11), FFP (8 vs. 4), and PLT (2 vs. 1) intraoperatively than the controls and displayed lower 30-day mortality (51 % vs. 66 %). After controlling for age, sex, mechanism of injury, Trauma and Injury Severity Score (TRISS), and 24-h blood product usage, a 74 % reduction in the odds ratio of mortality was found among patients in the TEP group. In a later study involving additionally 53 patients, Cotton also [73] reported that not only was 30-day survival higher in the TEP group compared to the controls but the incidence of pneumonia, pulmonary failure, and abdominal compartment syndrome was lower in the TEP patients. Also, the incidence of sepsis or septic shock and multiorgan failure was lower in TEP patients. In alignment with this, Duchesne et al. reported that in trauma patients undergoing damage control laparotomy, introduction of damage control resuscitation encompassing early administration of plasma and platelets together with RBC was associated with improved 30-day survival (73.6 % vs. 54.8 %, $p < 0.009$) when compared to patients treated with conventional resuscitation efforts [74]. A multicenter randomized control study evaluating the effect of different blood product ratios on survival in massively bleeding trauma patients will commence in the USA this year, and hopefully this will result in evidence for how best to resuscitate these patients with blood products (http://www.uth.tmc.edu/cetir/PROPPR/index.html).

2.6.5 Fresh Whole Blood

With the implementation of fractionated blood components, the routine use of fresh whole blood (FWB) for resuscitation of bleeding patients was abandoned in the civilian setting. In the combat setting, however, FWB has been used in situations where fractionated blood products and especially platelets were not available. In a report of US military patients in Iraq and Afghanistan from January 2004 to October 2007, those with hemorrhagic shock, a resuscitation strategy that included FWB was associated with improved 30-day survival (95 % vs. 82 %, $p = 0.002$) [75], and an ongoing trial is currently addressing this issue (www.clingovtrial.com/NCT01227005). It should be noted that administration of any blood product carries potential risks for the patient including viral and bacterial transmission, hemolytic transfusion reactions, transfusion-related acute lung injury, and immunomodulation and consequently transfusion of blood products should be reserved to patients who actually needs this therapy [76].

2.7 Goal-Directed Hemostatic Resuscitation with Transfusion Packages Together with VHA

Goal-directed treatment with blood products and antifibrinolytic pharmacological agents based on the result of the whole blood viscoelastic hemostatic assays (VHA), together with the clinical presentation, was introduced for more than 25 years ago in patients undergoing liver transplantation and cardiac surgery, and there are validated algorithms for how coagulopathy is identified and treated in patients with ongoing bleeding, based on VHA [77]. More than 25 studies encompassing more than 4,500 patients have evaluated VHA vs. conventional coagulation assays on bleeding and transfusion requirements in patients undergoing cardiac, liver, vascular, or trauma surgery and in patients requiring massive transfusion. These studies demonstrate the superiority of VHA in predicting the need for blood transfusion, and the VHA-based algorithm reduces the transfusion requirements and the need for redo surgery in contrast to the treatment based on conventional coagulation assays [49], and this was further corroborated in a recent Cochrane review [78].

We found that the implementation of goal-directed hemostatic resuscitation of massively bleeding patients, including trauma, based on the VHA reduced mortality by approximately 30 % in patients requiring more than 10 RBC in the first 24 h [77], and recently we reported that early hemorrhagic death in trauma patients was reduced by more than 40 % when a combination of transfusion packages and goal-directed hemostatic resuscitation was employed [79]. The systematic use of VHA to monitor and guide

transfusion therapy is furthermore endorsed by several recent international transfusion guidelines and teaching books [68, 69].

2.8 Hemostatic Agents

2.8.1 Antifibrinolytics

Hyperfibrinolysis contributes significantly to coagulopathy, and antifibrinolytic agents reduce the blood loss in patients with both normal and exaggerated fibrinolytic responses to surgery by preventing plasmin(ogen) from binding to fibrin and by preventing plasmin degradation of platelet glycoprotein Ib receptors [80]. In a placebo-controlled randomized study (CRASH-2) including 20,211 adult trauma patients, tranexamic acid as compared to placebo significantly decreased all-cause mortality from 16.0 to 14.5 %, $p = 0.0035$ [81]. We recommend monitoring of hemostasis with TEG to identify hyperfibrinolytic states in trauma patients and, consequently, targeted treatment with antifibrinolytic agents.

2.8.2 Recombinant Factor VIIa

Recombinant factor VIIa (rFVIIa) acts in pharmacological doses by enhancing thrombin generation on the activated platelets independent of factors VIII and IX and is currently approved for episodes of severe hemorrhage or perioperative management of bleeding in patients with congenital factor VII deficiency and hemophilia A or B with inhibitors [82]. Data from the CONTROL trial, a phase 3 randomized clinical trial evaluating the efficacy and safety of rFVIIa as an adjunct to direct hemostasis in major trauma, rFVIIa did not change mortality in patients with blunt (11.0 % (rFVIIa) vs. 10.7 % (placebo)) or penetrating (18.2 % (rFVIIa) vs. 13.2 % (placebo)) trauma [83]. In a recent review reporting on the rate of thromboembolic events in all published randomized placebo-controlled trials of rFVIIa use, Levi [84] reported that the rates of arterial thromboembolic events among all subjects were higher among those who received rFVIIa than

among those who received placebo (5.5 % vs. 3.2 %, $p=0.003$).

2.8.3 Fibrinogen Concentrate

Conversion of sufficient amounts of fibrinogen to fibrin is a prerequisite for clot formation, and reduction in the circulating level of fibrinogen due to consumption and/or dilution by resuscitation fluids induces coagulopathy [85]. It is, therefore, important to maintain an adequate fibrinogen level when continued bleeding is bridged by saline and/or colloid infusion or blood products (primarily RBC) without fibrinogen. Recent data indicate that coagulopathy induced by synthetic colloids such as HES may be reversed by the administration of fibrinogen concentrate [86]. A recent review only found four studies of poor quality assessing fibrinogen concentrate to bleeding surgical and trauma patients and concluded that randomized controlled trials of sufficient size and long-term follow-up need to be performed before such a practice can be recommended routinely [87]. The use of fibrinogen concentrate in patients with established hypofibrinogenemia, diagnosed by VHA (Functional Fibrinogen® or FibTEM®), in addition to a balanced administration of RBC, FFP, and platelets, may however contribute to faster achievement of a normal hemostasis in massively bleeding patients, and we recommend the use of fibrinogen concentrate according to TEG-guided algorithms in such patients.

2.8.4 Prothrombin Complex Concentrate

The four-factor PCC encompasses coagulation factors II, VII, IX, and X that all are essential for thrombin generation. Administration of PCC is indicated for the treatment of congenital coagulation disorders and to reverse orally administered anticoagulation by vitamin K antagonists [88], whereas experience with treatment of massive bleeding with PCC is lacking. Recently, Carvalho et al. reported that the administration of PCC to patients with massive bleedings had

beneficial effect on hemostasis and this warrants further investigation in a randomized controlled setting [89].

2.8.5 Factor XIII

Factor XIII is important for clot firmness by binding to platelets through the GPIIb/GPIIIa receptor and by cross-linking fibrin and increasing the resistance of the formed clot against fibrinolysis [90]. Notably, patients with "unexplained" intraoperative coagulopathies and, hence, bleeding demonstrate significantly less FXIII per unit thrombin available both before, during, and after surgery [91]. An increased tendency to postoperative bleeding has been observed, even at factor XIII activities as high as 60 % [92]. The role of FXIII administration to bleeding trauma patients however remains to be investigated in randomized clinical trials.

Conclusion

Viscoelastic whole blood assays, such as TEG and ROTEM, are advantageous for identifying coagulopathy and guide ongoing transfusion therapy. From the result of these assays, the implementation of a hemostatic control resuscitation strategy to massively bleeding patients seems both reasonable and lifesaving although data from prospective randomized controlled trials are lacking. Until a definite proof from such trials is available, retrospective data support a shift in transfusion medicine in regard to early and aggressive administration of plasma and platelets.

References

1. Lier H, Krep H, Schroeder S, Stuber F. Preconditions of hemostasis in trauma: a review. The influence of acidosis, hypocalcemia, anemia, and hypothermia on functional hemostasis in trauma. J Trauma. 2008;65:951–60.
2. Stern SA, Dronen SC, Birrer P, Wang X. Effect of blood pressure on hemorrhage volume and survival in a near-fatal hemorrhage model incorporating a vascular injury. Ann Emerg Med. 1993;22:155–63.

3. Dries DJ. Hypotensive resuscitation. Shock. 1996;6:311–6.
4. Dutton RP. Resuscitative strategies to maintain homeostasis during damage control surgery. Br J Surg. 2012;99 Suppl 1:21–8. doi:10.1002/bjs.7731.
5. American Society of Anesthesiologists Task Force on Perioperative Blood Transfusion and Adjuvant Therapies. Practice guidelines for perioperative blood transfusion and adjuvant therapies: an updated report by the American Society of Anesthesiologists Task Force on Perioperative Blood Transfusion and Adjuvant Therapies. Anesthesiology. 2006;105:198–208.
6. Chappell D, Jacob M, Hofmann-Kiefer K, Conzen P, Rehm M. A rational approach to perioperative fluid management. Anesthesiology. 2008;109:723–40.
7. Mittermayr M, Streif W, Haas T, Fries D, Velik-Salchner C, Klingler A, Oswald E, Bach C, Schnapka-Koepf M, Innerhofer P. Hemostatic changes after crystalloid or colloid fluid administration during major orthopedic surgery: the role of fibrinogen administration. Anesth Analg. 2007;105:905–17.
8. Knotzer H, Pajk W, Maier S, Dunser MW, Ulmer H, Schwarz B, Salak N, Hasibeder WR. Comparison of lactated Ringer's, gelatine and blood resuscitation on intestinal oxygen supply and mucosal tissue oxygen tension in haemorrhagic shock. Br J Anaesth. 2006;97:509–16.
9. Thorsen K, Ringdal KG, Strand K, Soreide E, Hagemo J, Soreide K. Clinical and cellular effects of hypothermia, acidosis and coagulopathy in major injury. Br J Surg. 2011;98:894–907.
10. Neal MD, Hoffman MK, Cuschieri J, Minei JP, Maier RV, Harbrecht BG, Billiar TR, Peitzman AB, Moore EE, Cohen MJ, Sperry JL. Crystalloid to packed red blood cell transfusion ratio in the massively transfused patient: when a little goes a long way. J Trauma Acute Care Surg. 2012;72:892–8.
11. Duchesne JC, Guidry C, Hoffman JR, Park TS, Bock J, Lawson S, Meade P, McSwain Jr NE. Low-volume resuscitation for severe intraoperative hemorrhage: a step in the right direction. Am Surg. 2012;78:936–41.
12. Nielsen VG. Colloids decrease clot propagation and strength: role of factor XIII-fibrin polymer and thrombin-fibrinogen interactions. Acta Anaesthesiol Scand. 2005;49:1163–71.
13. Hartog CS, Kohl M, Reinhart K. A systematic review of third-generation hydroxyethyl starch (HES 130/0.4) in resuscitation: safety not adequately addressed. Anesth Analg. 2011;112:635–45.
14. Hess JR. Massive transfusion for trauma: opportunities and risks. ISBT Science Series. 2008;3:197–201.
15. Wolberg AS, Meng ZH, Monroe III DM, Hoffman M. A systematic evaluation of the effect of temperature on coagulation enzyme activity and platelet function. J Trauma. 2004;56:1221–8.
16. Yoshihara H, Yamamoto T, Mihara H. Changes in coagulation and fibrinolysis occurring in dogs during hypothermia. Thromb Res. 1985;37:503–12.
17. Hess JR, Brohi K, Dutton RP, Hauser CJ, Holcomb JB, Kluger Y, Mackway-Jones K, Parr MJ, Rizoli SB, Yukioka T, Hoyt DB, Bouillon B. The coagulopathy of trauma: a review of mechanisms. J Trauma. 2008;65:748–54.
18. Djaldetti M, Fishman P, Bessler H, Chaimoff C. pH-induced platelet ultrastructural alterations. A possible mechanism for impaired platelet aggregation. Arch Surg. 1979;114:707–10.
19. Martini WZ, Holcomb JB. Acidosis and coagulopathy: the differential effects on fibrinogen synthesis and breakdown in pigs. Ann Surg. 2007;246:831–5.
20. Brohi K, Singh J, Heron M, Coats T. Acute traumatic coagulopathy. J Trauma. 2003;54:1127–30.
21. Brohi K, Cohen MJ, Ganter MT, Schultz MJ, Levi M, Mackersie RC, Pittet JF. Acute coagulopathy of trauma: hypoperfusion induces systemic anticoagulation and hyperfibrinolysis. J Trauma. 2008;64:1211–7.
22. Brohi K, Cohen MJ, Ganter MT, Matthay MA, Mackersie RC, Pittet JF. Acute traumatic coagulopathy: initiated by hypoperfusion: modulated through the protein C pathway? Ann Surg. 2007;245:812–8.
23. Johansson PI, Ostrowski SR. Acute coagulopathy of trauma: balancing progressive catecholamine induced endothelial activation and damage by fluid phase anticoagulation. Med Hypotheses. 2010;75:564–7.
24. Johansson PI, Stensballe J, Rasmussen LS, Ostrowski SR. A high admission syndecan-1 level, a marker of endothelial glycocalyx degradation, is associated with inflammation, protein C depletion, fibrinolysis, and increased mortality in trauma patients. Ann Surg. 2011;254:194–200.
25. Levi M, Toh CH, Thachil J, Watson HG. Guidelines for the diagnosis and management of disseminated intravascular coagulation. Br J Haematol. 2009;145:24–33.
26. Hess JR, Lawson JH. The coagulopathy of trauma versus disseminated intravascular coagulation. J Trauma. 2006;60:S12–9.
27. Johansson PI, Sørensen AM, Perner A, Welling KL, Wanscher M, Larsen CF, Ostrowski SR. Disseminated intravascular coagulation or acute coagulopathy of trauma shock early after trauma? An observational study. Crit Care. 2011;15:R272.
28. Gando S. Disseminated intravascular coagulation in trauma patients. Semin Thromb Hemost. 2001;27:585–92.
29. Schochl H, Frietsch T, Pavelka M, Jambor C. Hyperfibrinolysis after major trauma: differential diagnosis of lysis patterns and prognostic value of thrombelastometry. J Trauma. 2009;67:125–31.
30. Kashuk JL, Moore EE, Sawyer M, Wohlauer M, Pezold M, Barnett C, Biffl WL, Burlew CC, Johnson JL, Sauaia A. Primary fibrinolysis is integral in the pathogenesis of the acute coagulopathy of trauma. Ann Surg. 2010;252:434–42.
31. Budnitz DS, Lovegrove MC, Shehab N, Richards CL. Emergency hospitalizations for adverse drug events in older Americans. N Engl J Med. 2011;365:2002–12.

32. Wysowski DK, Nourjah P, Swartz L. Bleeding complications with warfarin use: a prevalent adverse effect resulting in regulatory action. Arch Intern Med. 2007;167:1414–9.

33. Oldgren J, Alings M, Darius H, Diener HC, Eikelboom J, Ezekowitz MD, Kamensky G, Reilly PA, Yang S, Yusuf S, Wallentin L, Connolly SJ. Risks for stroke, bleeding, and death in patients with atrial fibrillation receiving dabigatran or warfarin in relation to the CHADS2 score: a subgroup analysis of the RE-LY trial. Ann Intern Med. 2011;155:660–7, W204.

34. Huang J, Cao Y, Liao C, Wu L, Gao F. Apixaban versus enoxaparin in patients with total knee arthroplasty. A meta-analysis of randomised trials. Thromb Haemost. 2011;105:245–53.

35. Duggan ST. Rivaroxaban: a review of its use for the prophylaxis of venous thromboembolism after total hip or knee replacement surgery. Am J Cardiovasc Drugs. 2012;12:57–72.

36. Levi M, Eerenberg ES, Kampuisen PW. Anticoagulants. Old and new. Hamostaseologie. 2011;31:229–35.

37. Cotton BA, McCarthy JJ, Holcomb JB. Acutely injured patients on dabigatran. N Engl J Med. 2011;365:2039–40.

38. Lillo-Le Louët A, Wolf M, Soufir L, Galbois A, Dumenil AS, Offenstadt G, Samama MM. Life-threatening bleeding in four patients with an unusual excessive response to dabigatran: implications for emergency surgery and resuscitation. Thromb Haemost. 2012;108:583–5.

39. Boland M, Murphy M, Murphy M, McDermott E. Acute-onset severe gastrointestinal tract hemorrhage in apostoperative patient taking rivaroxaban after total hip arthroplasty: a case report. J Med Case Rep. 2012;6:129.

40. Ostrowski SR, Johansson PI. Endothelial glycocalyx degradation induces endogenous heparinization in patients with severe injury and early traumatic coagulopathy. J Trauma Acute Care Surg. 2012;73:60–6.

41. Rehm M, Bruegger D, Christ F, Conzen P, Thiel M, Jacob M, Chappell D, Stoeckelhuber M, Welsch U, Reichart B, Peter K, Becker BF. Shedding of the endothelial glycocalyx in patients undergoing major vascular surgery with global and regional ischemia. Circulation. 2007;116:1896–906.

42. Senzolo M, Coppell J, Cholongitas E, Riddell A, Triantos CK, Perry D, Burroughs AK. The effects of glycosaminoglycans on coagulation: a thromboelastographic study. Blood Coagul Fibrinolysis. 2007;18:227–36.

43. Spinler SA, Rees C. Review of prasugrel for the secondary prevention of atherothrombosis. J Manag Care Pharm. 2009;15:383–95.

44. Roberts HR, Hoffman M, Monroe DM. A cell-based model of thrombin generation. Semin Thromb Hemost. 2006;32 Suppl 1:32–8.

45. Fries D, Innerhofer P, Schobersberger W. Time for changing coagulation management in trauma-related massive bleeding. Curr Opin Anaesthesiol. 2009;22:267–74.

46. Murray D, Pennell B, Olson J. Variability of prothrombin time and activated partial thromboplastin time in the diagnosis of increased surgical bleeding. Transfusion. 1999;39:56–62.

47. Segal JB, Dzik WH. Paucity of studies to support that abnormal coagulation test results predict bleeding in the setting of invasive procedures: an evidence-based review. Transfusion. 2005;45:1413–25.

48. Salooja N, Perry DJ. Thrombelastography. Blood Coagul Fibrinolysis. 2001;12:327–37.

49. Johansson PI, Stissing T, Bochsen L, Ostrowski SR. Thrombelastography and tromboelastometry in assessing coagulopathy in trauma. Scand J Trauma Resusc Emerg Med. 2009;17:45.

50. Plotkin AJ, Wade CE, Jenkins DH, Smith KA, Noe JC, Park MS, Perkins JG, Holcomb JB. A reduction in clot formation rate and strength assessed by thrombelastography is indicative of transfusion requirements in patients with penetrating injuries. J Trauma. 2008;64:S64–8.

51. Park MS, Martini WZ, Dubick MA, Salinas J, Butenas S, Kheirabadi BS, Pusateri AE, Vos JA, Guymon CH, Wolf SE, Mann KG, Holcomb JB. Thromboelastography as a better indicator of hypercoagulable state after injury than prothrombin time or activated partial thromboplastin time. J Trauma. 2009;67:266–75.

52. Ostrowski SR, Sorensen AM, Larsen CF, Johansson PI. Thrombelastography and biomarker profiles in acute coagulopathy of trauma: a prospective study. Scand J Trauma Resusc Emerg Med. 2011;19:64.

53. Gaarder C, Naess PA, Frischknecht CE, Hakala P, Handolin L, Heier HE, Ivancev K, Johansson P, Leppaniemi A, Lippert F, Lossius HM, Opdahl H, Pillgram-Larsen J, Roise O, Skaga NO, Soreide E, Stensballe J, Tonnessen E, Tottermann A, Ortenwall P, Ostlund A. Scandinavian guidelines–"the massively bleeding patient". Scand J Surg. 2008;97:15–36.

54. Hess JR, Johansson PI, Holcomb JB. Trauma and massive transfusion. In: Mintz PD, editor. Transfusion therapy: clinical principles and practice. Bethesda: American Association of Blood Banks (AABB); 2010.

55. Holcomb JB, Minei KM, Scerbo ML, Radwan ZA, Wade CE, Kozar RA, Gill BS, Albarado R, McNutt MK, Khan S, Adams PR, McCarthy JJ, Cotton BA. Admission rapid thrombelastography can replace conventional coagulation test in the emergency department: experience with 1974 consecutive trauma patients. Ann Surg. 2012;256:476–86.

56. Hayward CP, Moffat KA, Raby A, Israels S, Plumhoff E, Flynn G, Zehnder JL. Development of North American consensus guidelines for medical laboratories that perform and interpret platelet function testing using light transmission aggregometry. Am J Clin Pathol. 2010;134:955–63.

57. Uijttewaal WS, Nijhof EJ, Bronkhorst PJ, Den Hartog E, Heethaar RM. Near-wall excess of platelets induced by lateral migration of erythrocytes in flowing blood. Am J Physiol. 1993;264:H1239–44.

58. Peyrou V, Lormeau JC, Herault JP, Gaich C, Pfliegger AM, Herbert JM. Contribution of erythrocytes to thrombin generation in whole blood. Thromb Haemost. 1999;81:400–6.
59. Valles J, Santos MT, Aznar J, Marcus AJ, Martinez-Sales V, Portoles M, Broekman MJ, Safier LB. Erythrocytes metabolically enhance collagen-induced platelet responsiveness via increased thromboxane production, adenosine diphosphate release, and recruitment. Blood. 1991;78:154–62.
60. Monroe DM, Hoffman M. What does it take to make the perfect clot? Arterioscler Thromb Vasc Biol. 2006;26:41–8.
61. Hardy JF, de Moerloose P, Samama CM. Massive transfusion and coagulopathy: pathophysiology and implications for clinical management. Can J Anaesth. 2006;53:S40–58.
62. Duchesne JC, Hunt JP, Wahl G, Marr AB, Wang YZ, Weintraub SE, Wright MJ, McSwain Jr NE. Review of current blood transfusions strategies in a mature level I trauma center: were we wrong for the last 60 years? J Trauma. 2008;65:272–6.
63. Holcomb JB, Wade CE, Michalek JE, Chisholm GB, Zarzabal LA, Schreiber MA, Gonzalez EA, Pomper GJ, Perkins JG, Spinella PC, Williams KL, Park MS. Increased plasma and platelet to red blood cell ratios improves outcome in 466 massively transfused civilian trauma patients. Ann Surg. 2008;248:447–58.
64. Maegele M, Lefering R, Paffrath T, Tjardes T, Simanski C, Bouillon B. Red-blood-cell to plasma ratios transfused during massive transfusion are associated with mortality in severe multiple injury: a retrospective analysis from the Trauma Registry of the Deutsche Gesellschaft fur Unfallchirurgie. Vox Sang. 2008;95:112–9.
65. Murad MH, Stubbs JR, Gandhi MJ, Wang AT, Paul A, Erwin PJ, Montori VM, Roback JD. The effect of plasma transfusion on morbidity and mortality: a systematic review and meta-analysis. Transfusion. 2010;50:1370–83.
66. Johansson PI, Oliveri R, Ostrowski SR. Hemostatic resuscitation with plasma and platelets in trauma. A meta-analysis. J Emerg Trauma Shock. 2012;5:120–5.
67. Johansson PI, Hansen MB, Sorensen H. Transfusion practice in massively bleeding patients: time for a change? Vox Sang. 2005;89:92–6.
68. Johansson PI, Stensballe J, Rosenberg I, Hilslov TL, Jorgensen L, Secher NH. Proactive administration of platelets and plasma for patients with a ruptured abdominal aortic aneurysm: evaluating a change in transfusion practice. Transfusion. 2007;47:593–8.
69. Inaba K, Branco BC, Rhee P, Blackbourne LH, Holcomb JB, Teixeira PG, Shulman I, Nelson J, Demetriades D. Impact of plasma transfusion in trauma patients who do not require massive transfusion. J Am Coll Surg. 2010;210:957–65.
70. Brown LM, Call MS, Margaret KM, Cohen MJ, Holcomb JB, Wade CE, Brasel KJ, Vercruysse G, MacLeod J, Dutton RP, Hess JR, Duchesne JC, McSwain NE, Muskat P, Johannigamn J, Cryer HM, Tillou A, Pittet JF, De Moya MA, Schreiber MA, Tieu B, Brundage S, Napolitano LM, Brunsvold M, Brunsvold M, Beilman G, Peitzman AB, Zenait MS, Sperry J, Alarcon L, Croce MA, Minei JP, Kozar R, Gonzalez EA, Stewart RM, Cohn SM, Mickalek JE, Bulger EM, Cotton BA, Nunez TC, Ivatury R, Meredith JW, Miller P, Pomper GJ, Marin B. A normal platelet count may not be enough: the impact of admission platelet count on mortality and transfusion in severely injured trauma patients. J Trauma. 2011;71:S337–42.
71. Snyder CW, Weinberg JA, McGwin Jr G, Melton SM, George RL, Reiff DA, Cross JM, Hubbard-Brown J, Rue III LW, Kerby JD. The relationship of blood product ratio to mortality: survival benefit or survival bias? J Trauma. 2009;66:358–62.
72. Cotton BA, Gunter OL, Isbell J, Au BK, Robertson AM, Morris Jr JA, Young PP, St Jacques P. Damage control hematology: the impact of a trauma exsanguination protocol on survival and blood product utilization. J Trauma. 2008;64:1177–82.
73. Cotton BA, Au BK, Nunez TC, Gunter OL, Robertson AM, Young PP. Predefined massive transfusion protocols are associated with a reduction in organ failure and postinjury complications. J Trauma. 2009;66:41–8.
74. Duchesne JC, Kimonis K, Marr AB, Rennie KV, Wahl G, Wells JE, Islam TM, Meade P, Stuke L, Barbeau JM, Hunt JP, Baker CC, McSwain Jr NE. Damage control resuscitation in combination with damage control laparotomy: a survival advantage. J Trauma. 2010;69:46–52.
75. Spinella PC, Perkins JG, Grathwohl KW, Beekley AC, Holcomb JB. Warm fresh whole blood is independently associated with improved survival for patients with combat-related traumatic injuries. J Trauma. 2009;66:S69–76.
76. Vamvakas EC, Blajchman MA. Transfusion-related mortality: the ongoing risks of allogeneic blood transfusion and the available strategies for their prevention. Blood. 2009;113:3406–17.
77. Johansson PI, Stensballe J. Effect of Haemostatic Control Resuscitation on mortality in massively bleeding patients: a before and after study. Vox Sang. 2009;96:111–8.
78. Afshari A, Wikkelso A, Brok J, Moller AM, Wetterslev J. Thrombelastography (TEG) or thromboelastometry (ROTEM) to monitor haemotherapy versus usual care in patients with massive transfusion. Cochrane Database Syst Rev. 2011;3:CD007871.
79. Johansson PI, Sørensen AM, Larsen C, Windeløv NA, Stensballe J, Perner A, Ostrowski SR. Low Hemorrhage-related mortality in trauma patients in a Level 1 Trauma Centre employing transfusion packages and early thrombelastography-directed hemostatic resuscitation with plasma and platelets. Transfusion. 2013. doi:10.1111/trf.12214. [Epub ahead of print]
80. Porte RJ, Leebeek FW. Pharmacological strategies to decrease transfusion requirements in patients undergoing surgery. Drugs. 2002;62:2193–211.

81. CRASH-2 Trial collaborators, Shakur H, Roberts I, Bautista R, Caballero J, Coats T, Dewan Y, El-Sayed H, Gogichaishvili T, Gupta S, Herrera J, Hunt B, Iribhogbe P, Izurieta M, Khamis H, Komolafe E, Marrero MA, Mejia-Mantilla J, Miranda J, Morales C, Olaomi O, Olldashi F, Perel P, Peto R, Ramana PV, Ravi RR, Yutthakasemsunt S. Effects of tranexamic acid on death, vascular occlusive events, and blood transfusion in trauma patients with significant haemorrhage (CRASH-2): a randomised, placebo-controlled trial. Lancet. 2010;376:23–32.

82. Johansson PI, Ostrowski SR. Evidence supporting the use of recombinant activated factor vii in congenital bleeding disorders. Drug Des Devel Ther. 2010;4:107–16.

83. Hauser CJ, Boffard K, Dutton R, Bernard GR, Croce MA, Holcomb JB, Leppaniemi A, Parr M, Vincent JL, Tortella BJ, Dimsits J, Bouillon B. Results of the CONTROL trial: efficacy and safety of recombinant activated factor VII in the management of refractory traumatic hemorrhage. J Trauma. 2010;69:489–500.

84. Levi M, Levy JH, Andersen HF, Truloff D. Safety of recombinant activated factor VII in randomized clinical trials. N Engl J Med. 2010;363:1791–800.

85. Hiippala ST, Myllyla GJ, Vahtera EM. Hemostatic factors and replacement of major blood loss with plasma-poor red cell concentrates. Anesth Analg. 1995;81:360–5.

86. Fenger-Eriksen C, Jensen TM, Kristensen BS, Jensen KM, Tonnesen E, Ingerslev J, Sorensen B. Fibrinogen substitution improves whole blood clot firmness after dilution with hydroxyethyl starch in bleeding patients undergoing radical cystectomy: a randomized, placebo-controlled clinical trial. J Thromb Haemost. 2009;7:795–802.

87. Meyer MAS, Ostrowski SR, Windeløv NA, Johansson PI. Fibrinogen concentrates for bleeding trauma patients – what is the evidence? Vox Sang. 2011; 101:185–90.

88. Pabinger-Fasching I. Warfarin-reversal: results of a phase III study with pasteurised, nanofiltrated prothrombin complex concentrate. Thromb Res. 2008;122 Suppl 2:S19–22.

89. Carvalho MC, Rodrigues AG, Conceicao LM, Galvao ML, Ribeiro LC. Prothrombin complex concentrate (Octaplex): a Portuguese experience in 1152 patients. Blood Coagul Fibrinolysis. 2012;23:222–8.

90. Lorand L. Factor XIII: structure, activation, and interactions with fibrinogen and fibrin. Ann N Y Acad Sci. 2001;936:291–311.

91. Wettstein P, Haeberli A, Stutz M, Rohner M, Corbetta C, Gabi K, Schnider T, Korte W. Decreased factor XIII availability for thrombin and early loss of clot firmness in patients with unexplained intraoperative bleeding. Anesth Analg. 2004;99:1564–9.

92. Chandler WL, Patel MA, Gravelle L, Soltow LO, Lewis K, Bishop PD, Spiess BD. Factor XIIIA and clot strength after cardiopulmonary bypass. Blood Coagul Fibrinolysis. 2001;12:101–8.

Diagnosis of Vascular Trauma

3

John Byrne and R. Clement Darling III

Contents

3.1 Introduction

In the past, imaging options in vascular trauma were limited and time-consuming. While "hard" signs of arterial and venous injuries still mandate immediate surgical treatment, exploratory laparotomy or thoracotomies are outmoded. Many patients are now treated endovascularly with, arguably, better outcomes. Good-quality imaging also prevents needless intervention. But not all modalities are equal and trauma surgeons should be aware of the limitations of each test.

Choice of imaging is dictated by anatomy. Duplex ultrasonography, no matter how expertly performed, will be of little use in chest trauma but is very helpful in patients with limb injuries; angiography, while useful in most territories, will not demonstrate isolated venous injuries and will be of no use in demonstrating soft tissue defects from ballistic injuries. Computerized tomographic angiography (CTA), in expert hands and with modern scanners, allows for both. As a result, it is rapidly becoming the investigation of choice in vascular trauma.

3.2 The Evolution of Vascular Imaging

Vascular imaging has evolved in recent years. Once, angiography in a radiology department was the gold standard. However, it is relatively slow and requires one physician and 2–3

R.C. Darling III, MD (✉)
J. Byrne, MCh, FRCSI (Gen)
Department of Surgery, Albany Vascular Group,
Albany Medical College, Albany, NY, USA

Division of Vascular Surgery,
Albany Medical Center Hospital,
Albany, NY 12208, USA
e-mail: darlingc@albanyvascular.com

A. Dua et al. (eds.), *Clinical Review of Vascular Trauma*,
DOI 10.1007/978-3-642-39100-2_3, © Springer-Verlag Berlin Heidelberg 2014

experienced paramedical personnel for each study. In mass trauma and battlefield situations, this is not feasible. Over the last two decades, three technological innovations have reduced dependency on catheter arteriography and relegated it to therapeutic interventions or rare diagnostic instances. First, computerized tomographic angiography (CTA) has become faster and more accurate. The standard CT scanner in most emergency rooms is now a 64-slice scanner, and scan time is only 1–2 min. Secondly, the increasing sophistication of ultrasound scanners and physician familiarity with them have led to focused assessment with sonography in trauma (FAST) becoming an extension of the stethoscope for many emergency room physicians [1]. Thirdly, many level 1 trauma centers now boast at least one "hybrid" operating room, which allows for

simultaneous open and endovascular treatment (Fig. 3.1).

3.3 Techniques

3.3.1 Chest Radiography

Simple anteroposterior chest radiographs may demonstrate signs of blunt aortic injury. The classic sign is a widened mediastinum. While this suggests bleeding, it is not specific to aortic injury. In 2011, Paterson and colleagues reviewed the available literature on imaging in vascular trauma and listed eight signs on chest X-ray of blunt aortic trauma (Table 3.1) [2]. A thoracic cavity to mediastinum ratio of 0.25 or an absolute mediastinal diameter of greater than 8 cm are markers of

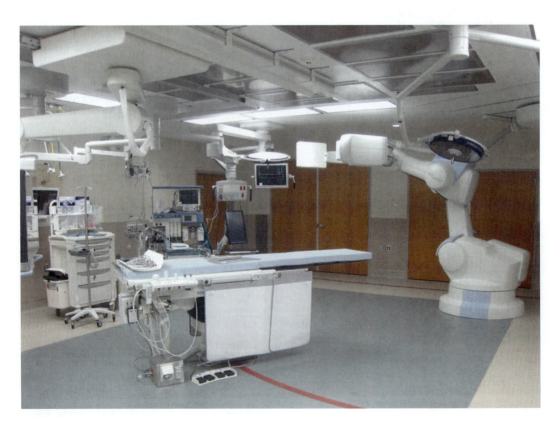

Fig. 3.1 Hybrid operating room

Table 3.1 Plain chest X-ray findings suggestive of blunt aortic trauma

Mediastinal widening
Aortopulmonary window opacification
Displacement of trachea/esophagus or nasogastric/ endotracheal tube to the left
Left mainstem bronchus displacement downwards
Rightward displacement of superior vena cava
Left apical cap
Left hemothorax
Markers of injury severity (first rib fracture, scapula fracture, paraspinal rib fractures, sternal fracture)

From Patterson et al. [2] with permission

injury. Chest X-ray was relatively sensitive with a high negative predictive value [3–6].

3.3.2 Ultrasound: Focused Assessment with Sonography in Trauma (FAST) and Duplex Ultrasonography

3.3.2.1 Theory

Modern ultrasound employs a "pulse-echo" technique with a brightness-mode (B-mode) display. Small pulses of ultrasound (sound waves above normal human hearing, i.e., 20,000 Hz or 20 KHz) are transmitted into the body. As ultrasound waves penetrate body tissues of differing densities and "acoustic impedances," some are reflected back as "echo signals" but most penetrate deeper or are absorbed. The amount of ultrasound or "echo" returned after hitting an object is called its "acoustic impedance." Lungs (mostly air) allow passage of almost all sound waves and have the lowest acoustic impedance; bone has the highest. The echo signals are processed to form "grayscale" (black and white) images.

Sound waves are described in terms of their frequency (cycles per second or hertz), wavelength (measured in millimeters), or amplitude (measured in decibels). Wavelength and frequency are inversely related. High-frequency sound has a short wavelength and vice versa. In medical devices, frequencies of 1–20 MHz are used. Selection of the correct ultrasound frequency for a given study is important. High-frequency ultrasound has high "axial resolution," which means it can easily distinguish two structures at different depths along the path of those sound waves. It also has narrower "beam width" which aids "lateral resolution" or ability to distinguish two objects lying side by side. Unfortunately, high-frequency ultrasound is also rapidly absorbed or "attenuated." So, it is most useful for superficial structures. Low-frequency/long-wavelength ultrasound, on the other hand, can penetrate more deeply due to a lower degree of attenuation and is better for deeper structures. Typically, a 2- or 3-MHz probe will be needed to examine the deep-lying aorta and iliac arteries, whereas a 5-MHz probe should image the infrainguinal vessels in normal-sized individuals. Higher-frequency probes (10–15 MHz) are used to image superficial nerves. Those used to ultrasound the anterior segment of the eye are 20–50 MHz.

As well as B-mode, modern units include pulsed-wave Doppler ultrasound to evaluate blood flow in arteries or veins (duplex ultrasonography). Christian Johann Doppler (1803–53) first described the "Doppler effect" in 1842. When a sound source moves towards a stationary receiver, the sound waves are crowded closer and closer together so that the wavelength is shorter and the frequency higher resulting in a higher pitch, e.g., a police siren approaching a pedestrian. The Doppler effect is used to determine the relative speed of an object to a sound source by bouncing sound waves off the object and measuring the shift in the frequency of the wave (also called the "Doppler shift"). Duplex ultrasonography is when pulsed Doppler is performed along with B-mode ultrasound because of its ability to measure flow as well as solid structures. Duplex can effectively image many vascular injuries such as arteriovenous fistulas, arterial disruption, intimal flaps, and pseudoaneurysms.

3.3.2.2 Equipment

Modern ultrasound units comprise a transducer probe, a central processing unit (CPU), display screen, and transducer pulse controls. The transducer probe sends and receives sound waves using *the piezoelectric effect*. In 1880, French physicists Jacques and Pierre Curie found that, in crystalline materials (e.g., quartz, ceramics, bone), mechanical pressure generates an electric charge. This is "reversible"—applying electrical charge to these crystals slightly alters their shape.

In a transducer probe, there are piezoelectric crystals (most commonly lead zirconate titanate or PZT). When current is applied to them, they change shape rapidly. These "vibrations" emit sound waves. Conversely, when these crystals are struck by sound waves such as those reflected back from a solid body, they generate electrical currents. Between the crystal and the skin is a "matching layer" of aluminum powder in epoxy resin or rubber that decreases the acoustic impedance difference between the crystal and the skin. An acoustic lens focuses emitted sound waves.

The central processing unit (CPU) generates the electric currents that cause vibrations in the transducer probe's crystals. It also processes the electrical pulses produced by the reflected sound waves and generates grayscale images on the monitor.

Finally, the transducer pulse controls alter the electrical currents generated by the CPU. This changes the frequency and duration of ultrasound pulses produced by the transducer probe. Three parameters that can be adjusted: depth, frequency, and "gain." The depth of tissue imaged can be adjusted on the machine by changing the frequency of the emitted ultrasound. Variable frequency probes allow such changes within a narrow range, e.g., 8–13 MHz. Ultrasound probes transmit ultrasound 1 % of time and "listen" for echoes 99 % of the time. Increasing the "gain" on the ultrasound machine increases signal amplification of the returning ultrasound to compensate for tissue attenuation.

3.3.2.3 Focused Assessment with Sonography in Trauma (FAST)

Focused assessment with sonography in trauma or "FAST scanning" is the practical application of B-mode ultrasound in trauma. It is used to detect free fluid in the peritoneal cavity following blunt abdominal trauma [7]. It has supplanted procedures such as "four-quadrant tap" and diagnostic peritoneal lavage (DPL) to diagnose intra-abdominal hemorrhage. It is noninvasive, is easily repeated, and is not hampered by previous laparotomy or thoracotomy scars. Using a 3.5-MHz probe, four areas (the four Ps) are examined: perihepatic, perisplenic, pelvic, and pericardium.

FAST scanning is easily taught. Shackford concluded that only ten scans were needed to become proficient [8]. The sensitivity of FAST ranges from 29 to 100 % and specificity from 94 to 100 % [8–14]. As it can be rapidly performed, many see the real role of FAST scanning as confirming the site of injury in a hemodynamically *unstable* patient. However, its role in the management of the hemodynamically *stable* patient with blunt abdominal trauma has been questioned, especially if CTA is readily available [9]. In the largest series, from Omaha, Nebraska, involving 2,980 patients, Natarajan reported a sensitivity of only 41 % in blunt abdominal trauma patients for FAST scanning (Table 3.2) [11]. The authors concluded that focused assessment with sonography for trauma in hemodynamically stable blunt trauma patients "seems not worthwhile" and that it should be reserved for hemodynamically unstable patients with blunt trauma. One might suggest that it will add little here, either, as these patients are going to the operating room regardless of their FAST scan findings. False negatives in FAST scanning are not confined to tyros. Even experienced operators may have a missed injury rate in these patients of 10 % [15]. Despite this, FAST scanning will continue to have a role. For most experienced emergency room physicians, it adds little time to assessment and will, more often than not, provide useful information.

3.3.2.4 Duplex Ultrasonography

While FAST scanning can be performed competently with relatively little training, duplex ultrasonography, especially in trauma patients, requires a much higher level of expertise. In trauma, duplex is used for extremity and cervical injuries and to follow conservatively managed injuries. But it is highly operator dependent and can be time-consuming. It is also limited by soft tissue defects, subcutaneous air, and casts applied to stabilize fractures or ligamentous injuries.

In the management of head and neck trauma, duplex is effective in screening for carotid and vertebral injury. In patients with penetrating neck

Table 3.2 Sensitivity and specificity of focused assessment with sonography in trauma (FAST)

Study	Number	Sensitivity (%)	Specificity (%)	NPV (%)
Smith (2013) [10]	166	90	100	N/A
Natarajan (2010) [11]	2,130	43	99	94
Gaarder (2009) [9]	104	62	96	89
Tsui (2008) [15]	242	86	99	98
Nural (2005) [79]	454	86.50	95.40	98.70
Dolich (2001) [80]	2,576	86	98	98
Becker (2010) [81]	3181	75	98	95
Kim (2012) [82]	240	61	96	83

injuries, it has been shown to have a 90.5–100 % sensitivity for detecting intimal flaps, dissections, occlusions, and pseudoaneurysms with a specificity of 85–100 % [16–19]. Important limitations, however, are an inability to image the distal internal carotid artery above the level of the mandible (zone III) and the common carotid artery proximal to the clavicle (zone I) [20]. Nonetheless, the Eastern Association for the Surgery of Trauma currently recommends that for hemodynamically stable patients, with penetrating zone II neck injuries, Duplex (and CTA) can safely replace conventional angiography [21]. This was based on several retrospective and prospective studies [16, 22, 23].

Initial reports on the use of duplex for extremity vascular injuries were encouraging. Knudson in 1993 reviewed his group's experience with 86 extremity injuries and found a 100 % true positive rate [23]. However, more recent assessments have been less enthusiastic. Felliciano in 2011 reported sensitivities in the 50–100 % range [24]. Unlike FAST scans, in most ERs, duplex is not an extension of the stethoscope and will not be available "out of hours."

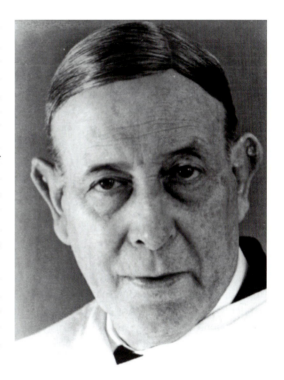

Fig. 3.2 Antonio Egas Moniz (1874–1955). Pioneer of angiography

3.3.3 Catheter Angiography

The first angiograms were hazardous affairs. In 1927, a "colorful" Portuguese physician Antonio Egas Moniz performed the first cerebral angiogram (Fig. 3.2) [25]. Moniz, who was (somewhat controversially) awarded the 1949 Nobel Prize for championing prefrontal lobotomy, performed a direct cutdown onto the carotid arteries to obtain exposure [26, 27]. He used strontium bromide as

the contrast agent. Four of the first six had complications and one died. In 1931, he began to use colloidal thorium oxide as his contrast agent, which unfortunately, as a perpetual α-particle emitter, is carcinogenic, and has a biological half-life of 500 years. In 1949, a patient shot him and he was wheelchair bound until his death in 1955. In 1929, Reynaldo Cid dos Santos performed the first aortogram, also in Lisbon [28]. He performed it with a long needle using surface anatomy landmarks. A safer technique for percutaneous femoral access was developed by Sven Ivar

Seldinger at the Karolinska Institute in Stockholm in 1953 [29]. Catheter-based interventions began with Charles Dotter in 1964, and coronary balloon angioplasty was first performed by Andreas Gruentzig in 1977 [30, 31].

3.3.3.1 Theory

Contrast media and fluoroscopy are the essentials of catheter angiography. Current contrast agents are iodine based. Iodinated contrast agents are either "ionic" or "nonionic." Ionic contrast agents were introduced in the 1930s. They have a high osmolality (osmoles per kilogram of solvent) and solubility but low viscosity. They are also known as high-osmolar contrast media (HOCM) as their osmolality is 7–8 times that of plasma. All are based on a benzene ring containing three iodine atoms, which dissociate in water into cations and anions, hence the term "ionic." They are hypertonic to enable them to achieve a high-enough concentration of iodine to provide intravascular contrast. However, such high osmolalities and viscosities (e.g., Hypaque has an osmolality of 1,500–1,700 mOsm/kg compared to 275–295 mOsm/Kg for human plasma) can cause vasodilatation, heat, pain, osmotic diuresis, and myocardial depression. Nonionic or iso-osmolar contrast media (IOCM) consist of two benzene rings, each with three iodine atoms, which are covalently bound and do not dissociate in water (hence "nonionic"). The osmolality of a typical nonionic contrast agent, such as Visipaque, is 300 mOsm/Kg. As a result, IOCMs have fewer side effects. Typically, ionic contrast agents will be associated with a 1:40,000 incidence of fatal anaphylaxis compared to 1:170,000 for nonionic contrast agents.

The second component is a fluoroscope with an image intensifier to display real-time X-ray images. A patient is placed between an X-ray source and a fluorescent screen (a transparent screen coated on one side with a phosphor that fluoresces when exposed to X-rays). The screen is coupled to an image intensifier (a vacuum tube device that converts low levels of light from the fluoroscope into visible light). A charge-coupled device (CCD) video camera converts the incoming light photons into digital images. Digital

flat-panel detectors are the modern incarnation of the image intensifier/video camera combination. Digital subtraction is where an initial mask image, containing bone, is taken, followed by a contrast study. The "mask" image is then removed from the subsequent images. There are two imaging modes on most contemporary machines: "fluoroscopy" and "acquisition" or "cine" mode. Fluoroscopy provides a real-time image of sufficient quality to guide catheter and wire placement. Typical frame rates are 3–5 frames per second. Acquisition (cine) mode, which is sometimes called "run" or "record" mode, generates much higher-quality images—at the expense of much higher radiation doses. A typical acquisition per-frame dose of radiation is 15 times that of fluoroscopy.

3.3.3.2 Equipment

The equipment for trauma angiography is no different from that required for elective angiography. For best results, especially if interventions are anticipated, these studies are best performed in a fully stocked interventional radiology suite (or hybrid room) with trained personnel.

3.3.3.3 Technique

In trauma patients, the likely point of access will be the common femoral artery. Local anesthesia over the common femoral artery is used with monitored sedation, if the patient is hemodynamically stable. In difficult cases, ultrasound guidance is useful to facilitate access. Either way, a Seldinger technique is used to access the artery. Aggressive hydration and use of half-strength contrast help to minimize renal insult in patients with chronic kidney disease (CKD). In elective patients with CKD, CO_2 angiography is useful but is unlikely to be as helpful in trauma due to its lack of fine detail.

3.3.3.4 Angiography in Vascular Trauma

Catheter angiography is still an excellent technique in vascular trauma. It is a dynamic study, so it will demonstrate hemorrhage and allow for deployment of covered stents or coils to staunch bleeding (Fig. 3.3).

9. Gaarder C, Kroepelien CF, Loekke R, Hestnes M, Dormage JB, Naess PA. Ultrasound performed by radiologists-confirming the truth about FAST in trauma. J Trauma. 2009;67(2):323–9.

10. Smith ZA, Wood D. Emergency focussed assessment with sonography in trauma (FAST) and haemodynamic stability. Emerg Med J. 2013 (Epub February 13, 2013).

11. Natarajan B, Gupta PK, Cemaj S, Sorensen M, Hatzoudis GI, Forse RA. FAST scan: is it worth doing in hemodynamically stable blunt trauma patients? Surgery. 2010;148(4):695–701.

12. Udobi KF, Rodriguez A, Chiu WC, Scalea TM. Role of ultrasonography in penetrating abdominal trauma: a prospective clinical study. J Trauma. 2001;50(3):475–9.

13. Brenchley J, Walker A, Sloan JP, Hassan TB, Venables H. Evaluation of focussed assessment with sonography in trauma (FAST) by UK emergency physicians. Emerg Med J. 2006;23(6):446–8.

14. Fleming S, Bird R, Ratnasingham K, Sarker SJ, Walsh M, Patel B. Accuracy of FAST scan in blunt abdominal trauma in a major London trauma centre. Int J Surg. 2012;10(9):470–4.

15. Tsui CL, Fung HT, Chung KL, Kam CW. Focused abdominal sonography for trauma in the emergency department for blunt abdominal trauma. Int J Emerg Med. 2008;1(3):183–7.

16. Bynoe RP, Miles WS, Bell RM, Greenwold DR, Sessions G, Haynes JL, Rush DS. Noninvasive diagnosis of vascular trauma by duplex ultrasonography. J Vasc Surg. 1991;14(3):346–52.

17. Kuzniec S, Kauffman P, Molnár LJ, Aun R, Puech-Leão P. Diagnosis of limbs and neck arterial trauma using duplex ultrasonography. Cardiovasc Surg. 1998;6(4):358–66.

18. Montalvo BM, LeBlang SD, Nuñez Jr DB, Ginzburg E, Klose KJ, Becerra JL, Kochan JP. Color Doppler sonography in penetrating injuries of the neck. AJNR Am J Neuroradiol. 1996;17(5):943–51.

19. Ginzburg E, Montalvo B, LeBlang S, Nunez D, Martin L. The use of duplex ultrasonography in penetrating neck trauma. Arch Surg. 1996;131(7):691–3.

20. LeBlang SD, Nunez Jr DB. Noninvasive imaging of cervical vascular injuries. AJR Am J Roentgenol. 2000;174(5):1269–78.

21. Tisherman SA, Bokhari F, Collier B, Cumming J, Ebert J, Holevar M, Kurek S, Leon S, Rhee P. Clinical practice guideline: penetrating zone II neck trauma. J Trauma. 2008;64(5):1392–405.

22. Demetriades D, Theodorou D, Cornwell E, Berne TV, Asensio J, Belzberg H, Velmahos G, Weaver F, Yellin A. Evaluation of penetrating injuries of the neck: prospective study of 223 patients. World J Surg. 1997;21(1):41–8.

23. Montalvo BM, LeBlang SD, Nuñez DB Jr, Ginzburg E, Klose KJ, Becerra JL, Kochan JP. Color Doppler sonography in penetrating injuries of the neck. AJNR Am J Neuroradiol. 1996;17(5):943–51.

24. Feliciano DV, Moore FA, Moore EE, West MA, Davis JW, Cocanour CS, Kozar RA, McIntyre Jr RC. Evaluation and management of peripheral vascular injury. Part 1. Western Trauma Association/critical decisions in trauma. J Trauma. 2011;70(6):1551–6.

25. Ferro JM. Egas Moniz (1874–1955). J Neurol. 2003;250(3):376–7.

26. Sassard R, O'Leary JP. Egas Moniz: pioneer of cerebral angiography. Am Surg. 1998;64(11):1116–7.

27. Raju TN. The Nobel chronicles. 1949: Walter Rudolf Hess (1881–1973); and Antônio Egas Moniz (1874–1955). Lancet. 1999;353(9160):1281.

28. Macedo MM. The "Portuguese school of angiography". Rev Port Cardiol. 1999;18 Suppl 1:I9–10.

29. Seldinger SI. Catheter replacement of the needle in percutaneous arteriography; a new technique. Acta Radiol. 1953;39(5):368–76.

30. Dotter CT, Krippaehne WW, Judkins MP. Transluminal recanalization and dilatation in atherosclerotic obstruction of femoral popliteal system. Am Surg. 1965;31:453–9.

31. Gruentzig AR. Percutaneous transluminal coronary angioplasty. Semin Roentgenol. 1981;16(2):152–3.

32. Endarterectomy for asymptomatic carotid artery stenosis. Executive Committee for the Asymptomatic Carotid Atherosclerosis Study. JAMA. 1995;273(18):1421–8.

33. North CM, Ahmadi J, Segall HD, Zee CS. Penetrating vascular injuries of the face and neck: clinical and angiographic correlation. AJR Am J Roentgenol. 1986;147(5):995–9.

34. Yang ST, Huang YC, Chuang CC, Hsu PW. Traumatic internal carotid artery dissection. J Clin Neurosci. 2006;13(1):123–8.

35. Miller PR, Fabian TC, Croce MA, Cagiannos C, Williams JS, Vang M, Qaisi WG, Felker RE, Timmons SD. Prospective screening for blunt cerebrovascular injuries: analysis of diagnostic modalities and outcomes. Ann Surg. 2002;236(3):386–95.

36. Eastman AL, Chason DP, Perez CL, McAnulty AL, Minei JP. Computed tomographic angiography for the diagnosis of blunt cervical vascular injury: is it ready for primetime? J Trauma. 2006;60(5):925–9.

37. Eastman AL, Muraliraj V, Sperry JL, Minei JP. CTA-based screening reduces time to diagnosis and stroke rate in blunt cervical vascular injury. J Trauma. 2009;67(3):551–6.

38. LaBerge JM, Jeffrey RB. Aortic lacerations: fatal complications of thoracic aortography. Radiology. 1987;165(2):367–9.

39. Frykberg ER, Dennis JW, Bishop K, Laneve L, Alexander RH. The reliability of physical examination in the evaluation of penetrating extremity trauma for vascular injury: results at one year. J Trauma. 1991;31(4):502–11.

40. AbuRahma AF, Robinson PA, Boland JP, Umstot RK, Clubb EA, Grandia RA, Kennard W, Bastug DF. Complications of arteriography in a recent series of 707 cases: factors affecting outcome. Ann Vasc Surg. 1993;7(2):122–9.

41. Egglin TK, O'Moore PV, Feinstein AR, Waltman AC. Complications of peripheral arteriography: a new system to identify patients at increased risk. J Vasc Surg. 1995;22(6):787–94.

42. Fruhwirth J, Pascher O, Hauser H, Amann W. Local vascular complications after iatrogenic femoral artery puncture. Wien Klin Wochenschr. 1996;108(7): 196–200.

43. Rose SC, Moore EE. Emergency trauma angiography: accuracy, safety, and pitfalls. AJR Am J Roentgenol. 1987;148(6):1243–6.

44. Itani KM, Burch JM, Spjut-Patrinely V, Richardson R, Martin RR, Mattox KL. Emergency center arteriography. J Trauma. 1992;32(3):302–7.

45. Cowper SE, Robin HS, Steinberg SM, Su LD, Gupta S, LeBoit PE. Scleromyxoedema-like cutaneous diseases in renal-dialysis patients. Lancet. 2000;356 (9234):1000–1.

46. Grobner T. Gadolinium—a specific trigger for the development of nephrogenic fibrosing dermopathy and nephrogenic systemic fibrosis? Nephrol Dial Transplant. 2006;12:3604–5.

47. Marckmann P, Skov L, Rossen K, et al. Nephrogenic systemic fibrosis: suspected causative role of gadodiamide used for contrast-enhanced magnetic resonance imaging. J Am Soc Nephrol. 2006;17:2359–62.

48. Ren X, Wang W, Zhang X, Pu Y, Jiang T, Li C. Clinical study and comparison of magnetic resonance angiography (MRA) and angiography diagnosis of blunt vertebral artery injury. J Trauma. 2007;63(6): 1249–53.

49. Ambrose J, Hounsfield G. Computerized transverse axial tomography. Br J Radiol. 1973;46(542):148–9.

50. Cormack AM. Representation of a function by its line integrals, with some radiological application. J Appl Phys. 1963;34(9):2722–7.

51. Radon J. Über die Bestimmung von Funktionen durch ihre Integralwurte längs gewisser Mannigfaltigkeiten, Ber. Verh. Sächs. Akad. Wiss. Leipzig, Math.-Nat. kl. 1917;69:262–77.

52. Berne JD, Norwood SH, McAuley CE, Villareal DH. Helical computed tomographic angiography: an excellent screening test for blunt cerebrovascular injury. J Trauma. 2004;57(1):11–9.

53. Wang AC, Charters MA, Thawani JP, Than KD, Sullivan SE, Graziano GP. Evaluating the use and utility of noninvasive angiography in diagnosing traumatic blunt cerebrovascular injury. J Trauma Acute Care Surg. 2012;72(6):1601–10.

54. Goodwin RB, Beery 2nd PR, Dorbish RJ, Betz JA, Hari JK, Opalek JM, Magee DJ, Hinze SS, Scileppi RM, Franz RW, Williams TD, Jenkins 2nd JJ, Suh KI. Computed tomographic angiography versus conventional angiography for the diagnosis of blunt cerebrovascular injury in trauma patients. J Trauma. 2009;67(5):1046–50.

55. Langner S, Fleck S, Kirsch M, Petrik M, Hosten N. Whole-body CT trauma imaging with adapted and optimized CT angiography of the craniocervical vessels: do we need an extra screening examination? AJNR Am J Neuroradiol. 2008;29(10):1902–7.

56. Malhotra AK, Camacho M, Ivatury RR, Davis IC, Komorowski DJ, Leung DA, Grizzard JD, Aboutanos MB, Duane TM, Cockrell C, Wolfe LG, Borchers CT, Martin NR. Computed tomographic angiography for the diagnosis of blunt carotid/vertebral artery injury: a note of caution. Ann Surg. 2007;246(4):632–43.

57. Múnera F, Soto JA, Palacio DM, Castañeda J, Morales C, Sanabria A, Gutiérrez JE, García G. Penetrating neck injuries: helical CT angiography for initial evaluation. Radiology. 2002;224(2):366–72.

58. Gracias VH, Reilly PM, Philpott J, Klein WP, Lee SY, Singer M, Schwab CW. Computed tomography in the evaluation of penetrating neck trauma: a preliminary study. Arch Surg. 2001;136(11):1231–5.

59. Mazolewski PJ, Curry JD, Browder T, Fildes J. Computed tomographic scan can be used for surgical decision making in zone II penetrating neck injuries. J Trauma. 2001;51(2):315–9.

60. Scaglione M, Pinto A, Pinto F, Romano L, Ragozzino A, Grassi R. Role of contrast-enhanced helical CT in the evaluation of acute thoracic aortic injuries after blunt chest trauma. Eur Radiol. 2001;11(12):2444–8.

61. Parker MS, Matheson TL, Rao AV, Sherbourne CD, Jordan KG, Landay MJ, Miller GL, Summa JA. Making the transition: the role of helical CT in the evaluation of potentially acute thoracic aortic injuries. AJR Am J Roentgenol. 2001;176(5):1267–72.

62. Ungar TC, Wolf SJ, Haukoos JS, Dyer DS, Moore EE. Derivation of a clinical decision rule to exclude thoracic aortic imaging in patients with blunt chest trauma after motor vehicle collisions. J Trauma. 2006;61(5):1150–5.

63. Mirvis SE, Shanmuganathan K, Miller BH, White CS, Turney SZ. Traumatic aortic injury: diagnosis with contrast-enhanced thoracic CT–five-year experience at a major trauma center. Radiology. 1996;200(2): 413–22.

64. Velmahos GC, Constantinou C, Tillou A, Brown CV, Salim A, Demetriades D. Abdominal computed tomographic scan for patients with gunshot wounds to the abdomen selected for nonoperative management. J Trauma. 2005;59(5):1155–61.

65. Inaba K, Barmparas G, Foster A, Talving P, David JS, Green D, Plurad D, Demetriades D. Selective nonoperative management of torso gunshot wounds: when is it safe to discharge? J Trauma. 2010;68(6):1301–4.

66. Berthet JP, Marty-Ané CH, Veerapen R, Picard E, Mary H, Alric P. Dissection of the abdominal aorta in blunt trauma: endovascular or conventional surgical management? J Vasc Surg. 2003;38(5):997–1004.

67. Franz RW, Shah KJ, Halaharvi D, Franz ET, Hartman JF, Wright ML. A 5-year review of management of lower extremity arterial injuries at an urban level I trauma center. J Vasc Surg. 2011;53(6):1604–10.

68. Wallin D, Yaghoubian A, Rosing D, Walot I, Chauvapun J, de Virgilio C. Computed tomographic angiography as the primary diagnostic modality in

penetrating lower extremity vascular injuries: a level I trauma experience. Ann Vasc Surg. 2011;25(5): 620–3.

69. Peng PD, Spain DA, Tataria M, Hellinger JC, Rubin GD, Brundage SI. CT angiography effectively evaluates extremity vascular trauma. Am Surg. 2008; 74(2):103–7.

70. Nitecki SS, Karram T, Ofer A, Engel A, Hoffman A. Vascular injuries in an urban combat setting: experience from the 2006 Lebanon war. Vascular. 2010; 18(1):1–8.

71. Hogan AR, Lineen EB, Perez EA, Neville HL, Thompson WR, Sola JE. Value of computed tomographic angiography in neck and extremity pediatric vascular trauma. J Pediatr Surg. 2009;44(6):1236–41.

72. Rieger M, Mallouhi A, Tauscher T, Lutz M, Jaschke WR. Traumatic arterial injuries of the extremities: initial evaluation with MDCT angiography. AJR Am J Roentgenol. 2006;186(3):656–64.

73. Hsu CS, Hellinger JC, Rubin GD, Chang J. CT angiography in pediatric extremity trauma: preoperative evaluation prior to reconstructive surgery. Hand (N Y). 2008;3(2):139–45.

74. Seamon MJ, Smoger D, Torres DM, Pathak AS, Gaughan JP, Santora TA, Cohen G, Goldberg AJ. A prospective validation of a current practice: the detection of extremity vascular injury with CT angiography. J Trauma. 2009;67(2):238–44.

75. Stengel D, Ottersbach C, Matthes G, Weigeldt M, Grundei S, Rademacher G, Tittel A, Mutze S, Ekkernkamp A, Frank M, Schmucker U, Seifert J. Accuracy of single-pass whole-body computed tomography for detection of injuries in patients with major blunt trauma. CMAJ. 2012;184(8):869–76.

76. Huber-Wagner S, Lefering R, Qvick LM, Körner M, Kay MV, Pfeifer KJ, Reiser M, Mutschler W, Kanz KG, Working Group on Polytrauma of the German Trauma Society. Effect of whole-body CT during trauma resuscitation on survival: a retrospective, multicentre study. Lancet. 2009;373(9673):1455–61.

77. Wurmb TE, Quaisser C, Balling H, Kredel M, Muellenbach R, Kenn W, Roewer N, Brederlau J. Whole-body multislice computed tomography (MSCT) improves trauma care in patients requiring surgery after multiple trauma. Emerg Med J. 2011;28(4):300–4.

78. Nural MS, Yardan T, Güven H, Baydin A, Bayrak IK, Kati C. Diagnostic value of ultrasonography in the evaluation of blunt abdominal trauma. Diagn Interv Radiol. 2005;11(1):41–4.

79. Dolich MO, McKenney MG, Varela JE, Compton RP, McKenney KL, Cohn SM. 2,576 ultrasounds for blunt abdominal trauma. J Trauma. 2001;50(1): 108–12.

80. Becker A, Lin G, McKenney MG, Marttos A, Schulman CI. Is the FAST exam reliable in severely injured patients? Injury. 2010;41(5):479–83.

81. Kim CH, Shin SD, Song KJ, Park CB. Diagnostic accuracy of focused assessment with sonography for

trauma (FAST) examinations performed by emergency medical technicians. Prehosp Emerg Care. 2012;16(3):400–6.

82. Hughes KM, Collier B, Greene KA, Kurek S. Traumatic carotid artery dissection: a significant incidental finding. Am Surg. 2000;66:1023–7.

83. Mutze S, Rademacher G, Matthes G, Hosten N, Stengel D. Blunt cerebrovascular injury in patients with blunt multiple trauma: diagnostic accuracy of duplex Doppler US and early CT angiography. Radiology. 2005;237:884–92.

84. Biffl WL, Egglin T, Benedetto B, Gibbs F, Cioffi WG. Sixteen-slice computed tomographic angiography is a reliable noninvasive screening test for clinically significant blunt cerebrovascular injuries. J Trauma. 2006;60:745–51.

85. Berne JD, Reuland KS, Villarreal DH, McGovern TM, Rowe SA, Norwood SH. Sixteen-slice multidetector computed tomographic angiography improves the accuracy of screening for blunt cerebrovascular injury. J Trauma. 2006;60:1204–9.

86. Utter GH, Hollingworth W, Hallam DK, Jarvik JG, Jurkovich GJ. Sixteen-slice CT angiography in patients with suspected blunt carotid and vertebral artery injuries. J Am Coll Surg. 2006;203:838–48.

87. Borisch I, Boehme T, Butz B, Hamer OW, Feuerbach S, Zorger N. Screening for carotid injury in trauma patients: image quality of 16-detector-row computed tomography angiography. Acta Radiol. 2007;48: 798–805.

88. Sliker CW, Shanmuganathan K, Mirvis SE. Diagnosis of blunt cerebrovascular injuries with 16-MDCT: accuracy of whole-body MDCT compared with neck MDCT angiography. AJR Am J Roentgenol. 2008;190:790–9.

89. Wick MC, Weiss RJ, Lill M, Jaschke W, Rieger M. The 'Innsbruck Emergency Algorithm' avoids the underdiagnosis of blunt cervical vascular injuries. Arch Orthop Trauma Surg. 2010;130:1269–74.

90. Gonzalez RP, Falimirski M, Holevar MR, Turk B. Penetrating zone II neck injury: does dynamic computed tomographic scan contribute to the diagnostic sensitivity of physical examination for surgically significant injury? A prospective blinded study. J Trauma. 2003;54:61–4.

91. Inaba K, Munera F, McKenney MG, Rivas L, Marecos E, de Moya M, et al. The nonoperative management of penetrating internal jugular vein injury. J Vasc Surg. 2006;43:77–80.

92. Inaba K, Munera F, McKenney M, Rivas L, de Moya M, Bahouth H, et al. Prospective evaluation of screening multislice helical computed tomographic angiography in the initial evaluation of penetrating neck injuries. J Trauma. 2006;61:144–9.

93. Downing SW, Sperling JS, Mirvis SE, Cardarelli MG, Gilbert TB, Scalea TM, et al. Experience with spiral computed tomography as the sole diagnostic method for traumatic aortic rupture. Ann Thorac Surg. 2001;72:495–501.

94. Cleverley JR, Barrie JR, Raymond GS, Primack SL, Mayo JR. Direct findings of aortic injury on contrast-enhanced CT in surgically proven traumatic aortic injury: a multi-centre review. Clin Radiol. 2002;57:281–6.

95. Chen MY, Miller PR, McLaughlin CA, Kortesis BG, Kavanagh PV, Dyer RB. The trend of using computed tomography in the detection of acute thoracic aortic and branch vessel injury after blunt thoracic trauma: single-center experience over 13 years. J Trauma. 2004;56:783–5.

96. Dyer DS, Moore EE, Ilke DN, McIntyre RC, Bernstein SM, Durham JD, et al. Thoracic aortic injury: how predictive is mechanism and is chest computed tomography a reliable screening tool? A prospective study of 1561 patients. J Trauma. 2000;48:673–83.

97. Ng CJ, Chen JC, Wang LJ, Chiu TF, Chu PH, Lee WH, et al. Diagnostic value of the helical CT scan for traumatic aortic injury: correlation with mortality and early rupture. J Emerg Med. 2006;30:277–82.

99. Soto JA, Múnera F, Morales C, Lopera JE, Holguín D, Guarín O, et al. Focal arterial injuries of the proximal extremities: helical CT arteriography as the initial method of diagnosis. Radiology. 2001;218: 188–94.

99. Busquéts AR, Acosta JA, Colón E, Alejandro KV, Rodríguez P. Helical computed tomographic angiography for the diagnosis of traumatic arterial injuries of the extremities. J Trauma. 2004;56:625–8.

100. Anderson SW, Foster BR, Soto JA. Upper extremity CT angiography in penetrating trauma: use of 64-section multidetector CT. Radiology. 2008;249: 1064–73.

Vascular Scoring Systems

4

Mark L. Shapiro

Contents

4.1 Introduction

Trauma scoring systems have been developed for tracking outcomes and developing standards in trauma centers. These standards allow groups like the American College of Surgeons Committee on Trauma (COT) to help develop measure and compare outcomes at trauma centers during the verification process. Injuries are applied to various scoring systems, and the predicted outcomes are measured against the actual outcomes to validate the scoring systems utilized. When applied to patients with concomitant vascular trauma, these scoring systems are poor predictors of outcome.

4.2 Abbreviated Injury Score

The Abbreviated Injury Score (AIS) is the basis from which most other trauma scoring systems are derived. First introduced in 1969 and updated in 1990, this anatomically oriented scoring system was developed by Copes et al. [1]. Injuries are scaled from one to six, with one being minor injuries, five being severe injuries, and six being unsurvivable trauma. The AIS forms the basis for other trauma scoring systems, such as the Injury Severity Score (ISS).

M.L. Shapiro, MD, FACS
Department of Trauma,
Duke University Medical Center,
Durham, NC, USA
e-mail: ml.shapiro@duke.edu

A. Dua et al. (eds.), *Clinical Review of Vascular Trauma*,
DOI 10.1007/978-3-642-39100-2_4, © Springer-Verlag Berlin Heidelberg 2014

4.3 Injury Severity Score

The Injury Severity Score (ISS) uses the AIS to assign points to six body regions: the head and neck, the face, the chest, the abdomen, the extremities, and the external regions. The top three scores are squared and added together, the sum of which equals the ISS. A score of 6 in any body region leads to an automatic total score of 75 no matter what the other body systems add up to; the overall range of scores falls between 0 and 75. The ISS has a positive correlation to overall morbidity and mortality and length of stay. However, this correlation falters in patients who have concomitant vascular injuries.

A specific organ injury scale (OIS) also exists for a variety of body systems. In general, the more severe the laceration, hematoma, or overall injury to the organ, the greater the score that is assigned. Grade I injuries are relatively minor, while grade V injuries may be lethal. Nonoperative, endovascular, and open surgical management decisions are occasionally based on the grade of injury to a particular organ system.

4.4 Glasgow Coma Score

The Glasgow Coma Score (GCS) sums the best eye response, verbal response, and motor response. The range is from 3 to 15, with higher scores correlated to improved morbidity and mortality. Scores over 13 are associated with the best outcome, those between 9 and 12 predict moderate neurological injury, and scores of 8 or less are associated with potentially severe neurological trauma. While the GCS has utility by itself, it is often used with the Revised Trauma Score (RTS) to better predict outcomes.

4.5 Revised Trauma Score

The RTS is a physiologic scoring system that is based on the GCS, systolic blood pressure, and respiratory rate. A score of 0 is assigned to any patient with a GCS of 3, no appreciable systolic blood pressure, or no spontaneous respiratory effort. A score of 1 assigned to patients with a GCS of 4 or 5, SBP under 50 mmHg, and a respiratory rate of 5 or lower. A score of 2 is assigned to patients with a GCS of 6, 7, or 8, SBP below 75 mmHg, and a respiratory rate below 10. A score of 3 is assigned to patients with a GCS between 9 and 12, SBP below 90 mmHg, and a respiratory rate of 30 or more. A score of 4 is assigned to patients with a GCS between 13 and 15, SBP over 90 mmHg, and a respiratory rate between 10 and 29 [2]. A formula is then used to derive the RTS and predict the overall likelihood of survival; higher numbers (closer to the maximum value of 7.8408) correspond to a greater probability of survival.

4.6 Trauma Injury Severity Score

Combining the anatomically based AIS system with the physiologically based RTS system, plus the patient's age, allows one to develop a score that corresponds well to overall survival following blunt or penetrating trauma [3]. Patients 55 years or older are less likely to survive following major trauma, according to the Trauma Injury Severity Score (TRISS). The calculation itself is complex and involves various lookup tables; a variety of online score calculators are available to aid in calculating the probability of survival [3].

4.7 Vascular Trauma Scoring Systems

The American Association for the Surgery of Trauma (AAST) has developed independent organ scoring systems that include vascular trauma. However, there is not yet a cohesive system that takes into account the OIS to predict overall morbidity and mortality. This issue was briefly addressed in the 1990s when a new scoring system known as the Physiological and Operative Severity Score for the Enumeration of Mortality and Morbidity (POSSUM) was attempted. When the POSSUM score was applied initially, results demonstrated a poor correlation to overall survival, with the score tending to overpredict mortality [4, 5]. A series of weighted cofactors were added by Prytherch et al. to generate the Portsmouth predictor equation (P-POSSUM), with somewhat improved mortality prediction [5]. The reliability of the P-POSSUM scoring system in predicting outcomes following vascular trauma improved when Wijesinghe et al. modified the method in which the values were applied [6].

Another modification was attempted around the same period by taking into account serum creatinine, age, GCS, hemoglobin, and EKG changes consistent with ischemia [4]. Known as the Hardman Index, this system had the same fundamental weakness as the original POSSUM calculator [4, 7]. Another attempt in 2008 using the National Trauma Data Bank (NTDB) identified 112 blunt pediatric arterial injuries in 103 pediatric patients (age <16 years). A trend toward increased mortality was found in patients with multiple arterial injuries $(P=0.49)$ and intra-abdominal venous injuries $(P=0.11)$ [8]. Mortality was greatest in patients with intra-abdominal arterial injuries and head trauma $(P=0.05)$, GCS <8 $(P=0.001)$, significant base deficit $(P=0.007)$, and cardiac arrest $(P<0.001)$. The authors concluded that increased mortality is likely to include a single vessel coupled with serious associated injury [8].

Loh et al. used a single-institution, retrospective evaluation to determine the effect of adding vascular injury to current trauma scoring systems [9]. One hundred patients, including 50 vascular trauma patients and 50 patients with no vascular trauma, were matched according to demographics, ISS, and TRISS. Of the vascular trauma patients, 72 % had an injury affecting a major vascular structure, of which 56 % of the total number of patients required an operative intervention. Mortality was somewhat higher for those patients who required operative intervention $(P>0.05)$; however, there was no statistical difference in overall mortality between the vascular trauma patients and those trauma patients without vascular injury regardless of the number of location of vascular injuries [9].

Vascular injuries appear to play a predominant role in morbidity and mortality in trauma patients with an RTS >5 or ISS >24. Traditional scoring systems in these patients underestimate mortality in patients with concomitant vascular injuries [9]. To some extent, this is also seen when evaluating extremity trauma with vascular involvement.

Conclusion

Few studies exist that discuss the impact of vascular trauma on overall morbidity and mortality as predicted by traditional scoring systems. Recent publications have identified weaknesses in vascular scoring systems when applied to survivability. Further studies need to be performed in order to determine whether vascular injuries truly impact survivability in comparison to nonvascular trauma. In the interim, a combination of traditional scoring systems in conjunction with best practices in vascular surgery should be used to properly manage vascular trauma patients and help prevent adverse outcomes.

References

1. Copes WS, Lawnick M, Champion HR, Sacco WJ. A comparison of Abbreviated Injury Scale 1980 and 1985 versions. J Trauma. 1988;28(1):78–86.
2. Champion HR, Sacco WJ, Carnazzo AJ, Copes W, Fouty WJ. Trauma score. Crit Care Med. 1981;9(9): 672–6.
3. Boyd CR, Tolson MA, Copes WS. Evaluating trauma care: the TRISS method. Trauma Score and the Injury Severity Score. J Trauma. 1987;27(4):370–8.
4. Neary WD, Crow P, Foy C, Prytherch D, Heather BP, Earnshaw JJ. Comparison of POSSUM scoring and the Hardman Index in selection of patients for repair of ruptured abdominal aortic aneurysm. Br J Surg. 2003;90(4):421–5.
5. Prytherch DR, Whiteley MS, Higgins B, Weaver PC, Prout WG, Powell SJ. POSSUM and Portsmouth POSSUM for predicting mortality. Physiological and Operative Severity Score for the enUmeration of mortality and morbidity. Br J Surg. 1998;85(9):1217–20.
6. Wijesinghe LD, et al. Comparison of POSSUM and the Portsmouth predictor equation for predicting death following vascular surgery. Br J Surg. 1998;85(2): 209–12.
7. Kurc E, Sanioglu S, Ozgen A, Aka SA, Yekeler I. Preoperative risk factors for in-hospital mortality and

validity of the Glasgow aneurysm score and Hardman index in patients with ruptured abdominal aortic aneurysm. Vascular. 2012;20(3):150–5.

8. Hamner CE, Groner JI, Caniano DA, Hayes JR, Kenney BD. Blunt intraabdominal arterial injury in pediatric trauma patients: injury distribution and markers of outcome. J Pediatr Surg. 2008;43(5): 916–23.

9. Loh SA, et al. Existing trauma and critical care scoring systems underestimate mortality among vascular trauma patients. J Vasc Surg. 2011;53(2): 359–66.

The Mangled Extremity

5

Andrew R. Burgess

Contents

A.R. Burgess, MD
Department of Orthopedic Surgery,
University of Texas, Houston, TX, USA
e-mail: andrew.r.burgess@uth.tmc.edu

5.1 Introduction

A polytraumatized patient with one or more mangled extremities presents challenges to the clinical team on multiple levels. The most sophisticated, resourced trauma facilities will have a team member familiar with the staging and management of severely injured extremities [1, 2].

5.2 Initial Management

A primary challenge is a rapid and accurate assessment of impaired extremities to ascertain if their complex of injuries is associated with patient survival (e.g., hemorrhage), and therefore needs immediate intervention, or can be temporized to urgent or delayed management. As the "ABCs" of ATLS protocols and evaluation of core issues proceed, extremities are evaluated for perfusion, neurological status, alignment (rapidly realigned, if necessary), and wound status (lacerations, de-gloving, nonviable tissue, contamination, etc.). Radiographic studies follow, and hard tissue injury correlated with wounds and vascular-neurological status, often resulting in a "zone of injury" paradigm.

If resources permit, *core* ATLS assessment coincides with *extremity* evaluation or just precedes it, permitting rapid formulation of an acute treatment plan, prioritization of lifesaving diagnostics and treatment interventions, and appropriately timed management of the injured extremity/extremities.

A. Dua et al. (eds.), *Clinical Review of Vascular Trauma*,
DOI 10.1007/978-3-642-39100-2_5, © Springer-Verlag Berlin Heidelberg 2014

Anatomical or system proximity to core injury may permit concurrent central and extremity peripheral diagnosis and treatment such as "runoff" vascular studies, soft tissue debridements of anatomically related truncal and extremity wounds, and CAT protocols. The ability of an experienced trauma team to coordinate the timing of diagnostic studies and operative interventions minimizes the overall time of workup and therapeutic intervention and the threat of complications associate with delay in either.

Soon after primary assessments and imaging, a logical plan for treatment is formulated with the "order of intervention" being the major factor, i.e., what delivers the best clinical value while minimizing risk. Examples may include treatment of compromised airway and pneumothorax and pelvic ring stabilization, followed by primary debridement of lower extremity wounds and spanning complex fractures with external fixation (e.g., damage control). Managed extremity/extremity-at-risk patients transferred to trauma centers as moving to a "higher level of care" are at risk of being initially underevaluated based on mechanism of injury, and all temporal issues related to extremity injury management need to be measured from initial event, and ABCs of evaluation repeated upon transfer and prior to definitive treatment at the accepting facility. Images do not necessarily need to be repeated, but by definition, the referring center is less experienced managing the polytraumatized patient.

Assuming the ABCs are completed, and management under way, the extremity is again rapidly aligned, pulses verified, and tourniquets adjusted, removed, and occasionally applied. This is an appropriate time for revascularization, be it using endovascular techniques or standard open repair. Shunts may be indicated in circumstances of life threatening core trauma, prolonged peripheral ischemia or gross contamination where definitive vascular repair in a contaminated and/or locally nonviable environment would be unwise.

5.3   Debridement

Preparation and draping of a mangled, fractured extremity presents challenges in handling, elevating, and maintaining alignment while completing preparation. The use of supplementary staff and atraumatic knots at uninjured digits permitting suspension while prepping the injured (and donor) extremity all aid in the task. If the presence of a vascular injury is noted at this time, a contralateral injured lower extremity may be prepped as a donor site for vein grafts, skin grafts, etc. Once prepped, sharp debridement of the wounds is completed, in the majority of cases by resection of a small border (1/8 to 1/4 in.) of skin and subcutaneous tissue surrounding the entire wound in large, circumferential sweeps, leaving bleeding edges, avoiding whittling the edges in multiple small cuts. Below the skin and subcutaneous tissue is usually contaminated or nonviable fat or muscle, both to be debrided aggressively, but with realization of functional role of the adjacent structures particularly neurovascular. Fasciotomies will be discussed separately, but as debridement progresses, any "compartmental releases" begun by the index injury should be completed.

Bone debridement is usually last of the primary surgical debridement. The surgeon should carefully assess osseous circulation, periosteal stripping, endosteal perfusion, and contamination status, as debridement continues, so that nonviable, contaminated bone might be aggressively debrided by resection, whereas viable, contaminated bone might be best served by scrubbing, low-pressure pulsed lavage, or high-volume gravity irrigation. All of the preceding steps are best accomplished if the fracture is temporarily redisplaced during the debridement, permitting the contaminated fracture fragments to face the surgical debridement techniques in the same orientation that occurred at the moment of injury.

Although restoration of perfusion is the primary goal in early management of the mangled extremity, the coordination, timing, and surgical field management are also critical because of the short-, mid-, and long-term complications of vascular repair and the effect timing, graft material, and completeness of debridement have on clinical outcome.

Very shortly after restoration of inflow, outflow integrity should be evaluated and approach to the extremity being rescued should include release of compartments, if indicated. In the case of the mangled extremity, release of all involved

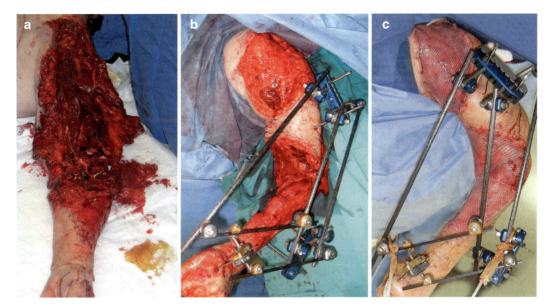

Fig. 5.1 (**a**) Photograph of a mangled left upper extremity following a motor vehicle collision. (**b**) Initial placement of an external fixator to stabilize the arm in a triangular fashion, following debridement and prior to vascular repair. (**c**) Early healing of left upper extremity after split-thickness skin grafting

and related compartments should be the default option. Extremely short-duration ischemia and anatomical compromises exposing vessels, nerves, or injured osseous structures are all circumstances that may indicate careful observation instead of fascial release, but with a low clinical tolerance to proceed.

5.4 Boney Fixation

Fixation of the skeletal elements centers around two issues: timing and implant choice. Timing of fixation really relates to "order of fixation." In ideal circumstances, moderate duration of ischemia and initial debridement can be coordinated with fracture/dislocation reduction and application of external fixation although traction or splinting may serve as an effective option. The use of plates is usually more time consuming but sometimes indicated in anatomic circumstances involving articular injury and non-anatomic circumstances such as surgeon familiarity or implant availability. Intramedullary nailing can be performed rapidly and may be applied in appropriate clinical situations, primarily with

vascular injury associated with diaphyseal fractures with an experienced team, prior to or immediately after restoration of perfusion.

Although rapid application with minimal additional dissection might be the primary concern when combined with vascular repair, implant selection should also be based on the need for re-debridement or reassessment for viability in circumstances with compromised and rapid initial treatment. This situation may demand reoperation and temporary re-displacement of the initial reduction to thoroughly assess contamination and viability, assure complete debridement, or prepare for local or free tissue coverage (Fig. 5.1).

5.5 Combined Vascular-Orthopedic Injuries: Orthopedic Management

In the developed world model in this decade, individuals are exposed to ever-increasing levels of energy when injured. Pedestrian injuries continue to be a large injury burden globally in both developed and more so in developing countries. Motor vehicle crash mitigation in developing countries has concentrated on protecting the head, abdomen, and thorax, resulting in high-energy extremity injuries attached to survivors who would previously not survive the same level of injurious energy. In a related demographic, our war fighters have the benefit of continual improvement in ballistic armor, primarily protecting the head and trunk of our combat troops.

At the same time, the level of serious extremity musculoskeletal/vascular injuries are increasing; the demographics, clinical experience, and changing technology have had a profound effect on the type and depth of experience of those physicians and surgeons responsible for diagnosing, treating, and rehabilitating combined vascular and musculoskeletal injury.

Today, fewer general surgery house staff have orthopedic rotations or basic clinical experience in the diagnosis of high-energy musculoskeletal injury, especially when combined with significant vascular injury. Vascular surgical training has recently focused on the endovascular treatment of both core and peripheral vascular pathology. A decade of conflict has exposed many of our war fighters to both central and peripheral vascular injury, resulting in a core of experienced general, vascular, and orthopedic military surgeons, familiar with severe extremity injuries, often in polytraumatized patients with issues of timing, severe contamination, and debridement. This has resulted in significant experience in some civilian trauma centers with senior or military veteran general/vascular clinicians familiar with the use of vascular shunts.

But the overall effect is many civilian centers have fewer clinicians with significant gross anatomical knowledge to diagnose, surgically approach, release associated compartments, and adequately debride associated soft tissue injury, especially without a former military surgeon on staff.

The environment surrounding combined musculoskeletal-vascular injury may be as important as the injury itself. Timely, accurate diagnosis and treatment is dependent on single versus mass casualties, isolated injury versus multiply injured patient, closed versus open injury, and penetrating versus blunt trauma. The most straightforward injury complex might be a low-velocity gunshot resulting in a midshaft long bone fracture and a single vessel injury and degree of collateral perfusion: the most challenging, a proximal extremity crush, blast, high-velocity skeletal/vascular disruption with a potentially viable distal extremity, further complicated by additional, and occasionally more life-threatening, injuries elsewhere [3].

5.6 Diagnosis

For purposes of this discussion, we will assume the patient has been appropriately assessed and managed at the scene with skilled extrication, splinting, and immobilization for transport. Further assessment during transport would include assessment of blood pressure and extremity perfusion, including color, temperature, and quality of pulse.

Emergency department assessment would repeat the basics of extremity assessment begun by EMS in a more controlled environment, X-rays and CAT studies, more precise alignment of associated fractures and dislocations, Doppler studies, and comparative pulses, including comparison with non-injured extremities. This workup will usually identify vascular pathology regarding location, whether it is presently hemorrhaging, and most importantly to the success of comanagement, the location of vascular injury in relationship to fracture pathology and significant soft tissue injury. The association of fracture/dislocation pattern, soft tissue pathology, and vascular injury type and location yields a concept long referred to as "zone of injury." Integration of zone of injury, mechanism, and time since injury and evaluation of the patient's overall status regarding associated injuries should form the basis of planning comanagement of the patient with combined orthopedic and vascular injury.

5.7 Transfer to Higher Level of Care

With these evaluations and patient stabilization under way in the context of the ABCs of trauma care, the management of the combined injury begins. Most levels of trauma care will know at any given time or immediately ascertain if the clinical resources needed to manage such combined injuries are available in an appropriate time context since time since injury is such a crucial factor. The need for timely treatment of life-threatening injury may have to take place at the initial receiving institution, further (but appropriately) delaying management of the vascular-compromised extremity.

The avoidable delays accompanying such circumstances will be minimized by a preestablished transfer agreement with trauma centers having established expertise in management of such injury available at all times.

5.8   Management of the Injury

In the best case scenario, these combined injuries would be isolated, transported and diagnosed rapidly, and have no open wounds or gross contamination or closely associated mass of nonviable soft tissue. The worst-case scenario is exemplified by extreme high-energy military blast wounds, occurring most frequently in multiply injured patients, often with multiple extremity injuries, with transport compromised by distance and time, and the vascular-orthopedic injury to be managed part of a grossly contaminated, mangled "zone of injury" (Fig. 5.1a). As would be expected, many of these military-type injuries as well as severe highway, industrial, and agricultural injuries with similar clinical presentations are best managed by early amputation, but a significant amount have potentially functional components distally and are candidates for vascular and concurrent orthopedic repair.

A typical scenario might involve a motorcycle crash or pedestrian bumper strike injury resulting in fracture of the proximal tibia (often segmental), a dislocated knee joint, and a distal femur fracture, either individually or in combination. Frequently these fracture patterns are associated with femoral or popliteal vascular injury, just proximal to, involving, or immediately distal to the trifurcation. Assuming transport and emergency department work-up are rapid, excluding other life-threatening injury, combined vascular-orthopedic treatment should commence. If it has been 2 h or less from injury to beginning treatment, one may suggest rapid transport to the operating theater; placement on an appropriate table, permitting vascular and orthopedic imaging; rapid careful prepping of the injured as well as the non-injured leg (expectantly managing donor needs); and proximal vascular control if hemorrhage is still active. In a closed injury, this author suggests rapid external fixation in the presence of skeletal instability, placed to permit uncompromised vascular access and to provide mechanical stability to the surgical field. This often accomplished in the scenario described, prior to vascular repair, simplifying and protecting the vascular procedure. It is appropriate to consider fasciotomy as a default component in the scenario described: they may be deemed unnecessary only if the leg has had a significant component of collateral flow or time from injury to revascularization has been short. It is common to underestimate the potential time from injury to restoration of flow even in the most experienced institutions, as these interventions are begun. If an endovascular repair is indicated, the sequence of vascular repair versus skeletal stabilization may be individualized.

A similar clinical situation, compromised by time (time of transport or diagnosis/management of other injuries), might best be managed by rapid placement of a shunt and fasciotomies to provide appropriate rapid revascularization prior to skeletal stabilization.

A second orthopedic-vascular indication for temporizing with a vascular shunt is the presence of a grossly contaminated wound or a large amount of devitalized muscle, bone, and/or associated soft tissue. Such situations require an extensive, thorough debridement of both bone and soft tissue throughout the zone of injury and are usually managed by secondary debridements prior to definitive closure with local or free tissue transfer (Fig. 5.1b, c). In these cases the shunt may be placed first if appropriate (occasionally in combination with a venous shunt), the fasciotomies may be incorporated in the wound extension/debridement, with conversion of shunt to definitive vascular repair done when wound status and skeletal stability are defined and maximized.

The most compromised management scenarios are in combat multiply injured patients, civilian polytrauma, or severe agricultural or industrial injury. As stated above, many of these are candidates for immediate amputation, but those "threshold" injuries, with a chance of functional salvage, are the most challenging cases for a damage control approach. In those situations, the patient is often placed on an operative table for chest or abdominal procedures which permits extremity imaging as discussed previously, but an approach often overlooked in the face of a life-threatening truncal or neurological injury. If the patient remains physiologically stable after treatment of more urgent injuries, the extremity vascular-orthopedic injury is reassessed, additional temporal factors considered, any incomplete diagnostics performed, and damage control attempted. In these conditions, the order of treatment is individualized, given the elapsed time, magnitude of soft tissue injury, and complexity of both vascular and skeletal pathology. In this circumstance fasciotomies are always performed and are generous to allow for unavoidably delayed revascularization.

5.9   Emergent Skeletal Stabilization

In the situations described above, external fixation is often the choice for skeletal stabilization in the presence of vascular injury (Fig. 5.1c). If time and wound conditions permit, it should be placed prior to definitive vascular repair. The goal is to have the extremity inflow reestablished between 4 and 6 h after injury. Simple, single-plane fixation is most useful, using half-pin constructs, spanning articular pathology (unless necessary to protect injured vessels, fresh shunts, or repairs).

The quality of anatomic reduction in these cases of combined injury is different from that which is acceptable in fracture surgery where the viability of the extremity is not a risk. General alignment of the limb is acceptable; small degrees of angulation, rotation, and shortening may be acceptable until the situation is clinically more stable. Any malreduced fracture segment which threatens the vascular repair is addressed, often with an individual pin or pins to assure position.

Fixator frames should be placed by a surgeon with a knowledge of vascular surgical approaches and obviously an understanding of the individual injury specifics, so that the components will not hamper access for vascular repair, protect the repair when complete, and aid in the acute post-op management of the extremity (permit wound access and soft tissue assessment, aid in gross positioning, as a "kick stand").

In addition, the orthopedic surgeon will allow for the eventual definitive skeletal management, usually an intramedullary nail for diaphyseal fractures or plates for intra-articular fractures. When considering a nail to follow, attention to detail to pin-site soft tissue management is critical to minimize late infection when converting from external fixation to definitive intramedullary nailing. Conversion from external fixation to more definitive methods should be considered soon after the extremity is deemed viable, sometimes within 48 h after initial treatment, although frequently up to 2 weeks following damage control. If conversion is delayed past 2 weeks, longer-term definitive use of the external fixator is considered. During any repeated visits to the operating room for any surgical procedures, the initial reduction may be adjusted to maximize precise anatomical alignment, especially if the external fixator may become the definitive fixation. In the case of a fracture pattern necessitating a plate for definitive open reduction and fixation, the placement of the initial fixator pins is accomplished by placing the initial pins as far from the eventual plate location as anatomy, injury pattern, and biomechanics permit. This is also to minimize pin tract location near the eventual dissection plane of the plate and thereby minimize delayed infection. The biomechanical compromises inherent in such long spanning fixators can be mitigated by choice of pin diameter and frame design.

5.10 Definitive Orthopedic Management

Usually external fixation is converted to intramedullary nails or screws when the extremity is considered stable with regard to both vascular and soft tissue status. The issues are primarily orthopedically centered with special consideration to the condition of any traumatic or surgical wounds, the status of external fixator pin sites, a review of the history of the vascular repair, its relationship to the initial zone of injury, and the anatomical routing of any grafts. The definitive fixation is completed as atraumatically as possible to mitigate any potential damage to the relatively immature status of the associated vascular repair. In the consideration of a dislocated knee, multiligamentous disruption is often a component; the timing and type of successful ligamentous repair are carefully considered in the face of accompanying vascular injury. High-energy injuries about the knee often require aggressive physical therapy, and the concerns of the vascular team should be integrated into the postoperative management protocol.

In certain femoral shaft fractures with associated vascular injury, the best damage control stabilization may be a rapidly inserted femoral nail, depending on injury profile, institutional assets, and the patient's pulmonary condition. These can occasionally be placed almost as rapidly as an external fixator. When done emergently, these injuries may require an additional visit to the operating theater to place more definitive locking screws and adjust the initial reduction.

5.11 Special Considerations

5.11.1 Scapulothoracic Dissociation of the Upper Extremity

Upper extremity vascular trauma diagnosis and management might begin with description of an entity that has become known over the last three decades as scapulothoracic dissociation [4, 5].

Although subclavian and proximal brachial vascular injury, in association with high-energy blunt trauma to the forequarter, has been described previously, there is a family of high-energy forequarter injuries, often avulsive in nature, that include disruption of vascular flow to the upper extremity, lateral displacement of the scapula, and disruption of the sternal-clavicular-acromial axis. The brachial plexus is frequently injured in this complex, resulting in abnormal neurological findings, frequently permanent.

The first AP chest film, which includes the shoulder, usually demonstrates a laterally displaced scapula and one or two of the following: a displaced, distracted clavicle fracture, a separated acromioclavicular joint, and a separated sternoclavicular joint (Fig. 5.2a). Many of these injury complexes include significant, additional distal injury to the arm or forearm. These injuries are often the result of ejection from a motorcycle with direct upper extremity contact with a fixed object or ejections, partial or full, from automobiles/trucks: they present with abnormal neurovascular findings frequently assigned to the more peripheral injury. Management of significant upper extremity injury with neurovascular findings should include early review of the chest film and radiographic assessment of the shoulder, noting signs of a traction-type injury. Any contrast study of the extremity vasculature should include the aorta and great vessels.

Early descriptions of the complex of neurovascular and the skeletal injuries described noted that the range of neurological injuries was broad, from complete avulsion of the plexus with no functional return to mild traction injuries followed by complete recovery.

Vascular injury pattern varies from complete avulsion of all associated vascular soft tissue requiring formal repair to intimal disruption manageable with endovascular methods (Fig. 5.2b–d). Degree of collateral circulation varies with the anatomic location of the primary vascular lesion (Fig. 5.2b).

While the exact musculoskeletal, vascular, and neural components of the injury complex may differ slightly, the challenges in recognition, diagnosis, timing, and type of treatment

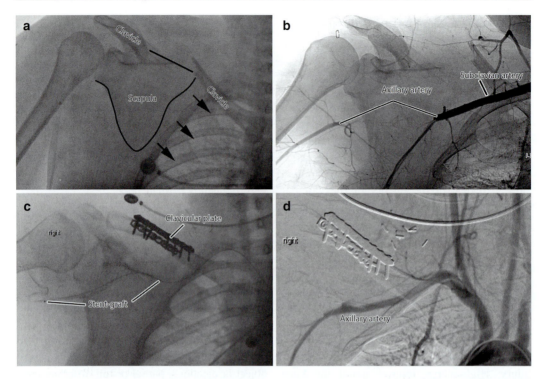

Fig. 5.2 (**a**) The first AP chest film, which includes the shoulder, demonstrating a laterally displaced scapula and a displaced, distracted clavicle fracture. (**b**) Arteriogram in a patient with scapulothoracic dissociation demonstrating abrupt cessation of flow within the right axillary artery near the lateral border of the first rib. (**c**) Placement of clavicular plates to reappose the fractured clavicle and a wire with an undeployed stent graft going across the previously disrupted axillary artery. (**d**) Completion arteriogram demonstrating patent axillary artery

should be realized by experienced clinicians. The author believes that management of high-energy blunt injury to the upper extremity and/or shoulder-forequarter region should include scapulothoracic dissociation in the differential diagnosis.

Conclusion

Overall management of the mangled extremity requires rapid revascularization coupled with aggressive debridement. Fasciotomy should be generous in nature to ensure optimum flow. Multifunctional fixation, anatomic reduction, and appropriate wound access with elevation of the extremity are tenants in orthopedic management in trauma that includes bony and vascular injury.

References

1. de Mestral C, Sharma S, Haas B, Gomez D, Nathens AB. A contemporary analysis of the management of the mangled lower extremity. J Trauma Acute Care Surg. 2013;74(2):597–603.
2. Fleming ME, Watson JT, Gaines RJ, O'Toole RV, Extremity War Injuries VII Reconstruction Panel. Evolution of orthopaedic reconstructive care. J Am Acad Orthop Surg. 2012;20 Suppl 1:S74–9.
3. Ellington JK, Bosse MJ, Castillo RC, MacKenzie EJ, LEAP Study Group. The mangled foot and ankle: results from a 2-year prospective study. J Orthop Trauma. 2013;27(1):43–8.
4. Oreck SL, Burgess A, Levine AM. Traumatic lateral displacement of the scapula: a radiographic sign of neurovascular disruption. J Bone Joint Surg Am. 1984;66(5):758–63.
5. Witz M, Korzets Z, Lehmann J. Traumatic scapulothoracic dissociation. J Cardiovasc Surg (Torino). 2000;41(6):927–9.

Fasciotomy

6

Andrew R. Burgess and Abdul Aziz

Contents

A.R. Burgess, MD (✉)
Department of Orthopedic Surgery,
University of Texas-Houston, Houston, TX, USA
e-mail: andrew.r.burgess@uth.tmc.edu

A. Aziz, MBChB
Department of Trauma and Orthopaedic Surgery,
Queens Medical Centre, Nottingham, UK

6.1 Introduction

The clinical presentations that may occur necessitating upper extremity fasciotomy include both blunt and penetrating injury, include isolated injury, or as one of several injuries in a polytraumatized patient [1, 2]. In addition, rapid transport to a center familiar with such injury versus delay in discovery, transport, or a patient transferred to a higher level of care, all contribute to the approach to fasciotomies, as does the role of fascial release following revascularization.

6.2 Surgical Approach to the Arm

Most surgical approaches should begin with a curvilinear approach over the volar forearm, with marking the incision extensions to be made distally to decompress the carpal tunnel and proximally to extend into the medial aspect of the arm/biceps with attention to crossing the antecubital fossa in a "z" or transverse incision with release of the lacertus fibrosis of the biceps insertion, also in the antecubital approach (Fig. 6.1). Approach to the deeper volar structures should include decompression of the mobile wad, medial flexor mass, and the deeper layers of digital flexors and pronators. After central volar decompression, including the lacertus fibrosus, overall wound assessment

Fig. 6.1 (**a**) Reverse Henry incision and brachial artery exposure. (**b**) Close-up of incision with nearby neurovascular structures. (**c**) Photograph of patient with reverse Henry incision. The carpal tunnel aspect is often included. A proximal incision lateral to the biceps is used for direct access to the brachial artery. The antecubital crease is crossed transversely, followed by a curvilinear incision over the wrist. The lacertus fibrosis (bicipital aponeurosis) is released at the elbow, followed by the mobile wad and forearm muscles. The medial flexor wad and digital flexors are also released. The dorsum of the forearm and carpal tunnel are also released if necessary

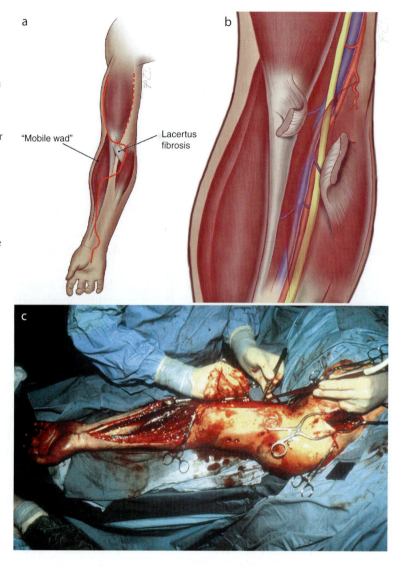

will determine the need for further proximal extension of the forearm volar incision and/or distal decompression of the carpal tunnel (and occasionally Guyen's Canal), and the necessity of dorsal decompression should be determined last, as dorsal decompression is often unnecessary as pattern of injury plus volar decompression often decompress the dorsal structures of the forearm.

The muscles of the hand are then assessed and interossei and thenar decompression as necessary.

6.2.1 Step-by-Step Fasciotomy of the Upper Extremity (Fig. 6.1)

1. Inscribe Henry incision of forearm.
2. Include carpal tunnel aspect if necessary; center of wrist to space between middle and ring, favoring ring finger aspect.
3. Proximal incision lateral to biceps for direct access to brachial artery joins incision from proximal repair; requires primary closure or protected VAC.

4. Cross antecubital crease transversely; direction depending on proximal incision option.
5. Curvilinear incision over wrist to create radial artery protective flap.
6. Release lacertus fibrosis (bicipital aponeurosis) at elbow, between biceps tendon.
7. Release mobile wad; brachioradialis, extensor carpi radialis longus and brevis.
8. Release medial flexor wad.
9. Release superficial and deep digital flexors.
10. Assess need for carpal tunnel and dorsal forearm release, often unnecessary.
11. Release dorsum of forearm and carpal tunnel.

Final assessment prior to applying dressings includes a reassessment of proximal structures. The biceps and brachialis can be decompressed with a proximal extension of the fasciotomy over the medial biceps. Occasionally the triceps need to be released through a separate dorsal approach. Deltoid release is on a case by case basis.

There are several options for wound management, and, as of the writing of this chapter, vacuum-assisted wound management is one of the more frequently used in North American trauma centers. One must carefully protect the neurovascular structures prior to application, occasionally the carpal tunnel can be closed prior to dressing application.

6.3 Orthopedic Fixation in Combination with Vascular Repair

Skeletal fixation choices will also depend on time since injury, associated contamination, location of fracture as well as relation to vascular repair, and other injuries to the same patient. Vascular repair and fasciotomies are usually stabilized relative to the fracture or dislocation associated with the vascular injury. Fixation methods must allow access to the fasciotomy to allow for inspection and dressing changes. Subclavian and proximal brachial arterial injuries usually do not benefit skeletal fixation as fixation of the proximal humerus is complex and time consuming.

At the time of this writing, our preference for fasciotomy coverage and closure is early VAC dressings, delayed primary closure, and split thickness skin graft if necessary. Free tissue transfer is used if the upper extremity is deemed salvageable and fasciotomy position is concurrent with wounds of the arm or forearm [3].

6.4 Fasciotomy of the Thigh

Fasciotomies of the lower extremity in a civilian trauma practice are primarily indicated to treat conditions of the leg, usually associated with blunt or penetrating trauma affecting the extremity between knee and ankle. Most discussion on indications, anatomy, and technique centers on pathology affecting this area. The buttock, thigh, and foot require fascial release less often, and indications for release in some of these areas are evolving topics of discussion.

Fasciotomy of the buttock is rarely indicated in blunt trauma, occasionally suspected with both direct injury and developing signs such as decreasing sciatic function, observed directly. There are few cases described involving vascular injury to the area resulting in contained hemorrhage into muscle bellies or fascial planes that yield compartment syndrome-like symptoms. If encountered, it may be secondary to a named vessel hemorrhage related to a superior gluteal branch. Useful fasciotomies to this area can be performed through a Kocher-Langenbach approach.

The thigh rarely needs decompression because the anatomy provides significant space to contain moderate amounts of hemorrhage (Fig. 6.2). There are instances of direct vascular trauma, high-energy crush, prolonged entrapment, or extreme positioning. The thigh has three anatomic compartments, two of which can be decompressed through the same skin incision, after which the third is reevaluated for need of decompression. Upon deciding to release the fascia of the thigh, an anterior lateral incision of at least 20 cm is made over the anterolateral thigh with a slight lateral bias. The incision permits inspection of the quadriceps fascia which is then released.

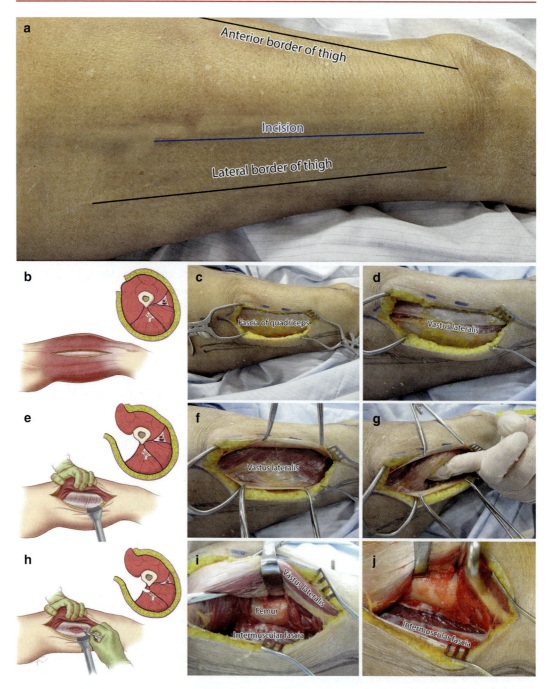

Fig. 6.2 Lateral thigh fasciotomy and key steps for release of intermuscular fascia (**a–j**). After making an incision midway between the anterior and lateral border of the thigh (**b**, **c**), the fascia of the quadriceps is incised and released (**d**). The vastus lateralis is rolled anteriorly to expose the intermuscular fascia (**e–g**). This fascia is then incised 1 cm from the femur in order to avoid the perforating vessels (**h–j**). The hamstrings are released and the medial compartment reassessed. The adductors may be released if necessary using a longitudinal 5 cm incision

Following this, the quadriceps is rotated anteriorly, exposing the longitudinal intermuscular fascia separating the lateral quadriceps from the posterior hamstring compartment. This fascia is incised for at least 20 cm, being careful to dissect at least 2–3 cm from the bone, avoiding perforating vessels. The viability of the muscles of both compartments is assessed, nonviable muscle removed, and attention turned to the adductor compartment. Depending on the site of original pathology in the thigh, the release of both the quadriceps and hamstring compartments often decreases pressure indirectly, making adductor fascial release unnecessary.

6.4.1 Step-by-Step Fasciotomy of the Thigh (Fig. 6.2)

1. Incise thigh midway between anterior and lateral border
2. Release fascia of quadriceps
3. Roll vastus lateralis anteriorly, exposing intermuscular fascia
4. Incise intramuscular fascia, 1 to 3 cm from femur, avoiding perforators
5. Digitally release hamstrings
6. Reassess medial compartment
7. Release adductors, if necessary
8. Longitudinal, 5 cm incision

6.5 Fasciotomy of the Lower Leg (Figs. 6.3, 6.4, and 6.5)

The leg, from knee to ankle, is the most frequent anatomic location to require fasciotomy in a typical North American Trauma Center. The injury may be the result of blunt or penetrating trauma and may or may not include named vascular injury. Associated vascular injury may or may not have collateral flow, be an isolated injury, or part of a multi injury scenario. In addition, the patient may present soon after injury to an institution able to diagnose and perform compartmental release or may arrive after prolonged transport or as a transfer to a level of greater care. With regard to diagnostics, the physical exam of a conscious patient is the most valuable diagnostic tool with pain on passive stretch, or pain out of proportion, increasing while observed being the most sensitive to experienced clinicians. Obviously, an unconscious patient, an altered sensorium, and a patient under anesthesia present challenging diagnostic situations. A patient known to be

dysvascular for more than 2 h should have a fasciotomy concurrent with or prior to vascular repair.

Both one- and two-incision techniques are described; most traumatologists prefer the two-incision variant to guarantee release of the four compartments of the leg. Many legs requiring compartmental release in conjunction with treatment of vascular injury have relatively recognizable anatomic landmarks, even though injured. The two-incision technique maximizes the release of all compartments and maximizes the orientation of the operating surgeon to named compartment identification, location of critical neurovascular structures, occasionally necessary in a grossly disrupted injury as a result of blast, severe motorcycle, pedestrian, or industrial/agricultural injury.

The lateral leg incision is often described along a longitudinal line bisecting the tibial crest and the cutaneous position of the fibula (Figs. 6.3 and 6.4). This permits access to both the anterior and lateral compartments of the leg (and serves as access to complete the single incision technique) but is usually modified by experienced extremity trauma surgeons in two ways. The generous starting incision is made about 2 cm posterior to the usually described position, favoring the lateral compartment; the anterior skin flap is then swept anteriorly from the subcutaneous tissue, exposing the bulging muscle bellies of both anterior and lateral compartments. The intermuscular septum can often be palpated with some certainty as this flap is retracted.

A subcutaneous incision is then completed perpendicular to and across the intermuscular septum. This is completed gently, with minimal pressure, allowing the swollen muscle bellies to protrude somewhat, and confirming the location of the intermuscular septum. The septum is plucked like a guitar string and longitudinal compartmental release incisions made from that point, starting in the anterior compartment 1 cm from the septum anteriorly, and then lateral compartment release longitudinally, beginning at least 1 cm posteriorly to the septum. Both longitudinal releases made via this lateral approach start just off the intermuscular septum and progress both proximally and distally with the surgical scissor points directed obliquely away from the septum.

Fig. 6.3 (**a**) Cross-sectional view and line demonstrating site of incision to make lateral lower leg fasciotomy for release of anterior and lateral compartments. (**b**) Stylized view on a cadaveric specimen. *Black line* at top is tibial crest, dashed *black line* at bottom marks site of fibula, dotted *black line* in center is midway between tibial crest and fibula, and *blue line* marks site of incision. This incision is made 1–2 cm posterior to the dotted *black line*. (**c**) Exposure of anterior and lateral compartments divided by the intermuscular septum

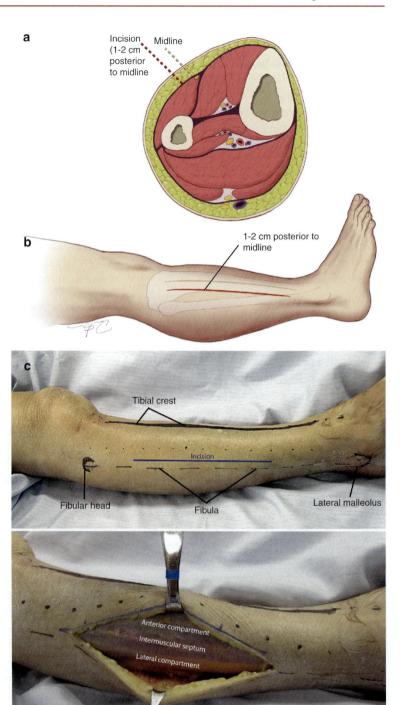

a

Incision (1-2 cm posterior to midline   Midline

b

1-2 cm posterior to midline

c

Tibial crest

Fibular head   Fibula   Lateral malleolus

Anterior compartment
Intermuscular septum
Lateral compartment

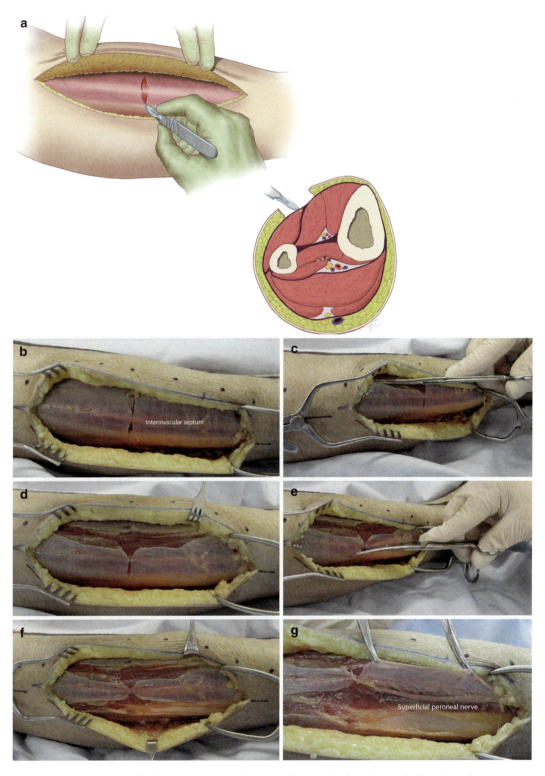

Fig. 6.4 Lateral lower leg fasciotomy incision and key steps for release of anterior and lateral compartments (**a–g**). Start with a 3 cm incision transverse to septum (**b**), and then create anterior compartment fasciotomy with scissors pointed anterior (**c, d**). Create lateral compartment fasciotomy with scissors pointed posterior (**e, f**). Verify superficial peroneal nerve in lateral compartment (**g**)

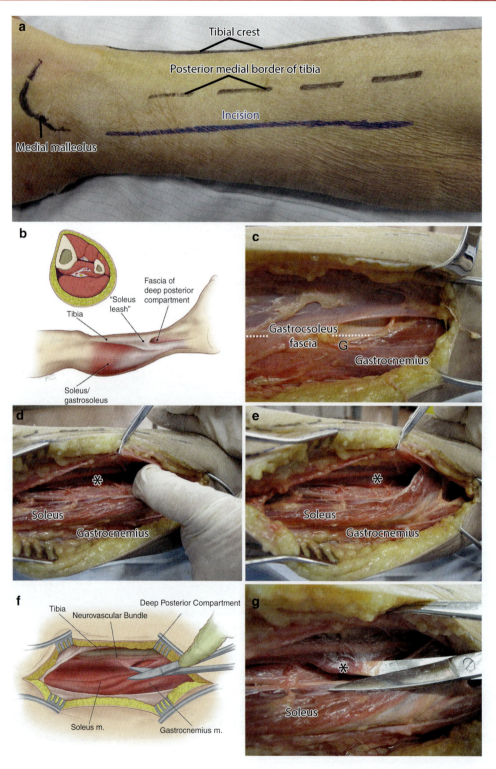

Fig. 6.5 Medial lower leg fasciotomy incision and key steps for release of superficial and deep compartments (**a**–**g**). Identify posterior medial boarder of tibia (**a**), make a 20 cm skin incision 2 cm posterior to the border (**b**, **c**), and identify the fascia of the gastrocsoleus muscle belly (**b**, **c**). After incising through the fascia, identify the distal attachment of the soleus and the soleus fascia (also known as the soleus leash) (**d**, **e**). Release the soleus leash and expose the true fascia of the deep compartment. Longitudinally release the investing fascia of the deep posterior compartment (**f**, **g**). *Asterisk* marks location of deep posterior compartment

good communication regarding the role of endovascular management for these severely injured patients, as some injuries may be more expeditiously managed by open surgery [3].

Of paramount importance to the rapid repair of vascular injuries is the ability to quickly convert between open and endovascular surgery. Traditionally, endovascular procedures have been performed in imaging suites remote from the operating room, with poor lighting and limited room to set up an open surgical case. Hybrid endovascular suites in the operating room environment help obviate these issues, and provided both vascular and trauma surgeons the ability to perform complex hybrid endovascular procedures without excessive delay (Fig. 7.1). These hybrid suites are particularly important in cases where it is important to determine location and extend of major vascular injuries in order to expeditiously deploy large covered endografts to stabilize the patient and prevent further bleeding. By having the ability to move from an endovascular to open surgical approach and vice versa,

the surgeon afforded the flexibility to provide to gain arterial or venous access and deliver the best of both vascular and trauma surgical care in a single operating suite. Additionally, performing these cases in a hybrid operating room, as opposed to an interventional radiology suite or cardiology catheterization laboratory, provides an extra layer of comfort for trauma surgeons, vascular surgeons, and anesthesiologists as a result that any and all necessary instruments, medications, and personnel support are present and immediately available the operating team.

7.2.3 Radiation Safety

Critically ill patients are exposed to numerous safety hazards [4]. The introduction of endovascular techniques to the care of trauma patients of necessity exposes patients and the interventional operating team to the effects of ionizing radiation, which can accumulate quickly in patients with multiple injuries which necessitates the need

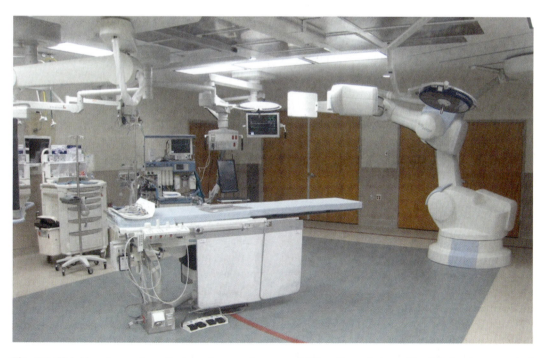

Fig. 7.1 Hybrid endovascular suite in main operating room. The floating table is fully capable of accommodating mounted retraction systems and has all movement capabilities (i.e., airplane, Trendelenburg) as standard operating room tables

for multiple procedures and prolonged operative procedure times. Dose-dependent effects of ionizing radiation exposure include hypothyroidism, cataract formation, alopecia, and hematologic and solid organ malignancies [4]. All members of the interventional or operative team participating in endovascular procedures should wear wraparound lead aprons, thyroid shields, and lead-lined radiation protective glasses or goggles. It is underappreciated that the majority of radiation exposure during endovascular cases comes from beam scatter from the patient, not from the imaging device itself, and patterns of exposure can be unpredictable. Real-time monitoring of radiation dose exposure is important and each member should wear two radiation monitoring badges. One badge should be worn outside the neck collar at the level of the thyroid and the second badge should be worn inside the lead apron at waist level. Of particular importance in these procedures is minimizing exposure by proper use of collimation of the x-ray beam, intermittent rather than continuous fluoroscopy use, and use of last image hold techniques [5]. Additionally, it is important to keep the image detector of the C-arm as close to the patient as possible to minimize the scattering of the x-ray beam, which is the most common source of radiation exposure in these procedures.

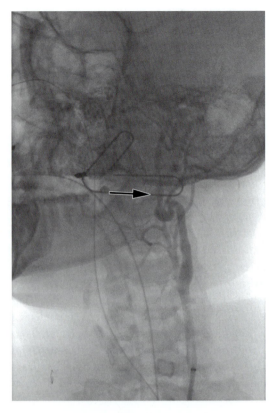

Fig. 7.2 Penetrating injury to the distal left internal carotid artery with false aneurysm formation (*arrow*)

7.3 Specific Management Principles

7.3.1 Head and Neck

Endovascular management of carotid and vertebral artery trauma has been documented for several years. One of the earliest reports of this examined numerous methods to treat traumatic carotid and vertebral lesions with embolization therapy, including the use of detachable balloons, liquid tissue adhesives, microcoils, and pieces of silk suture [6]. A large variety of lesions were treated, including carotid-cavernous fistulas, dural fistulas, and direct penetrating arteriovenous fistulas. Five out of 234 patients experienced strokes. The number of patients requiring

open surgical therapy was not reported. Since that time, numerous case reports and series have documented techniques of management of carotid and vertebral artery injuries, all in a selective fashion. Herrera reported 36 cases of penetrating cervical carotid trauma treated with endovascular management over a 12-year period with successful repair in 34 cases [7]. No randomized trials have been reported, and long-term results are not available. Endovascular stent grafts have also been used for the treatment of traumatic jugular-carotid fistulas, to repair true and false aneurysms of the carotid arteries and to repair iatrogenic carotid injuries [8–10].

The distal internal carotid artery is an ideal location for application of endovascular management due to its difficult surgical access. Figure 7.2 is the initial angiogram of patient that presented to our institution with hemorrhage from the distal internal carotid artery as the result of a transcervical gunshot wound. The patient was brought to

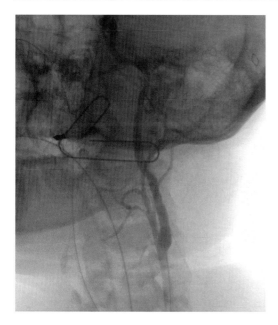

Fig. 7.3 Successful exclusion of internal carotid penetrating injury with Viabahn (W.L. Gore, Flagstaff, AZ) covered stent

the hybrid operating room for an initial attempt at endovascular exclusion, with left neck exploration planned if unable to cross the lesion with a wire. The lesion was successfully excluded with a covered endograft (Fig. 7.3), with a total procedure time from femoral arterial puncture to lesion exclusion of 22 min. The patient did not require neck exploration; he did have a tracheostomy post-procedurally for airway management and was discharged home on postoperative day #19.

Blunt carotid injury is a potentially devastating condition that is notoriously difficult to diagnose, and the management of which remains controversial [11]. Patients with internal carotid dissection that either becomes symptomatic (transient ischemic attack [TIA], stroke, amaurosis) or worsens during surveillance are candidates for endovascular stenting. These patients are required to take antiplatelet agents (clopidogrel and aspirin) both pre- and post-procedurally, and this may be impractical in the setting of concomitant major trauma to other organ systems. Likewise, the natural history of stents in the internal carotid arteries of young patients is not clearly defined. When carotid stenting is required due to

symptomatic dissections, or worsening dissection during surveillance, it should be done with embolic protection and with pre-procedural administration of antiplatelet medications. Although the use of embolic protection devices in these patients is controversial, they should be used when possible until more data are available for review [11].

7.3.2 Thoracic Aortic Injury

Blunt injury to the thoracic aorta is a highly lethal injury resulting in approximately 8,000 deaths in the United States annually [12, 13]. It is the second most common cause of trauma-related death, behind intracranial hemorrhage. Most patients who sustain this type of injury die at the scene with less than 25 % surviving long enough to be evaluated at a hospital [14]. Of those who present to the hospital with blunt aortic injury (BAI), up to 50 % die within 24 h [15].

Traumatic aortic injuries range from small defects in the intimal layer to complete transection of the artery, typically just beyond the origin of the left subclavian artery (LSA). Several classification schemes have been proposed based on radiologic imaging in an attempt to grade the various types of aortic defects according to severity of injury, which can be used to guide therapy. The Society of Vascular Surgery in their 2011 practice guidelines endorsed the classification scheme published by Azizzadeh [16]. In this scheme there are four grades of aortic injury, ranging in severity from grade I (intimal tear) to grade IV (free rupture) (Fig. 7.4).

Prior to the endovascular era, a majority of aortic injuries were repaired via a conventional surgical approach consisting of a left thoracotomy with or without cardiopulmonary bypass. Open repair for traumatic aortic injuries historically has been associated with a mortality rate approaching 30 % and a paraplegia rate of 16 % [17, 18]. The first thoracic endovascular aortic repair (TEVAR) was described in 1997 and, since then, has become the preferred technique to repair BAI [19]. TEVAR has proven to be a durable repair option for these critically ill patients

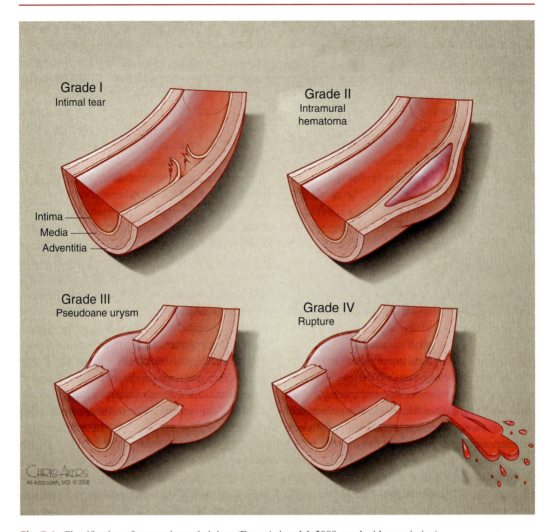

Fig. 7.4 Classification of traumatic aortic injury (From Azizzadeh 2009, used with permission)

and eliminates the morbidity associated with cross clamping of the aorta and the need for cardiopulmonary bypass required for an open repair. Although better tolerated by patients, TEVAR still carries a risk of spinal cord ischemia, stroke, and other complications that are associated with open repair.

There have not been randomized trials comparing open versus endovascular repair of traumatic aortic injury, but there have been several single institution reports as well as meta-analyses of the literature comparing the two procedures. In 2012, Risenman and colleagues reported their institutional experience over a 20-year period comparing 60 open repairs to 26 endovascular repairs [20]. They concluded that patients undergoing endovascular repair had a significantly lower intraoperative mortality rate (0 % vs. 18 %) and overall hospital mortality rate (12 % vs. 37 %) compared to open surgical repair [20]. Rousseau and colleagues reported their 22-year experience which revealed mortality and paraplegia rates of 21 and 7 %, respectively, in 28 patients undergoing open repair versus 0 % mortality and paraplegia rate in 29 patients undergoing endovascular repair of BAI [21]. Ott and colleagues reported an 11-year retrospective study comparing 12 open procedures to 6 endovascular procedures [18]. Mortality and paraplegia rates were 17 and 16 %, respectively, for the open group versus 0 % mortality and paraplegia rate for the endovascular group. In a recent meta-analysis, Tang et al. reviewed 33 published articles including 699 procedures (TEVAR – 370; open – 329) which showed a significantly lower rate of mortality (7.6 % vs. 15.2 %), paraplegia (0 % vs. 5.6 %), and stroke (0.85 % vs. 5.3 %) in patients who underwent TEVAR compared to open repair [22]. Collectively, outcomes from these reports and others have provided compelling data which has led to endovascular repair of traumatic aortic injury becoming the mainstay of therapy.

Traumatic aortic injuries should be suspected in trauma patients who present with mechanism of injury consistent with rapid deceleration. Historically, aortic injuries were suggested by abnormal chest x-rays and confirmed with arch aortography; however, with the improvements in high-resolution computed tomography scanners, they have been replaced by CTA as the preferred method of diagnosis. In addition, CTA imaging is instrumental in procedural planning.

Once an aortic injury has been confirmed, strict blood pressure control should be obtained. A goal systolic pressure between 100 and 120 mmHg and a heart rate of 60–80 is ideal. Multiple studies have shown that aggressive blood pressure and heart rate control is associated with improved outcomes in those suffering BAI [21, 23, 24]. In a review by Hemmila, it was shown that antihypertensive therapy started at the time of aortic injury diagnosis reduced the risk of aortic rupture to less than 1.5 % in patients whose aortic repair was delayed due to other life-threatening injuries taking precedence [25].

Approximately 10 % of patients with traumatic aortic injuries have grade I aortic injuries also referred to as minimal aortic injury [26]. These injuries can be managed with observation with the expectation that these injuries will heal spontaneously. These patients do however require serial imaging to monitor for injury progression. Grade II through IV aortic injuries should be repaired urgently within 24 h of diagnosis unless there are other more life-threatening cranial or intra-abdominal injuries which require more emergent intervention. In these patients, aortic

repair can be delayed but should be performed prior to discharge [12, 27]. Hemmila reported that delay in surgical repair for traumatic aortic injury beyond 16 h was not associated with an increased risk of mortality [25].

Since there is a potential risk of paralysis associated with the repair of the thoracic aorta, some have advocated the placement of spinal drains prior to intervention. The use of spinal drainage for the management of spinal cord ischemia during TEVAR for aneurysmal disease has been routine; however, no data exist on the prophylactic use for traumatic injuries. Spinal cord ischemia following TEVAR occurs in only 3 % of patients due to the limited coverage of the thoracic aorta [28]. Because of the low risk of ischemia and the risk of epidural hematoma during placement in coagulopathic trauma patients, the Society for Vascular Surgery in their most recent consensus guidelines has recommended against the routine placement of spinal drains and stated that they should only be placed if symptoms of spinal cord ischemia develop [27].

There are multiple thoracic endovascular grafts currently available for the use in the treatment of aneurysmal disease of the thoracic aorta. Only the Gore TAG device (W.L. Gore and Associates, Flagstaff, AZ) has FDA approval for use in the treatment of aortic transection in patients with traumatic aortic injuries. Despite not having FDA approval, the other devices have been used to treat these injuries in an off label manner with equal success.

TEVAR can be performed under local or general anesthesia in the endovascular suite or an operating room with access to proper imaging equipment. Unless contraindications exist, general anesthesia is preferred in order to better control the patient's respirations during digital subtraction angiography acquisition and graft deployment. Depending on surgeon preference, the procedure is performed by obtaining bilateral or single femoral artery access. If bilateral access is obtained, one side is accessed percutaneously to advance a marking catheter which is used to obtain imaging as well as to guide graft positioning. The other access site, which is achieved either open or percutaneously, is used to advance

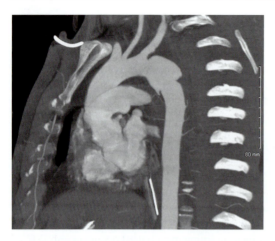

Fig. 7.5 CT reconstruction of a grade III aortic injury in a patient following a fall from a third story building

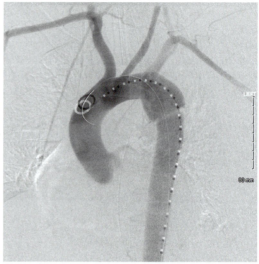

Fig. 7.6 Diagnostic aortogram demonstrating grade III pseudoaneurysm associated with BAI

and deploy the endograft. If single femoral access is used, both the marking catheter and device are advanced through the same sheath using a buddy wire technique. The selection of femoral access is not only determined by physician preference but is also based on the femoral and iliac anatomy. Preoperative CT can aid in planning as to which femoral/iliac artery is better suited for the large sheath needed to deliver the endovascular device (Fig. 7.5). Patients with severe bilateral iliac occlusive disease may require a surgical conduit to be sewn onto the iliac artery or abdominal aorta proximal to the occlusion in order to advance and deploy the graft.

Once access has been obtained, an arch angiogram is performed. This is done to not only to identify the area of injury but also to identify the origin of the great vessels and to appropriately size the graft (Fig. 7.6). With the currently available endografts, aortic sizes ranging from 18 to 42 mm can be treated. It is currently recommended that the implanted device be oversized by approximately 10 % for the treatment of BAI in order to ensure adequate graft apposition to the aortic wall and to prevent graft migration [29].

Following graft selection, the patient is systemically anticoagulated with heparin. Due to the often associated injuries acquired from the accident, full-dose anticoagulation is often contraindicated. In these situations it is recommended to anticoagulate with a reduced heparin

dose. In the event that there is no contraindication to anticoagulation, full-dose heparin (80–100 units/kg) should be given intravenously. The device is then advanced over a stiff wire to the desired position. It is our practice to repeat an angiogram prior to deployment of the endograft in order to confirm correct positioning (Fig. 7.7). Once in the appropriate position, the graft is deployed under fluoroscopic guidance. Some surgeons advocate the use of decreasing the mean blood pressure pharmacologically during graft deployment to maximize the precision of deployment. A completion angiogram is then performed to confirm graft placement, to assure there is good apposition between the graft and the aortic wall, and to confirm that there is no endoleak present (Fig. 7.8). Post deployment balloon angioplasty is not routinely performed unless there is incomplete graft apposition at the proximal landing zone or there is a type I endoleak present.

The majority of the aortic injuries occur within the first few centimeters distal to the origin of the LSA. In 30 % of TEVAR cases the LSA is covered in order to achieve a proximal seal [28]. This can be done safely with few adverse events except in individuals with documented stenosis or occlusion of the right vertebral artery or those who have previously undergone coronary bypass

Fig. 7.7 Repeat aortogram identifying the origin of the great vessels prior to endograft deployment

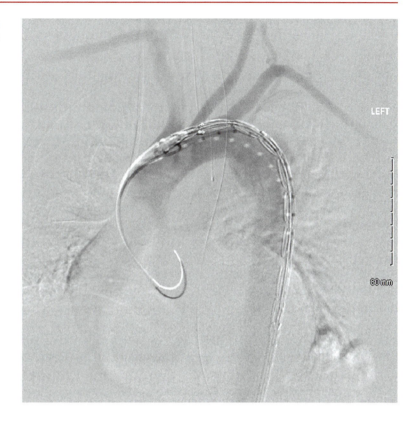

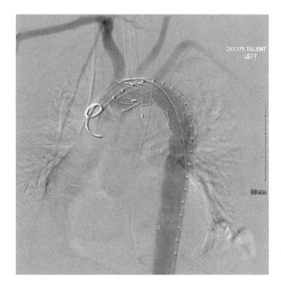

Fig. 7.8 Completion angiogram demonstrating successful exclusion of pseudoaneurysm. In order to obtain a seal, the origin of the left subclavian artery (LSA) was covered. The LSA is visualized due to retrograde flow

grafting using the left internal mammary artery. In these situations revascularization of the left subclavian artery should be performed with a carotid-subclavian bypass prior to implantation of the endograft. All other patients should be selectively revascularized if they develop vertebrobasilar insufficiency or symptomatic left upper extremity arterial insufficiency.

Patients who sustain BAI require routine long-term follow-up imaging to either ensure that their aortic defect has resolved (i.e., grade I injuries) or to monitor their endovascular repair and assure that the endograft does not migrate or collapse. Although there are no published follow-up guidelines, patients with grade I injuries identified on initial imaging have a repeat CTA at 7 days, 30 days, 6 months, 1 year, and every other year thereafter, until there is resolution of their injury [29]. In patients with grade II–IV injuries, who received a TEVAR, follow-up imaging is done at 1, 6, and 12 months and then yearly for the first 5 years [29]. After this follow-up schedule is relaxed and extended to every 2–3 years with noncontrast CT scans. This is done in attempt to limit the cumulative radiation exposure, given the often young age of this patient population.

7.3.3 Abdominal and Pelvic Vascular Trauma

Abdominal vascular injuries may be the result of either trauma that occurs outside the hospital or iatrogenic trauma. Iatrogenic trauma can occur during vascular access procedures (i.e., inappropriately high puncture for femoral artery/vein cannulation resulting in external iliac injury) or during operations for other conditions. Numerous publications have documented the utility of endovascular management of injuries sustained in the course of operations on the lumbar spine, where large vascular structures need to be mobilized to facilitate spine exposure [30–33]. Injuries can occur to the abdominal aorta, inferior vena cava, iliac arteries, and/or iliac veins. The high likelihood of legal action from patients with these complications managed with open reconstruction makes the use of endovascular techniques particularly inviting [30]. Injuries to these large vessels can be managed by deployment of covered endografts and can be applied to venous and arterial injuries [31–33]. These techniques involve access of either the ipsilateral or contralateral common femoral artery, placement of a wire across the lesion, and deployment of a covered stent with gentle balloon dilation to seal the proximal and distal ends of the stent. Injuries at the aortic or caval bifurcations may require a "kissing" stent technique to prevent a unilateral stent from deploying too high above the bifurcation with occlusion of flow through the contralateral vessel.

Injuries to abdominal and pelvic vessels occurring pre-hospital tend to occur in patients with massive concomitant injuries and present with very high injury severity scores (ISS) [34, 35]. Endovascular management may be life-saving to these patients. However, there are no randomized controlled trials demonstrating differences in outcomes in patients managed with endovascular or open surgery for these injuries.

Patients with injuries to the abdominal aorta and iliac arteries may be well suited to endovascular management with covered endografts. The largest reported series of blunt abdominal aortic injury (BAAI) showed an overall mortality of 32 % associated with this injury, with most

deaths occurring during the initial operation [35]. Endovascular management was used in 21 % of the patients in this series and techniques included use of aortic cuffs, bifurcated endografts, and hybrid procedures with aortic debranching and endograft placement. In this series, the patients undergoing the most complex endovascular interventions all died, consistent with increasing severity of vascular, and other associated, injuries [35].

Increasing complexity of injury may be associated with a higher rate of technical failure when endovascular techniques are employed. A review of 16 patients from 2004 to 2006 at a single institution revealed a technical success rate of 75 % for endovascular management of retroperitoneal vascular trauma which included internal iliac artery injuries, renal artery injuries, and abdominal aortic injuries [34]. Embolization was used as therapy for the majority of patients, consistent with most of the injuries being related to internal iliac artery branches. In a review of blunt abdominal aortic injuries, de Mestral found that 69 % of 436 patients survived to hospital discharge with non-operative therapy, consistent with reports of similar management of patients with blunt thoracic aortic injury as discussed previously [36]. Additionally, patients in this series had a higher mortality rate with associated injuries to the lumbar spine, small bowel, colon, liver, pancreas, and kidney. While endovascular management is particularly attractive for patients with severe multisystem trauma, the risk of these procedures may not justify an aggressive early management approach in individuals that may have other overriding management priorities.

Figure 7.9 shows the initial CT scan of a patient admitted after a car crash with multiple severe injuries. False aneurysm of the abdominal aorta was identified, and after stabilization he was taken to the hybrid endovascular suite for exclusion which was accomplished with two Gore Excluder (W.L. Gore, Flagstaff, AZ) proximal aortic cuffs via a small left groin cutdown (Fig. 7.10). The patient subsequently sustained a stroke due to an initially undiagnosed bilateral blunt internal carotid dissection. He is now well 3 years after his injury and living independently at home, with surveillance CT scans showing

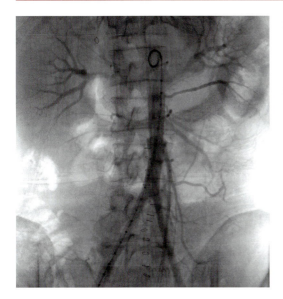

Fig. 7.9 Blunt abdominal aortic injury with pseudoaneurysm

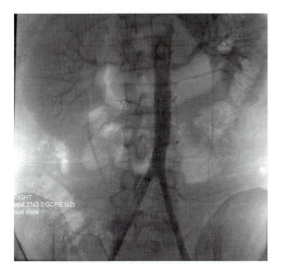

Fig. 7.10 Successfully excluded pseudoaneurysm

resolution of the false aneurysm and no evidence of stent migration or endoleak.

7.3.4 Peripheral Arterial Trauma

Injuries to extremity vessels are often well suited to endovascular repair. This management style remains controversial as these injuries are also ideally suited for open surgical repair. Numerous recent case studies and case series have been published regarding the endovascular management of peripheral arterial trauma, for both upper and lower extremity injuries [37–46]. No prospective randomized trials comparing open and endovascular surgery for these injuries have to date been reported. These injuries may be either acquired from trauma in the pre-hospital setting or may be iatrogenic due to attempts at vascular access.

In the setting of iatrogenic vascular injury, endovascular management principles depend on the location of the injury and whether there is still access to the injured vessel at the time of diagnosis. When a vessel is inadvertently catheterized during attempts at central access, several methods of management are available. Percutaneous vascular closure devices can be utilized if the size of the access catheter does not exceed the instructions for use (IFU) for the device. Examples include the suture-mediated, passive or active gel-based or anchor-based closure devices. These devices all have unique deployment mechanisms and vascular and trauma surgeons performing endovascular procedures for traumatic injuries should have mastery knowledge of each device. These devices can be used to repair injuries to the subclavian artery, femoral artery, and in selected cases of carotid artery puncture when open surgical repair is deemed to be too hazardous to consider for an individual patients. Our group has likewise utilized this approach in the case of a central line placed into the arch of the thoracic aorta of a frail elderly patient, with excellent results. These devices all have a learning curve for both selection and reference vessel use and should not be used in the emergency setting without extensive prior experience.

In cases of iatrogenic trauma where access has been lost, or cases of blunt or penetrating trauma to peripheral vessels, the decision to employ endovascular techniques as opposed to open surgery can be difficult. Endovascular management is very attractive in patients where access to vessels is difficult or time consuming (i.e., subclavian and proximal axillary artery, proximal common carotid artery, retrogeniculate popliteal artery). As with any method of endovascular treatment, the only absolute contraindication to proceeding with repair is inability to cross the injury with a wire. Technical success has been excellent in these maneuvers. Trellopoulos reported 18 cases of arterial injuries treated endovascularly with a 100 % technical success rate [44]. All patients were in shock at the time of treatment, and the mortality rate was 17 %. While selection does remain an issue, the most recent review of the NTBD by Worni showed that 5.9 % of 8,977 patients underwent endovascular repair of their peripheral (upper and lower extremity) arterial injuries [47]. The patients undergoing endovascular therapy had more severe associated injuries, more preexisting comorbid conditions, and were more likely to be in shock, and despite this, patients undergoing endovascular repair had fewer complications and a shorter hospital stay [47]. While this review suffers from the typical drawbacks of retrospective studies involving administrative databases, it nonetheless highlights the fact that endovascular repair is becoming more frequent and more accepted as an alternative to open surgery in certain injured patients.

Vascular access is an important issue when dealing with these injuries. While transfemoral access is the traditional method of access for most endovascular procedures, arm access is an excellent alternative in patients with central upper extremity arterial injuries. Access to the upper extremity arteries may be obtained either percutaneously (radial or brachial approach) or with a cutdown and direct repair of the arteriotomy. No published studies exist regarding the use of radial artery access for vascular trauma, though the radial artery is a frequent access site for percutaneous coronary intervention (PCI). The size of the required access sheath is a very important consideration – very large sheaths for covered endografts may mandate open exposure and direct repair when brachial access is considered and may make radial access impossible. In experienced hands, sheath sizes up to 28 F may be accommodated by the common femoral artery with percutaneous closure (often by partially deploying closure devices prior to sheath access, known as the "preclose" technique); however, contralateral lower extremity access using a sheath larger than 9–10 F directed over the aortic bifurcation can be extremely challenging,

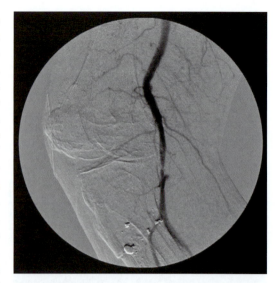

Fig. 7.11 Gunshot wound to the retrogeniculate popliteal artery

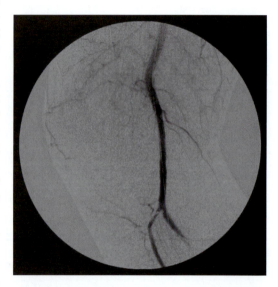

Fig. 7.12 Successful exclusion of popliteal injury with covered stent graft

requiring antegrade access for endovascular treatment of lower extremity injuries.

Figure 7.11 shows the popliteal artery injury of a 72-year-old male which was accidentally self-inflicted. His foot was pulseless on arrival and there was active hemorrhage from behind the knee. The injury was successfully repaired with a covered stent from an ipsilateral superficial femoral artery cutdown (Fig. 7.12). Postoperatively pulses were restored and he was discharged home

Fig. 7.13 Ruptured subclavian artery after clavicular fracture (*arrow* shows free extravasation)

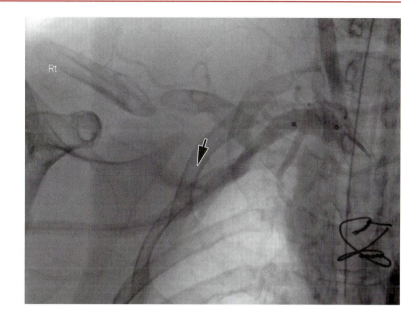

Fig. 7.14 Successful exclusion of subclavian injury with covered stent, delivered from ipsilateral brachial artery approach

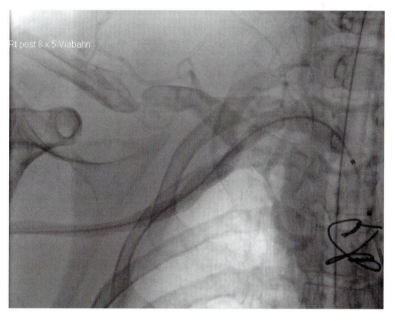

on postoperative day #3. Figure 7.13 shows a subclavian artery rupture from a clavicular fracture with active extravasation. The patient was hypotensive and obtunded on arrival, was morbidly obese, and had undergone renal transplantation several years prior to this incident. Figure 7.14 shows exclusion of the injury from an ipsilateral brachial artery cutdown with delivery of a covered stent. The patient was discharged home on postoperative day #3 with normal pulses and no wound complications.

Conclusion

The management of vascular trauma is undergoing an evolution toward endovascular techniques of management, particularly for blunt arterial injuries. These techniques are generally well tolerated, and safety depends on multiple factors including patient stability, associated injuries, vascular access requirements, and experience of the operating surgeon. Endovascular management may be used as a bridge to surgical therapy in critically ill, unstable patients as procedure times may be faster. Vascular surgeons play an important role in this process, as they have a unique understanding of every aspect of both endovascular therapy and open surgical management of vascular trauma. Quality imaging equipment, readily available supplies, and experienced support staff are crucial to technical success in these interventions. Long-term follow-up is required as with any vascular procedure, and the natural history of these interventions in young patients has yet to be defined.

References

1. Avery LE, Stahlfeld KR, Corcos AC, et al. Evolving role of endovascular techniques for traumatic vascular injury: a changing landscape? J Trauma. 2012;72:41–7.
2. Burkhardt GE, Rasmussen TE, Propper BW, et al. A national survey of evolving management patterns for vascular injury. J Surg Educ. 2009;66:239–47.
3. Kalish J. Selective use of endovascular techniques in the management of trauma. Semin Vasc Surg. 2011;23:243–8.
4. Rossi PJ, Edmiston Jr CE. Patient safety in the critical care environment. Surg Clin North Am. 2012;92:1369–86.
5. Ketteler ER, Brown KR. Radiation exposure in endovascular procedures. J Vasc Surg. 2011;53:35s–8.
6. Higadisha RT, Halbach VV, Tsai FY, et al. Interventional neurovascular treatment of traumatic carotid and vertebral artery lesions: results in 234 cases. AJR Am J Roentgenol. 1989;153:577–82.
7. Herrera DA, Vargas SA, Dublin AB. Endovascular treatment of penetrating traumatic injuries of the extracranial carotid artery. J Vasc Interv Radiol. 2011;22:28–33.
8. Faure E, Canaud L, Marty-Ane C, Alric P. Endovascular repair of a left common carotid pseudoaneurysm associated with a jugular-carotid fistula after gunshot wound to the neck. Ann Vasc Surg. 2012;26:1129e13–6.
9. Pulli R, Dorigo W, Alessi Innocenti A, et al. A 20-year experience with surgical management of true and false internal carotid artery aneurysms. Eur J Vasc Endovasc Surg. 2013;45(1):1–6. doi: 10.1016/j.ejvs.2012.10.011. Epub 2012 Nov 11.
10. Leopoldo M, Sarac TP. Hybrid stent-graft repair of an iatrogenic complex proximal right common carotid artery injury. Ann Vasc Surg. 2012;26:574e1–7.
11. Cohen JE, Gomori JM, Itshayek E, et al. Single-center experience on endovascular reconstruction of traumatic internal carotid artery dissections. J Trauma. 2012;72:216–21.
12. Nagy K, Fabian T, Rodman G, et al. Guidelines for the diagnosis and management of blunt aortic injury: an EAST Practice Management Guidelines Work Group. J Trauma. 2000;48:1128–43.
13. Starnes B. Treating blunt aortic injuries with endografts: pros and cons of a meta-analysis. Semin Vasc Surg. 2010;23:176–81.
14. Fabian TC, Richardson JD, Croce MA, et al. Prospective study of blunt aortic injury: multicenter trial of the American Association for the Surgery of Trauma. J Trauma. 1997;42:42374–83.
15. Jameison WR, Janusz MT, Gudas VM, et al. Traumatic rupture of the thoracic aorta: third decade of experience. Am J Surg. 2002;183:571–5.
16. Azizzadeh A, Keyhani K, Miller III CC, et al. Blunt traumatic aortic injury: initial experience with endovascular repair. J Vasc Surg. 2009;49:1403–8.
17. Cowley RA, Turney SZ, Hankins JR, et al. Rupture of thoracic aorta caused by blunt trauma. A 15-year experience. J Thorac Cardiovasc Surg. 1990;100:652–60.
18. Ott MC, Stewart TC, Lawlor DK, et al. Management of blunt thoracic aortic injuries: endovascular stents versus open repair. J Trauma. 2004;56:565–70.
19. Semba CP, Kato N, Kee ST, et al. Acute rupture of the descending thoracic aorta: repair with use of endovascular stent-grafts. J Vasc Interv Radiol. 1997;8:337–42.
20. Riesenman PJ, Brooks JD, Farber MA. Acute blunt traumatic injury to the descending thoracic aorta. J Vasc Surg. 2012;56:1274–80.
21. Rousseau H, Dambrin C, Marcheix B, et al. Acute traumatic aortic rupture: a comparison of surgical and stent-graft repair. J Thorac Cardiovasc Surg. 2005;129:1050–5.
22. Tang GL, Tehrani HY, Usman A, et al. Reduced mortality, paraplegia, and stroke with stent graft repair of blunt aortic transections: a modern meta-analysis. J Vasc Surg. 2008;47:671–5.
23. Akins CW, Buckley MJ, Daggett W, et al. Acute traumatic disruption of the thoracic aorta: a ten-year experience. Ann Thorac Surg. 1981;31:305–9.
24. Pate JW, Fabian TC, Walker W. Traumatic rupture of the aortic isthmus: an emergency? World J Surg. 1995;19:119–25.
25. Hemmila MR, Arbabi S, Rowe SA, et al. Delayed repair for blunt thoracic aortic injury: is it really equivalent to early repair? J Trauma. 2004;56:13–23.
26. Malhotra AK, Fabian TC, Croce MA, et al. Minimal aortic injury: a lesion associated with advancing diagnostic techniques. J Trauma. 2001;51:1042–8.
27. Lee WA, Matsumura JS, Mitchell RS, et al. Endovascular repair of traumatic thoracic aortic injury: clinical practice guidelines of the Society of Vascular Surgery. J Vasc Surg. 2011;53:187–92.
28. Murad MH, Rizvi AZ, Malgor R, et al. Comparative effectiveness of the treatments for aortic transection: a systematic review and meta-analysis. J Vasc Surg. 2011;53:193–9.

29. Farber MA, Mendes RR. Endovascular repair of blunt thoracic aortic injury: techniques and tips. J Vasc Surg. 2009;50:683–6.

30. Hans SS, Shepard AD, Reddy P, et al. Iatrogenic arterial injuries of spine and orthopedic operations. J Vasc Surg. 2011;53:407–13.

31. Zahradnik V, Kashyap VS. Alternative management of iliac vein injury during anterior lumbar spine exposure. Ann Vasc Surg. 2012;26:277e15–8.

32. Canaud L, Hireche K, Joyeux F, et al. Endovascular repair of aorto-iliac artery injuries after lumbar-spine surgery. Eur J Vasc Endovasc Surg. 2011;42:167–71.

33. Jin SC, Park SW, Cho DS. Management of proximal iliac artery injury during lumbar discectomy with stent graft. J Korean Neurosurg Soc. 2012;51:227–9.

34. Boufi M, Bordon S, Dona B, et al. Unstable patients with retroperitoneal vascular trauma: an endovascular approach. Ann Vasc Surg. 2011;25:352–8.

35. Shalhub S, Starnes BW, Tran NT, et al. Blunt abdominal aortic injury. J Vasc Surg. 2012;55:1277–86.

36. de Mestral C, Dueck AD, Gomez D, et al. Associated injuries, management, and outcomes of blunt abdominal aortic injury. J Vasc Surg. 2012;56:656–60.

37. Valentin MD, Tulsyan N, James K. Endovascular management of traumatic axillary artery dissection: a case report and review of the literature. Vasc Endovascular Surg. 2004;38:473–5.

38. Shalhub S, Starnes BW, Hatsukami TS, et al. Repair of blunt thoracic outlet arterial injuries: an evolution from open to endovascular approach. J Trauma. 2011;71:E114–21.

39. Franz RW, Skytta CK, Shah KJ, et al. A five-year review of management of upper-extremity arterial injuries at an urban level I trauma center. Ann Vasc Surg. 2012;26:655–64.

40. Piffaretti G, Tozzi M, Lomazzi C, et al. Endovascular treatment for traumatic injuries of the peripheral arteries following blunt trauma. Injury. 2007;38:1091–7.

41. Maleux G, Herten P, Vaninbroukx J, et al. Value of percutaneous embolotherapy for the management of traumatic vascular limb injury. Acta Radiol. 2012;53:147–52.

42. Franz RW, Shah KJ, Halaharvi D, et al. A 5-year review of management of lower extremity arterial injuries at an urban level I trauma center. J Vasc Surg. 2011;53:1604–10.

43. Xiong J, Liu M, Liu X, et al. A retrospective study on endovascular management of iatrogenic vascular injuries. Vascular. 2012;20:65–71.

44. Trellopoulos G, Georgiadis GS, Aslanidou EA, et al. Endovascular management of peripheral arterial trauma in patients presenting in hemorrhagic shock. J Cardiovasc Surg. 2012;53:495–506.

45. Leong BDK, Naresh G, Hanif H, et al. Endovascular management of axillosubclavian artery injuries: report of three cases. Surg Today. 2012. doi:10.1007/s00595-012-0330-6.

46. de Troia A, Tecchio T, Azzarone M, et al. Endovascular treatment of an innominate artery iatrogenic pseudoaneurysm following subclavian vein catheterization. Vasc Endovascular Surg. 2011;45:78–82.

47. Worni M, Scarborough JE, Gandhi M, et al. Use of endovascular therapy for peripheral arterial lesions: an analysis of the National Trauma Data Bank from 2007 to 2009. Ann Vasc Surg. 2013;27(3):299–305. doi: 10.1016/j.avsg.2012.04.007. Epub 2012 Sep 9.

Part II

Cerebrovascular and Upper Extremity

Walter Biffl, Ruth L. Bush, Sapan S. Desai,
and Justin L. Regner

Carotid and Vertebral Injuries

8

Jeremy S. Juern and Karen J. Brasel

Contents

J.S. Juern, MD
Department of Trauma and Critical Care,
Medical College of Wisconsin, Milwaukee, WI, USA

K.J. Brasel, MD, MPH (✉)
Division of Trauma and Critical Care,
Department of Surgery, Medical College of Wisconsin,
Milwaukee, WI, USA
e-mail: kbrasel@mcw.edu

8.1   Introduction

Presentation of carotid and vertebral artery trauma ranges from an obvious exsanguinating penetrating injury to an asymptomatic small intimal tear from blunt trauma. The former is clearly dealt with in the operating room. Management of the latter can be uncertain and controversial. This chapter will discuss both penetrating and blunt carotid and vertebral artery trauma.

8.2   Anatomy

Proper management of carotid and vertebral artery trauma begins with an appreciation of key anatomic landmarks. The course of the carotid artery occurs through the anterior cervical triangle of the neck, while that of the vertebral artery is through the transverse foramina of the cervical vertebrae before entering the vertebral canal in a course that is largely parallel to that of the carotid artery. The anterior cervical triangle of the neck is bounded by the sternocleidomastoid muscle, inferior border of the mandible, and anterior midline of the neck. The anterior cervical triangle can be further subdivided into four additional triangles, of which the carotid triangle is the most important. The carotid triangle is bounded by the sternocleidomastoid muscle, superior belly of the omohyoid muscle, and posterior belly of the digastric muscle. Within this triangle is the bifurcation of the common carotid artery into the external and internal carotid

A. Dua et al. (eds.), *Clinical Review of Vascular Trauma*,
DOI 10.1007/978-3-642-39100-2_8, © Springer-Verlag Berlin Heidelberg 2014

Fig. 8.1 The major vessels of the head and neck. The arch of the aorta gives rise to the innominate, left common carotid, and left subclavian arteries. The innominate bifurcates to form the right common carotid and right subclavian arteries. The common carotid artery bifurcates to form the left internal carotid and left external carotid

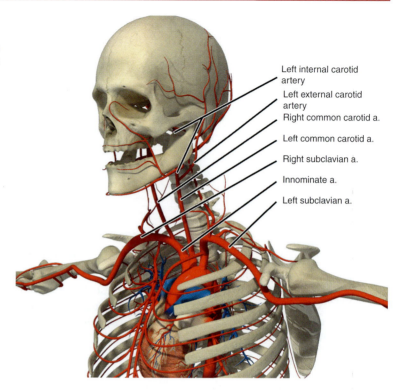

Left internal carotid artery

Left external carotid artery

Right common carotid a.

Left common carotid a.

Right subclavian a.

Innominate a.

Left subclavian a.

arteries, internal jugular vein, vagus nerve, and hypoglossal nerve.

The arch of the aorta gives rise to the innominate artery, left common carotid artery, and left subclavian artery (Fig. 8.1). The innominate artery bifurcates into the right common carotid artery and right subclavian artery. The left common carotid artery travels near the recurrent laryngeal nerve and thoracic duct before entering the carotid triangle. The common carotid arteries are enclosed by the carotid sheath, which also includes the internal jugular vein and vagus nerve. The common carotid artery bifurcates into the external and internal carotid arteries.

The external carotid artery is located medial and anterior to the internal carotid artery and terminates as the maxillary artery and superficial temporary artery. Additional branches include the superior thyroid artery, facial artery, occipital artery, and posterior auricular artery. Located posterior to the external carotid artery is the glossopharyngeal nerve [1]. The external carotid artery is the primary blood supply to the face,

but due to the presence of extensive collaterals from the contralateral side, ligation of the external carotid artery can often be completed with impunity.

The internal carotid artery can be divided into seven distinct segments according to the Bouthillier classification: the cervical, petrous, lacerum, cavernous, clinoid, supraclinoid, and terminal segments [2]. At the bifurcation of the common carotid artery is the carotid bulb, which contains the carotid sinus and carotid body. The carotid sinus contains chemoreceptors that detect carbon dioxide and acidosis. The carotid body contains mechanoreceptors and baroreceptors that lead to bradycardia and vasodilation when stimulated. The internal carotid artery is the primary blood supply to the brain; ligation of the internal carotid artery can lead to stroke in up to 40 % of patients due to an incomplete circle of Willis [1].

The vertebral artery is the first branch of the subclavian artery and provides circulation to the posterior brain and collateral flow via the circle of Willis. The vertebral artery initially travels anterior to the transverse process of C7 (segment V1) and then within the transverse foramina until it reaches C1 (segment V2). It then travels posterior to the arch of the atlas (segment V3), enters the vertebral canal (segment V4) then passes through the foramen magnum where the vertebral arteries combine to form the basilar artery. In rare circumstances, the vertebral artery may terminate directly into the posterior inferior cerebellar artery, a condition known as PICA syndrome. Ligation of the vertebral artery in this case may lead to infarction of the posterior inferior cerebellum [1].

8.3 Penetrating Injuries to the Vascular Structures of the Neck

It is impossible to talk about penetrating vascular trauma of the neck region without discussing also the evaluation and management of aerodigestive injuries. Therefore, these injuries will also be mentioned in this focus on penetrating vascular trauma.

8.3.1 Evaluation

All patients with penetrating trauma to the neck must be treated initially according to the principles of Advanced Trauma Life Support (ATLS):

- **A**irway: The airway must be patent and the patient must be able to control it. If not, the patient will require oral endotracheal intubation; depending on the injury, cricothyroidotomy may be necessary, or if the trachea has been severed, a tube can be inserted into it. The threshold for airway control must be lower in the setting of neck trauma, as progressive soft tissue swelling or expanding hematoma may compromise the patency of the airway.
- **B**reathing: Injuries to the neck can also cause injury to the pleura; therefore, pneumothorax must be ruled out by physical exam and chest x-ray if needed.
- **C**irculation: Take note of pulses, but especially with penetrating neck injuries, stop the bleeding by applying direct pressure to the area.
- **D**isability: Assess the ability to move all four extremities and Glasgow Coma Score (GCS). It is crucial to know if a patient already demonstrates signs or symptoms of ischemic neurologic deficit.

After this primary survey is completed, the secondary survey is performed, noting which zone of the neck the injury is located. A laceration must traverse the platysma muscle to be classified as a true penetrating injury. If the injury does not traverse the platysma, it is considered a superficial injury and no further evaluation needs to be done. Penetrating injuries to the anterior neck between the sternocleidomastoid muscles are more likely to cause significant vascular or aerodigestive injury as compared to the side and posterior portions of the neck. The anterior neck between the sternocleidomastoid muscles is divided into three zones. Beginning caudad, zone 1 is from the sternal notch and clavicles to the cricoid cartilage (Fig. 8.2). Zone 2 is from the cricoid cartilage to the angle of the mandible. Important structures at risk in both zones 1 and 2 are the trachea, esophagus, and carotid and vertebral arteries. Zone 3 is from the angle of the mandible to the base of the skull. Important structures at risk in zone 3 are the carotid and vertebral arteries.

8.3.2 History and Exam

Important subjective findings of penetrating neck trauma are pain, dysphagia, and change in voice. Objective findings specific for vascular injury are active hemorrhage, hematoma, and presence of a bruit. Objective findings specific for a trachea or esophagus injury are crepitus, air coming from the wound, and subcutaneous emphysema. These findings are traditionally characterized as "soft" or "hard" signs of injury. Hard signs include active bleeding or shock from blood loss, expanding or pulsatile hematoma, air bubbling through the injury site, hemoptysis, and/or extensive subcutaneous emphysema. Hard signs indicate a surgical emergency and thus mandate immediate operation.

Fig. 8.2 The three zones of the neck. Zone I is located below the cricoid cartilage. Zone II is located between the cricoid cartilage and the angle of the mandible. Zone III is located above the angle of the mandible. Injury to zone I occurs in about 18 % of patients with neck trauma, zone II injuries occur in 47 %, and zone III injuries occur in 19 %

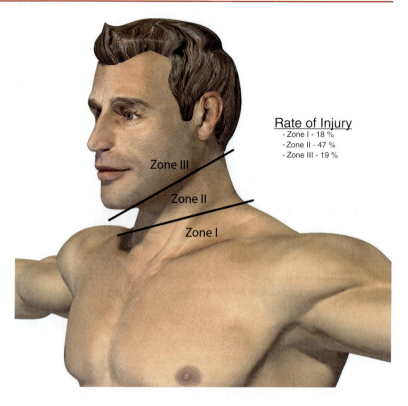

Soft signs include dysphagia, voice change, venous oozing, and nonexpanding or nonpulsatile hematoma. Soft signs may be safely observed, at least for a short time to allow for further evaluation with imaging and procedures.

8.3.3 Initial Imaging

Initial imaging may or may not be indicated. A chest x-ray may be performed to look for a pneumothorax or other injury. Plain films of the neck are rarely done and will only be useful if a fracture of the cervical spine is suspected. Patients with "hard" signs for neck injury will require an immediate chest x-ray to evaluate for thoracic trauma and assist with operative planning and treatment. Plain films of the neck are rarely performed but are useful to rule out a fracture of the cervical spine and assist with cervical collar removal to facilitate positioning and neck exploration. Penetrating injury with "soft" signs for cervical injury will best be evaluated by computed tomography angiography (CTA) of the neck.

8.3.4 Management

Any patient with penetrating neck trauma to any zone with hard signs of vascular injury should go immediately to the operating room for neck exploration. Hard signs by definition indicate an injury that requires surgical repair. However, there is a possible exception to this. If a patient has a penetrating injury to zones 1 and 3 and if the patient is not in shock, a CTA of the neck and upper chest may show a "road map" of injury to better plan the operative approach.

Patients with soft signs or no signs at all can be managed in a few different ways. A traditional algorithm called for all zone 2 injuries to be explored in the operating room. This approach is based partially on the fact that injuries in zone 2 are amenable to straightforward, though not mandatory exploration, unlike zones 1 and 3 which are not as easily explored. In this algorithm, zone 1 injuries are evaluated by CTA to evaluate for a great vessel injury in the chest or in the carotid arteries in the neck, followed by whatever combination of esophagoscopy, bronchoscopy, and esophagram is necessary to evaluate for an aerodigestive injury. Finally, zone 3 injuries are worked up by CTA to evaluate the vasculature; there is no need to evaluate the aerodigestive structures here because it is only the oropharynx there and it is not under any pressure because it is superior to the cricopharyngeus.

Tracheal injury can be evaluated by physical exam or bronchoscopy. Esophageal injury can be evaluated by barium esophagram and/or esophagoscopy. Recent literature highlights the accuracy of either study alone—i.e., endoscopy for intubated patients and esophagography for awake patients [3]. Arterial vascular injury is best evaluated by CTA, preferably a minimum of 64 slices. CTA has also been used to evaluate for aerodigestive injuries. One prospective study found that CTA was 100 % sensitive and 97.5 % specific for detecting clinically significant aerodigestive or vascular injuries [4].

8.3.5 Management of Specific Penetrating Vascular Injuries

8.3.5.1 Venous
At neck exploration, bleeding from the external or internal jugular veins is common and these vessels may be ligated with impunity. If the internal jugular vein has a minor injury, then consider repair via lateral venorrhaphy with 5-0 or 6-0 Prolene. If both jugular veins are injured, consider repairing one of the injured vessels not associated with a carotid artery repair suture line.

8.3.5.2 Carotid Artery Injuries
Injuries to the carotid artery are subdivided into the common carotid, external carotid, and internal carotid artery. In general, injuries to the carotid artery can be dealt with using ligation, primary repair, patch, or interposition grafting. Surgical exposure of the common carotid, external carotid, and internal carotid arteries can be accomplished via a longitudinal incision anterior to the medial border of the sternocleidomastoid muscle after positioning the patient supine with a roll under the shoulder to extend the neck and the head turned away from the site of injury (Fig. 8.3).

The dissection continues through the platysma, then the SCM is retracted laterally. The carotid sheath is identified and incised, with the internal jugular vein retracted laterally. The site of injury of the carotid artery should be identified and proximal and distal control established. Clamping of the vessels should proceed first with the internal carotid artery, followed by the common carotid and external carotid arteries to avoid dislodging plaque into the brain. If the patient's other injuries permit, therapeutic heparin should be administered prior to clamping these vessels.

Injuries involving the internal carotid artery may require extensive dissection into the superior portion of the neck. Better visualization can be achieved by dividing the posterior belly of the digastric and nasotracheal intubation to permit subluxation of the mandible. One of several cerebral protective adjuncts should be utilized whenever blood flow through the internal carotid artery is impeded to identify cerebral ischemia; otherwise, the mandatory use of shunting should be considered. Patients with a back pressure less than 40 mmHg, electroencephalogram changes, changes in neurologic status during awake surgery, or changes in cerebral oximetry are candidates for shunt placement. Extensive exposure of the external carotid artery is rarely necessary, as this vessel can simply be ligated at its takeoff from the common carotid artery in cases where extensive bleeding is present. In cases involving extensive bleeding from the carotid vessels, the use of a temporary occlusive balloon can achieve hemostasis while a more through exposure is completed. Endovascular stent placement across lesions of the common carotid and/or internal carotid arteries can also be completed in selected patients, although long-term results in trauma patients are not available. Exposure of the internal and external jugular veins can also be accomplished in a similar manner.

Trauma to the V1 segment of the vertebral artery may best be treated with ligation of the vertebral artery. A transverse supraclavicular incision at the base of the neck can be made to expose the subclavian artery. The dissection is carried to the subclavian artery by separating the two heads of the sternocleidomastoid muscle,

Fig. 8.3 Incision for neck exploration. A longitudinal incision turned posterior under the ear is made medially along the anterior border of the sternocleidomastoid

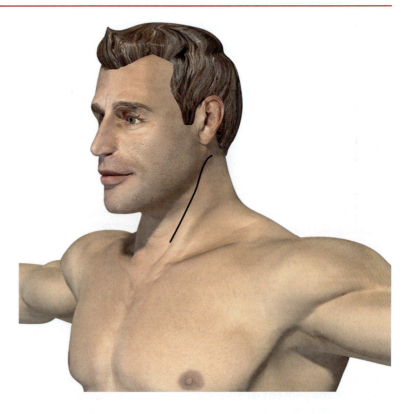

dividing the omohyoid muscle, and identifying the scalenus anticus. The vertebral artery will travel in conjunction with its vertebral vein at this location, and the vessel may be ligated after confirming a satisfactory collateral supply from the contralateral vertebral artery and ruling out PICA syndrome via cerebral arteriography.

Trauma to the V2 segment of the vertebral artery is difficult to repair and often involves ligation of the vessel at the base of the neck. Trauma to the V3 segment can be investigated by completing an incision similar to that of a carotid exposure, with the superior extent being just inferior to the earlobe. The digastric muscle and the proximal portion of the levator scapulae are divided to expose the transverse process of C1, at which point the V3 portion of the vertebral artery can be identified. Trauma to the V4 portion of the vertebral artery is typically self-limiting due to its course within the bony portion of the skull.

Common Carotid Artery (CCA)

Proximal and distal control can be gained on the common carotid artery in the neck for zone 2 injuries. Zone I injuries involve the most proximal portion of the common carotid artery and may require a median sternotomy to gain vascular control of its most proximal portion. Control of both the left and right proximal common carotid arteries can be gained by extending the anterior SCM incision to a median sternotomy. The right common carotid originates from the innominate artery (brachiocephalic trunk), which is the first and most anterior vessel off the aortic arch. The left common carotid artery originates directly from the aorta as the arch begins to transverse posteriorly and is just posterior to the brachiocephalic artery. The vagus nerve will descend left lateral along the common carotid artery and is at risk of injury with proximal control. There should be a low risk of significant cerebral ischemia and stroke with clamps only on the CCA because of collateral flow from the contralateral cerebral hemisphere via the external carotid artery and circle of Willis. The area of the injury must be defined and debrided back to normal healthy intima. Options for repair are primary repair, patch angioplasty, or interposition graft. If an interposition graft is needed, reversed saphenous vein graft is the preferred conduit, although

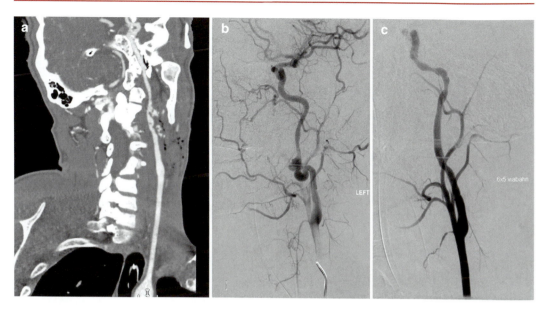

Fig. 8.4 (**a**) CT angiogram reformatted image of a gunshot wound to the left internal carotid artery. (**b**) Angiogram of the same injury showing pseudoaneurysm and extravasation. (**c**) Angiogram after placement of a covered stent

prosthetic use with expanded polytetrafluoroethylene (ePTFE) has been described.

Internal Carotid Artery (ICA)

Attaining proximal and distal control on the internal carotid artery (ICA) increases the risk of stroke, although this will be low in a young trauma patient. Just as for the CCA, repair can be done primarily either with a patch or with an interposition graft. Additionally, similar to the CCA, autogenous conduit with reversed saphenous vein is recommended. Another alternative that may be appropriate for the right situation is transposition of the ECA to the ICA [5].

Intraluminal shunting of the internal carotid artery in trauma is rarely reported. Most trauma patients are young and do not have the extensive atherosclerosis that make shunting so important in elective carotid surgery. However, if back bleeding from the distal internal carotid artery is not vigorous, this may need to be considered.

Zone III ICA injuries can be the most challenging to approach and repair. The ICA enters the skull base to become the middle cerebral artery. Obtaining distal control in zone III as the ICA nears the skull base is difficult in a bloody field. One option is to carefully pass a #3 or #4 balloon embolectomy catheter into the distal ICA

to obtain intraluminal control. Another option is inserting a 5 ml Foley balloon catheter into the external wound and inflating it until hemorrhage ceases. Once distal control is obtained, a decision must be made regarding continued balloon tamponade, operative repair, or endovascular intervention [6]. Continuing balloon tamponade (either intraluminal or external) has the equivalent outcome as ligation of the distal ICA. Therefore, evidence of cerebral ischemia must be assessed by EEG, head CT, or neurologic exam. If cerebral ischemia is present, operative repair or endovascular intervention will be urgently necessary. Operative repair may entail the assistance of a multidisciplinary team of neurosurgery, otolaryngology, and oromaxillofacial surgery. Subluxation or osteotomy of the mandible will be needed to expose this distal ICA [7]. Endovascular techniques are particularly well suited to this area of the body, and using a "hybrid" operating room that allows for both open and endovascular treatment modalities will be advantageous. Alternatively, the availability of fluoroscopy in a standard operating room is satisfactory as well. Endovascular options include placement of a covered stent or coil embolization of the ICA. Figure 8.4 is a case of a gunshot wound to zone III with a distal ICA injury that

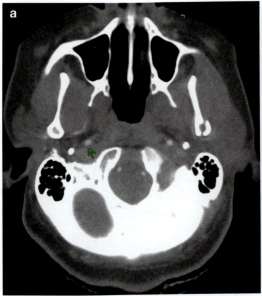
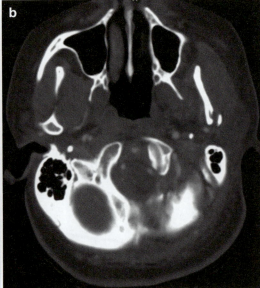

Fig. 8.5 A 27-year-old female in a motorcycle crash with a mandible fracture and C7 transverse process fracture. (**a**) CT angiogram of the neck was obtained showing narrowing of the distal right ICA. She was started on a heparin drip. (**b**) CT angiogram 10 days later showed progression to a grade III injury. The pseudoaneurysm was subsequently embolized

was taken to a "hybrid" room and treated with a covered stent.

For the patient with a penetrating injury to the carotid artery and a neurologic deficit, a decision must be made as to whether to repair the injury and restore flow or ligate the vessel. In general, for patients presenting acutely, repair the injury and restore flow. For patients that present in a delayed fashion with an established stroke on head CT, ligation is appropriate [8]. Revascularization in this situation may convert an ischemic stroke into a hemorrhagic stroke (Fig. 8.5).

External Carotid Artery (ECA)

An isolated external carotid artery injury can be ligated with impunity.

8.3.5.3 Vertebral Artery

An incision along the anterior border of the sternocleidomastoid from sternal notch to mastoid process will allow exposure of the entire length of the vertebral artery. The route utilized to gain access to the vertebral artery depends on the position of the injury whether low or high in the neck [9]. Lower down, the trachea and esophagus are retracted medially to expose the vertebral artery. The vertebral arteries originate from their respective subclavian arteries. The origins are medial and slightly posterior to the thyrocervical trunk. Care must be taken not to injure the thoracic duct on the left side or the phrenic nerves (anterior to the anterior scalene) on either side [9]. If the injury is more distally located on the vertebral artery, the mandible may need to be subluxed or an osteotomy performed of the mandible just as in a distal ICA injury. Once the artery is exposed, sutures may be passed around the vessel for ligation, ideally both proximally and distally. In one series of 43 cases of vertebral artery trauma, 15 % of those treated with proximal vascular control alone had postoperative complications [10]. The transverse foramen may need to be opened to help with exposure. Other open approaches involve placing clips on the vessel proximally and distally, or filling the transverse foramen with bone wax has also been reported. A final approach is packing the neck and using endovascular techniques to embolize the vertebral artery. This is another example where using a "hybrid" operating room will avoid having to transport the patient to a different room or one needs to have access to portable fluoroscopy.

8.4 Vascular Injury from Blunt Trauma

This discussion will focus on the workup and management of injuries to the carotid and vertebral arteries from blunt trauma. The carotid and vertebral arteries will commonly be grouped together as the term "cerebrovascular." All clinicians that treat blunt trauma must keep in the mind that the most feared and devastating complication of a blunt cerebrovascular injury (BCVI) is stroke.

8.4.1 Exam and Screening

Similar to penetrating neck trauma, a careful neurologic exam is crucial to detect deficits. Special note must be made of the patient's level of consciousness as well as motor strength in all four extremities. The challenge of BCVI is screening and detection; one must have a high level of suspicion in blunt traumatic accidents.

A major question is: "Who should be screened" for BCVI? Table 8.1 is a summary of the signs/symptoms and risk factors from the Western Trauma Association (WTA) and the Eastern Association for the Surgery of Trauma (EAST) guidelines [11, 12]. In addition, a recent meta-analysis found that patients with cervical spine and thoracic injuries had significantly greater likelihoods of BCVI [13]. Because of the many screening criteria, there must be an appropriately low threshold for screening for BCVI.

8.4.2 Imaging

CT angiography (minimum of 16 slices) of the neck is the preferred imaging modality. The injuries are graded as 1–5 (Table 8.2). Conventional contrast angiography was used more frequently in the past but has been superseded by CTA because of availability as well as its lower complication profile. Magnetic resonance angiography (MRA) does not have the required sensitivity and specificity necessary to accurate detect BCVI [12]. Duplex ultrasonography (US) is of limited value because of the inability to visualize near the skull

Table 8.1 Screening criteria for BCVI: combination of WTA (Biffl et al. [11]) and EAST (Bromberg et al. [12]) guidelines

Signs/symptoms of BCVI
Arterial hemorrhage
Cervical bruit
Expanding cervical hematoma
Focal neurologic deficit
Stroke
Neurologic deficit that is inconsistent with the head CT
Risk factors for BCVI
High energy mechanism with:
Le Fort II or III facial fractures
Basilar skull fracture with carotid canal involvement
Traumatic brain injury with DAI and GCS <6
Any fracture C1-3, any cervical body or transverse foramen fracture or subluxation
Near hanging with anoxia
Clothesline-type injury or seat belt abrasion with swelling, pain, or altered MS

Table 8.2 Grading of BCVI (Biffl et al. [11])

Grade	Description
I	Luminal irregularity or dissection with <25 % luminal narrowing
II	Dissection or intramural hematoma with ≥25 % luminal narrowing, intraluminal thrombosis, or raised intimal flap
III	Pseudoaneurysm
IV	Occlusion
V	Transection with free extravasation

base where many of these blunt cerebrovascular injuries occur. Neither MRA nor duplex US is recommended as the sole modality for screening for BCVI [12].

8.4.3 Management

The goal of management of BCVI is prevention of vascular thrombosis. The injury disrupts the laminar blood flow and the resulting vascular narrowing and turbulent flow can lead to thrombosis. Anticoagulation is the cornerstone of pharmacotherapy. The choices for antithrombotic therapy are either anticoagulation using heparin/warfarin or antiplatelet agents including aspirin (ASA) 325 mg daily or clopidogrel 75 mg daily. Note that most of these injuries occur near or in the skull base and are therefore surgically inaccessible. However, if a lesion is surgically accessible, consideration can be given to operative repair.

8.4.4 Contraindications to Antithrombotic Therapy

Patients with BCVI frequently have other injuries (i.e., traumatic brain injury, pelvic hematoma) that may prevent the use of antithrombotics in the short term or longer. Factors that must be taken into account when choosing anticoagulation vs. antiplatelet therapy are existence and type of other injuries, time course needed for further operations, and reversibility of the agent chosen. Therefore, heparin infusion may be useful initially because of its short half-life and ability to be reversed. At other times, aspirin by itself may be useful in patients who cannot be anticoagulated with heparin/warfarin.

8.4.4.1 The Case for Antithrombotic Therapy

One review of 114 patients with blunt carotid injuries had 73 patients that received antithrombotic therapy and none developed a stroke. In 41 patients who did not receive antithrombotic therapy of any type, 19 patients (46 %) developed neurologic ischemia [14]. From this data and many other studies, it is clear that antithrombotic therapy is essential to decrease the risk of stroke.

8.4.4.2 The Case for Anticoagulation with Heparin Products

One study of 171 patients with BCVI found no significant difference in healing or progression between heparin/warfarin and antiplatelet therapy. However, the authors felt that heparin may be better at improving the neurologic outcome in patients with ischemic deficits and also may be better at preventing stroke in asymptomatic patients [15].

8.4.4.3 The Case for Antiplatelet Therapy by Itself

There has never been a prospective randomized trial of heparin vs. antiplatelet therapy. Based on the retrospective studies available, antiplatelet therapy is as effective as anticoagulation.

8.4.4.4 The Case for Equivalence

One review of 422 BCVIs showed equivalent injury healing rates and injury progression rates between heparin, aspirin, and aspirin/clopidogrel [16]. Another study of 110 consecutive patients found that antiplatelet therapy and anticoagulation are equally effective [17]. Further research, such as a prospective randomized controlled trial, would help to elucidate the best antithrombotic treatment strategy for BCVI.

8.4.5 Specific Management Recommendations Based on Grade

8.4.5.1 Grades I and II

Antithrombotic therapy is needed. From the data, either heparin/warfarin can be used or aspirin or clopidogrel (not both; nor should heparin/warfarin be used along with aspirin or clopidogrel). To date, no definitive advantage has been shown in asymptomatic patients for one over the other.

The patient should then have the arterial injury reimaged in 7–10 days to see if the grade I or II injury has progressed to a grade III injury or if the lesion has healed. One study of 171 patients showed that 57 % of grade I injuries and 8 % of grade II injuries healed on follow-up imaging, which allowed cessation of pharmacotherapy. Conversely, 8 % of grade I and 43 % of grade II injuries progressed to pseudoaneurysm (grade III) [15]. Figure 8.3 is an example of a grade I injury that progressed to a grade III.

8.4.5.2 Grade III

This is a pseudoaneurysm where not only the intima is disrupted but also the elastic layers of the artery. The resulting disruption is high risk for developing thrombosis and further dissection. These patients should receive antithrombotic therapy to prevent stroke. While endovascular stenting has been promoted to prevent rupture of the pseudoaneurysm, there are no controlled data demonstrating a benefit. Some centers have reported relatively high complication rates, while others have reported good safety results [17].

8.4.5.3 Grade IV

An occluded artery should be treated with antithrombotics because there is still the risk of stroke. One review had a stroke incidence of 50 % for blunt carotid injury (BCI) and 28 % in blunt vertebral injury (BVI) when they were untreated [15].

8.4.5.4 Grade V

There is no treatment for carotid artery transection. These are fatal injuries with a 100 % risk of devastating stoke [15].

Conclusions

Cerebrovascular trauma, both penetrating and blunt, will continue to be a challenge for trauma surgeons and others who are confronted with these injuries. Two controversies that will persist for years to come are the best management algorithm for penetrating neck trauma (particularly zone 2 injuries) and anticoagulation vs. antiplatelet therapy for BCVI. Although these injury patterns are quite different, treatment principles are the same: cessation of hemorrhage, prevent of stroke, and location of all associated injuries.

References

1. Desai SS, Lidsky M, Pascarella L, Shortell CK. Surgical principles in clinical review of vascular surgery. In: Desai SS, Shortell CK, editors. Surgisphere Corporation. 1st ed. 2011.
2. Bouthillier A, van Loveren HR, Keller JT. Segments of the internal carotid artery: a new classification. Neurosurgery. 1996;38(3):425–32; discussion 432–3.
3. Rathlev NK, Medzon R, Bracken ME. Evaluation and management of neck trauma. Emerg Med Clin North Am. 2007;25(3):679–94, viii.
4. Inaba K, Branco BC, Menaker J, et al. Evaluation of multidetector computed tomography for penetrating neck injury: a prospective multicenter study. J Trauma. 2012;72(3):576–84.
5. Galante JM, London JA, Pevec WC. External-internal carotid artery transposition for repair of multiple pseudoaneurysms from penetrating injury in a pediatric patient. J Pediatr Surg. 2009;44:E27–30.
6. Van Waes OJ, Cheriex KCAL, Navasaria PH, van Riet PA, Nicol AJ, Vermeulen J. Management of penetrating neck injuries. Br J Surg. 2012;99 Suppl 1: 149–54.
7. Kumins NH, Tober JC, Larsen PE, Smead WL. Vertical ramus osteotomy allows exposure of the distal internal carotid artery to the base of the skull. Ann Vasc Surg. 2001;15:25–31.
8. Feliciano DV. Management of penetrating injuries to carotid artery. World J Surg. 2001;25:1028–35.
9. Landreneau RJ, Weigelt JA, Meier DE, Snyder WH, Brink BE, Fry WJ, McClelland RN. The anterior operative approach to the cervical vertebral artery. J Am Coll Surg. 1995;180:475–80.
10. Reid JDS, Weigelt JA. Forty-three cases of vertebral artery trauma. J Trauma. 1988;28(7):1007–12.
11. Biffl WL, Cothren CC, Moore EE, et al. Western trauma Association critical decisions in trauma: screening for and treatment of blunt cerebrovascular injuries. J Trauma. 2009;67(6):1150–3.
12. Bromberg WJ, Collier BC, Diebel LN, et al. Blunt cerebrovascular injury practice management guidelines: the eastern association for the surgery of trauma. J Trauma. 2010;68(2):471–7.
13. Franz RW, Willette PA, Wood MJ, Wright ML, Hartman JF. A systematic review and meta-analysis of diagnostic screening criteria for blunt cerebrovascular injuries. J Am Coll Surg. 2012;214:313–27.
14. Cothren CC, Moore EE, Biffl WL, et al. Anticoagulation is the gold standard therapy for blunt carotid injuries to reduce stroke rate. Arch Surg. 2004;139(5):540–5.
15. Biffl WL, Ray CE, Moore EE, et al. Treatment-related outcomes from blunt cerebrovascular injuries; importance of routine follow-up arteriography. Ann Surg. 2002;235(5):699–706.
16. Cothren CC, Biffl WL, Moore EE, Kashuk JL, Johnson JL. Treatment for blunt cerebrovascular injuries: equivalence of anticoagulation and antiplatelet agents. Arch Surg. 2009;144(7):685–90.
17. Edwards NM, Fabian TC, Claridge JA, Timmons SD, Fischer PE, Croce MA. Antithrombotic therapy and endovascular stents are effective treatment for blunt carotid injuries: results from longterm followup. J Am Coll Surg. 2007;204:1007–15.

Axillary and Brachial Injuries

9

Neal C. Hadro and Ronald I. Gross

Contents

N.C. Hadro, MD (✉)
Department of Surgery, Tufts University School
of Medicine, Baystate Vascular Services, Boston,
MA, USA

Division of Vascular Surgery,
Baystate Medical Center, Springfield, MA, USA
e-mail: neal.hadromd@baystatehealth.org

R.I. Gross, MD
Division of Trauma and Emergency Surgery,
Department of Surgery, Tufts University School
of Medicine, Boston, MA, USA

Division of Trauma, Acute Care Surgery
and Surgical Critical Care, Baystate Medical Center,
Springfield, MA, USA

9.1   Introduction

While the extremities are frequently subject to both blunt and penetrating mechanisms of trauma, associated vascular injuries are not common and isolated vascular injuries are very rare. When vascular injuries do occur in modern trauma practice, successful revascularization with limb salvage is almost routine, and ischemic limb loss has become the rare exception. Despite success in arterial repair, desirable outcomes with regard to extremity function and disability more often depend on successful identification and treatment of the frequent coexisting injuries to the bone, nerves, and soft tissue. The typical wounding mechanisms, mobility of the extremities, superficial location of vascular structures, and their intimate relationship with the adjacent bone and major motor neurons create a unique challenge that is best served by a collaborative model of multidisciplinary care.

Historically, the management of extremity vascular trauma was focused solely on hemorrhage control with styptics, compression, and ligation as a means to save life. In the Civil War, there were no options for arterial repair, and injury such as these often resulted in amputation with an associated 10–40 % mortality [1]. While there were sporadic reports from military conflict across the globe regarding arterial repair, including Carleton Mathewson's circa World War II vintage repair of a brachial artery in 1938, it was Carl Hughes in the Korean conflict who reliably demonstrated that arteries and veins could be successfully repaired even in less than ideal circumstance [2]. Refined

A. Dua et al. (eds.), *Clinical Review of Vascular Trauma*,
DOI 10.1007/978-3-642-39100-2_9, © Springer-Verlag Berlin Heidelberg 2014

surgical technique and innovations in patient transport and resuscitation have delivered us to a contemporary period where successful limb salvage following upper extremity trauma is greater than 92 %, as outlined in a review of 16 published series of upper extremity vascular trauma [3]. Through the years, major innovations from military and civilian experience that have delivered such outstanding success with limb salvage include arterial repair over ligation, enhanced resuscitation and transport programs, improved antimicrobial therapy, digital fluoroscopic imaging, noninvasive duplex imaging, computed tomographic angiography, microvascular techniques, appreciation of the impact of vein repair and timely fasciotomy, contemporary endovascular techniques, and novel wound care products and systems to simplify complex wound care such as the vacuum-assisted closure (VAC) device.

From a comparison of extremity arterial injuries using the National Trauma Data Bank, upper and lower extremity trauma patients have distinct modes of presentation and outcomes [4]. In a review from the National Trauma Data Bank of 8,311 extremity trauma cases, there were 63 % upper and 36 % lower extremity injuries with the majority (62 %) of upper extremity injuries from a penetrating mechanism and the majority (56 %) of the lower extremity injuries from blunt trauma [4]. Upper extremity trauma patients generally have a lower injury severity score, lower amputation rate, and lower overall mortality when compared to lower extremity injured patients [4]. Upper extremity injuries are more frequently from a penetrating mechanism than blunt etiologies. They are usually associated with lower-velocity missiles and a smaller region of injury than lower extremity injuries [4]. Associated injuries are more frequent with blunt trauma as opposed to penetrating mechanisms, and the incidence of coexisting orthopedic, neurologic, and soft tissue injury can be a defining characteristic of the regional population served. From trauma bank literature, there are more penetrating than blunt injuries when comparing military with civilian trauma and more blunt than penetrating comparing rural catchment centers with urban populations [4].

Contemporary review of the literature highlights the success of upper extremity limb salvage.

Franz et al. presented their series of 159 patients managed in a multidisciplinary fashion combined within a review of several large contemporary series of arterial injuries [3]. These patients represented 0.74 % of their admissions, and 78.5 % had concomitant additional nonvascular injuries, including 55 % with nerve injury. While the majority of injuries involved the distal portion of the arm, proximal injuries were associated with higher injury severity scores, more often the result of blunt force, and associated with additional nonvascular injuries and a longer intensive care unit stay. Major amputation rate across all series was only 2.2 % with a 97.8 % limb salvage rate. In a review of 58 patients by Ergunes et al. with a 77 % incidence of penetrating brachial artery injuries over an 8-year period, there was a 24 % rate of concomitant nerve injuries with a 35 % rate of long-term disability associated with nerve injury [5]. Locker et al. reported on 89 arterial injuries over a 20-year period from blunt trauma. Injuries reported included 72 % orthopedic, 43 % nerve, and 17 % venous injuries. Blunt axillary artery lesions had a 100 % incidence of additional nonvascular injuries. In this series, limb salvage was 98 % successful with only 2 late amputations due to uncontrolled infection [6].

Contrasting that series of blunt trauma is a review by Gill et al. of civilian penetrating axillary artery injuries [7]. They reported 100 % limb salvage with major morbidity related to brachial plexus injury. Seventy-nine percent of patients suffered stab or gunshot wounds with 22 % presenting with hypotension, 77 % were hemodynamically stable, and 23 % suffered prehospital mortality. In the series, 26 % required emergency exploration for bleeding or ischemia, and more than one-third had additional brachial plexus, axillary vein, or intrathoracic injuries. Lastly, in a large series reported by Zellweger et al. from South Africa of 124 brachial artery injuries with the majority from a penetrating mechanism, there was a 21 % rate of post-op complications with the majority (11.3 %) comprised of soft tissue infection [1]. Also reported were causalgia and ongoing muscle necrosis after fasciotomy, and only one out of 73 interposition grafts thrombosed [1].

9.2   Anatomic Considerations

The anatomy of the axillary and brachial arteries is relevant to both the diagnosis and management of upper extremity trauma (Fig. 9.1). Both segments have intimate relationships with neighboring major nerves and venous structures. Proximally, the neurovascular bundles within the shoulder are well protected and fixed in position, thus more vulnerable to blunt than penetrating trauma. The force required for injury usually underscores a forceful blow, thus a more severely injured patient. The superficial nature of the more distal extremity segment, the brachial artery, enhances vulnerability to penetrating mechanisms which are usually isolated and collateral damage localized (Fig. 9.2).

The axillary artery is defined anatomically by the lateral margin of the first rib proximally and lateral edge of the teres major muscle distally. In its proximally protected location surrounded by the chest wall and pectoral and shoulder muscles, the axillary artery is protected from penetrating injury. Due to its anatomical location, the axillary artery may present a formidable challenge to the operative surgeon seeking direct surgical exposure for proximal control. The remainder of the mid- and distal axillary artery becomes more superficial and easily accessible heading toward the axilla. The pectoralis minor muscle serves as the gateway to the midaxillary artery and is draped over the anterior surface of the vessel. Along the length of the artery from proximal to distal are an increasing number of branch arteries to the chest wall and shoulder. Intimately associated with the third portion of the axillary artery are the major nerves to the arm, shoulder, and pectoral muscles. This close relationship underscores the likelihood of combined neurovascular injuries with wounding as well as inherent challenges in rapid, efficient exposure and repair without causing unnecessary iatrogenic injury.

The brachial artery runs with the median nerve along the anterior compartment of the arm. The profunda brachial branch joins the radial nerve and penetrates an intermuscular septum laterally becoming the radial collateral artery which is an important proximal collateral to the forearm following injury below the level of the mid-biceps. This important

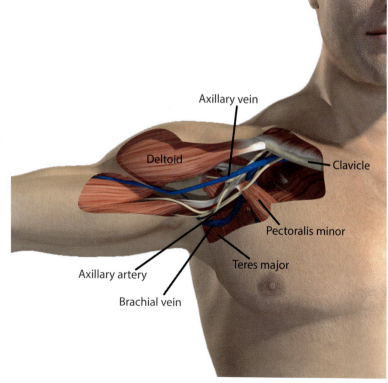

Fig. 9.1 The axillary artery is defined anatomically by the lateral margin of the first rib proximally and lateral edge of the teres major muscle distally. In its proximally protected location surrounded by chest wall, pectoral, and shoulder muscles, the axillary artery is protected from penetrating injury. The pectoralis minor muscle serves as the gateway to the midaxillary artery and is draped over the anterior surface of the vessel. Intimately associated with the third portion of the axillary artery are the major nerves to the arm, shoulder, and pectoral muscles

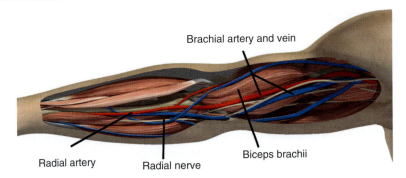

Brachial artery and vein

Radial artery   Radial nerve   Biceps brachii

Fig. 9.2 The brachial artery runs with the median nerve along the anterior compartment of the arm. The profunda brachial branch joins the radial nerve and penetrates an intermuscular septum laterally becoming the radial collateral artery which is an important proximal collateral to the forearm following injury below the level of the mid-biceps

collateral may support distal viability in the setting of major arterial injury and allow time for more serious associated injuries to be addressed. The superior ulnar collateral artery accompanies the ulnar nerve at mid-brachium and penetrates the intermuscular septum medially. The brachial artery is accompanied by two veins: the basilic which is superficial at the antecubital level and then penetrates the fascia to join the brachial vein and the brachial vein with its numerous deep and superficial anastomoses which unite at the level of the lateral border of the teres major to become the axillary vein.

A timeless adage still holds that standard vessel exposure should not be altered or compromised by traumatic wounds with the principles of proximal and distal control obtained whenever possible in the safest and most familiar manner. The most proximal axillary artery beneath the clavicle and adjacent to the first rib presents a major problem for hasty exposure such that a more traditional proximal mediastinal or intrathoracic subclavian exposure might be suitable. In a modern practice, these morbid exposures lend themselves more appropriately to the promise and benefit of rapid and less invasive endovascular control such as balloon occlusion from brachial or femoral access. The Seldinger technique is used to access the femoral artery with a steep left anterior oblique projection of the chest and opacification of the aortic arch to demonstrate the origins of the great vessels. Depending on laterality, the innominate or left subclavian may be cannulated with the appropriate preformed catheter and selective hydrophilic glide wire and advanced toward the site of injury. Next, an exchange made for a stiffer support wire and a long, large-diameter

sheath to support the appropriate diameter compliant occlusion balloon. This balloon can be gently inflated under fluoroscopy with the use of a stopcock to maintain inflation and arrest inflow. In special circumstances, the use of a long sheath near the site of injury may also afford the option of covered stent placement to seal extravasation, close an arteriovenous fistula, cover a pseudoaneurysm, or permit coil embolization of bleeding branch vessels.

The remainder of the mid- and distal axillary artery is more classically exposed with an incision two fingerbreadths below mid-lateral clavicle. This separates the underlying pectoralis major fibers with the neurovascular bundle beneath the clavipectoral fascia. Wider arterial exposure may be facilitated by dividing the attachment between the pectoralis minor and the coracoid process. The more distal axillary artery can be approached with an axillary incision and retraction of the lateral pectoralis border medially and coracobrachialis superiorly. In this position, the median nerve is encountered and needs to be gently mobilized. Being a superficial artery in the brachium lends the brachial artery to an easy exposure along the medial groove between the biceps and the triceps. The basilic vein, brachial vein, and median nerve must be identified and protected particularly during a hasty exposure to control bleeding.

9.3 Treatment Algorithm

The first decision confronting the attending surgeon is immediate surgery versus delay for additional imaging. For high-velocity blunt trauma and particularly with proximal upper extremity injury, there is a significant concurrence of associated head and neck, intrathoracic, and abdominal injury that may supersede extremity care. Following the basic tenets of advanced trauma life support protocols, resuscitation and triage and after addressing immediate life-threatening injuries affecting airway, breathing and circulation, attention is turned to the injured extremity. The first priority is life-sustaining hemorrhage control, the second goal relieving ischemia, and lastly stabilizing measures to mitigate future disability with a goal of restoring meaningful limb function beyond basic limb salvage. This includes orthopedic stabilization and repair, nerve repair and adequate soft tissue coverage combined with appropriate antibiotic usage, and a comprehensive and compulsive wound care plan with early and aggressive physical and occupational therapy.

From a purely vascular standpoint, the presenting symptoms of upper extremity vascular injury dictate triage and are divided into hard signs that mandate immediate exploration and softer signs that may beg additional investigation for diagnosis and prognosis and even afford the option of less invasive endovascular intervention or selective nonsurgical observation. The well-known hard signs include active hemorrhage, expanding hematoma, pulseless extremity, or frank ischemia as manifest clinically by pain, pallor, paresthesia, paralysis, poikilothermy, and pulselessness. These patients manifesting hard signs are prepared and taken immediately to the operating room for proximal and distal control of the injury site and exploration and repair of the artery. For the most proximal injuries at the clavicle level and a relatively stable patient, it is expected that intraoperative angiography with endovascular means for proximal control of bleeding through balloon occlusion with an option for definitive endovascular repair should be in the armamentarium of a modern vascular surgeon or collaborating interventional radiologist. The large diameter and fixed location of the subclavian-axillary vessels and their privileged location that challenges safe exposure make this area fruitful for endovascular endeavors and quite distinct from the more superficial and smaller-diameter arterial tree beyond the mobile shoulder and elbow joints.

A more stable patient without frankly ischemic signs may demonstrate softer signs of vascular injury such as an ominous mechanism or proximity of the wound to a major artery, large non-expanding hematoma, high-velocity missile, abnormalities in noninvasive perfusion measurement, bruit or thrill, suspicious mechanism with additional associated factors such as a major fracture or soft tissue injury that affects accuracy of serial examination or multiple sites of injury such as a shotgun blast that raises a high probability or suspicion with uncertainty about the location of the most critical vascular lesion. While traditional contrast-enhanced angiography has been the gold standard and affords opportunity for intervention with coil embolization and covered stent placement or at a minimum proximal control with endoluminal balloon occlusion, the ability to rapidly acquire high-specificity diagnostic imaging with spiral CT angiography has been a game changer as a rapid screening test and plays a major role in the management of multi-trauma patients. In particular, high-resolution diagnostic CT angiography is very useful when there are additional complex orthopedic and soft tissue injuries to be evaluated outside the limited view of angiography which only shows intraluminal blood flow and vessel wall contour. CT angiography also allows grading of injury and thereby allows triage decisions in addition to planning revascularization with conduit assessment and required exposure (Fig. 9.3).

The CT exam requires a clinically stable patient who does not have hard signs of vascular injury that would mandate immediate attention and treatment. Furthermore, CTA technology is widely available, and other than contrast exposure is noninvasive with rapidly available images and information. The images provide necessary detail about the associated orthopedic and soft tissue injuries that would not be delineated by angiography alone. The argument against CTA is that it is purely diagnostic and often a significant contrast exposure in a frequently hypovolemic or hypotensive patient at risk for contrast nephropathy. Conversely, angiography is not always available and may take time to assemble a team in addition to its invasive nature. Angiography, particularly with highly selective views, can be done with

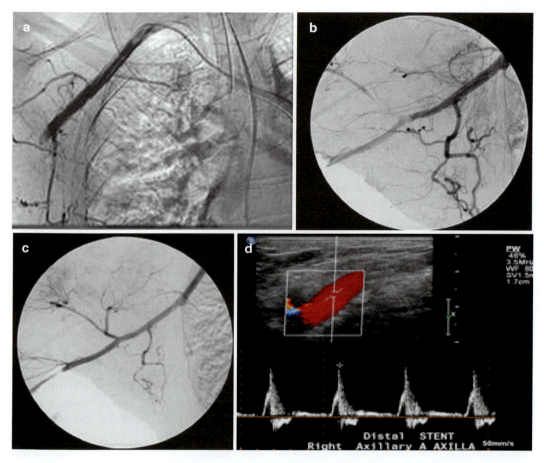

Fig. 9.3 (**a**) A 46-year-old male pedestrian struck with skull fracture, subarachnoid bleed, shoulder dislocation, lumbar fracture, and open tibia-fibula fracture. The hand ischemic in ICU. (**b**) Follow-up images after placement of 6×40 self-expanding stent. (**c**) A 52-year-old male fell 5 ft onto outstretched arm with shoulder dislocation. Unable to pass guidewire due to extrinsic compression. Treated successfully with vein graft from axillary artery to brachial artery (Courtesy of Dr. Hao Wu). (**d**) Duplex images of stent at 1-year post procedure

much less iodinated contrast than CT angiography, offer directly measurable physiologic information regarding direction of flow and pressure gradients, and permit coil embolization of bleeding lesions.

9.4   Surgical Repair

In the operating suite, consideration must be given to wide prepping of the patient to allow vein harvest for possible interposition grafting or at least vein patch repair of the injured vessel. Choices for conduit include great saphenous vein, basilic or cephalic vein, cryopreserved vein, and antibiotic-impregnated prosthetic graft. Once proximal and distal control is successfully obtained, the area of

injury can be explored with meticulous sharp dissection. In the presence of major hematoma, the extravasated blood usually has accomplished much of the tissue dissection. Care should be taken to avoid directly entering the hematoma until safe proximal control can be obtained above the wound site. With an isolated penetrating injury and long period of anticipated ischemia, systemic heparin may be administered once control is obtained. Otherwise, local infusion into the artery with a syringe of heparinized saline followed by passage of a balloon embolectomy catheter to clear the vessel of acute thrombus should be the initial steps prior to definitive repair.

For focal injuries, the vessel should be mobilized, the injured wall debrided to normal artery, and decision made regarding direct repair, primary anastomosis, vein patch angioplasty, or interposition grafting with adequately size-matched autologous vein. A wall injury less than one-third of the circumference can potentially be primarily repaired if the final diameter post repair is not reduced. This is best done with interrupted 5-0, 6-0, or 7-0 nonabsorbable monofilament suture. Intimal disruption requires a more extensive arteriotomy for proper visualization and intimal debridement and tacking with vein patch repair of the arteriotomy. It is essential that the arteriotomy extend beyond the level of intimal repair so that the suture line of the vein patch is not directly over the intimal tacking sutures which could lead to narrowing, flow disturbance, and acute thrombosis. Primary anastomotic repair may be required and acceptable if after adequate debridement the vessel can be approximated without either tension or luminal compromise. Permanent monofilament suture that is 5-0 or 6-0 is often employed, and an interrupted suture repair is favored for smaller-caliber arteries to prevent narrowing or cicatrix formation.

Additionally, the young trauma patient frequently exhibits severe reactive vasospasm that is unique to healthy non-atherosclerotic vessels and compounded by hypothermia and hypovolemia, so adjuvant intra-arterial nitroglycerin or papaverine boluses may be helpful to overcome high-resistant outflow following repair. A final option, rarely employed but essential in the hypothermic, acidotic, and coagulopathic patient, is vessel ligation and a deliberate choice of life over limb. This is a rare scenario and interestingly with the rich collateral circulation of the shoulder and proximal profunda brachial branches may be tolerable until a delayed secondary repair is possible.

Vein injuries are also frequently coexisting with arterial injuries; however, with the redundant venous drainage of the arm, these injuries are usually ligated with impunity unless an easy lateral suture repair option exists or a major outflow vein such as the proximal axillary or subclavian is involved. Another concern is the high incidence of failed venous repair with venous thrombosis and potential pulmonary embolism.

9.5   Multidisciplinary Care

Given the frequency of coexisting injuries and overriding impact on functional outcomes and salvage, it is prudent to approach patients whenever possible in a multidisciplinary manner through early collaboration with orthopedics, plastics, hand and neurosurgery. The success of upper extremity revascularization is high, and it is the coexisting orthopedic, soft tissue, and nerve injuries that are the true determinants of functional outcomes. Excluding ischemia, acute limb loss is frequently from overwhelming and uncontrolled secondary infection so adequate debridement of nonviable tissue and appropriate coverage of vascular and orthopedic repair is essential. Unstable fractures may require stabilization before repair such that ultimate reduction does not strain the vascular repair and length of conduit for bypass can be precisely determined. In this case, communication and intraoperative collaboration between vascular and orthopedic surgeon are essential.

In an "ortho-first" scenario, rapid temporary perfusion with placement of a simple shunt is often necessary. The shunt should be matched to the artery size and secured with Rummel tourniquets or Javid clamps with the vascular surgeon in attendance during orthopedic manipulation and fracture stabilization followed by prompt vascular repair once orthopedic stabilization is complete. Major nerve injuries are best served by immediate repair when patient stability permits, revascularization and orthopedic stabilization are completed, and a qualified specialist is available. The definitive repair is often performed by a plastic and reconstructive specialist or hand surgeon and often under microscope guidance. If delayed repair is required, particularly in the setting of major soft tissue damage or patient instability, the identifiable nerve endings should at least be tagged with nonabsorbable suture to aid identification during secondary exposure, and consultation with the reconstructive surgeon at some point during the initial presentation is best.

Finally, it is essential that all nonviable soft tissue is debrided to avoid secondary infection while allowing a viable solution for adequate coverage of exposed vascular, neurologic, and orthopedic repair. This may require local tissue rotation, myoplasty, free-flap coverage, synthetic dermal substitutes combined with a VAC device, and ultimate skin grafting procedures that once again make collaboration with a skilled plastic surgeon invaluable.

9.6 Fasciotomy Use

At the conclusion of the initial operation, it is essential to assess the need for decompressive fasciotomy. Fascial compartment pressures can be elevated from reperfusion edema after prolonged ischemia, local hematoma or extensive soft tissue swelling from crush injury, major fractures, or the concussive blast from a high-velocity missile. Given the significant risk for permanent disability from a missed decompression and irreversible neuromotor injury and with the advent of wound VAC therapy to simplify postoperative wound management, the threshold for decompression and fascial release should be low. Pressure measurements may be helpful when physical exam is equivocal or unreliable, particularly in an intubated and sedated patient who cannot articulate pain or allow a reliable physical exam. Although an objective measurement, compartment pressures may still require some subjective interpretation within the clinical context of patient mean arterial pressure, central venous pressure, concurrent use of vasopressors, and resuscitation status. Ultimately, any suspicion of present or pending compartment syndrome is best acted upon early in the hospital course, and the threshold for decompressive fasciotomy should be very low.

Compartment syndrome is uncommon in the upper arm, while the forearm is extremely vulnerable as the anterior interosseous artery, which has no collaterals, supplies the deep volar compartment. The true incidence of compartment syndrome associated with upper extremity vascular injury is unknown, presenting between 2 and 29 % in a review of brachial artery injuries combined with a series of 139 patients complied by Kim et al. In this series there were three statistically significant predictors of compartment syndrome after brachial artery injury including intraoperative blood loss, combined injuries, and open fractures [8]. Typically, a dorsal and volar incision is required on the forearm. The volar incision is curvilinear across the elbow and wrist joints, meandering from the medial side above the antecubital crease, migrating nearly transverse across the elbow crease, and travelling down the ulnar side of the forearm. The volar incision releases the flexor compartment and dorsal incision releases the extensors. The volar incision should release the median, radial, and ulnar nerves, and a deeper intramuscular incision will release the deep flexor muscles. Frequently, a carpal tunnel release must be performed as an extension of the volar incision.

9.7 Pediatric Upper Extremity Injury

Any discussion linking upper extremity trauma and vascular injury would be incomplete without mentioning the distinct entity of pediatric elbow fracture or more precisely supracondylar fracture of the humerus. This is one of the most common fractures in children and a 3–14 % risk of associated vascular injury with a high risk of ischemic-related long-term damage that includes neurologic injury, Volkmann's contracture, and amputation as the worst possible outcome [9]. A lengthy review of the literature by Griffin et al. advocated selective management, while a small series over an 8-year period that felt any pulseless hand following fracture repair must be explored to prevent devastating complications or long-term disability [10]. The close proximity of neurovascular structures to the elbow joint makes these structures vulnerable to forces of stretch or entrapment by bone fragments or repair wires. Management begins with fracture stabilization and specific attention to the pulse exam before and after reduction.

The obviously ischemic hand requires immediate brachial exploration and repair. The standard treatment is exploration with brachial thrombectomy and assessment of damage (Fig. 9.4). The artery is small and easily prone to spasm. Repair options include intimal examination with local repair through the arteriotomy and primary closure, vein patch angioplasty, resection with tension-free primary anastomosis, or vein interposition graft with saphenous vein or local basilic vein. Interrupted 6-0, 7-0, or even

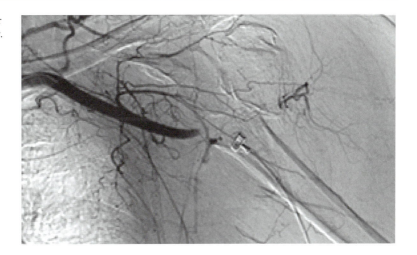

Fig. 9.4 C-arm images after over-the-wire thrombectomy. Residual dissection flap noted

8-0 suture is required under loupe or microscope magnification depending on the size of the artery.

In addition to the technical challenges imposed by miniature size and vasospastic reactivity of pediatric arterial repair, there is a unique subgroup whose management remains open to some lively debate in the literature. This group is the pediatric supracondylar fracture patient with a distinctly pink and pulseless hand postreduction. This patient has a clearly viable limb yet no palpable pulses; only continuous Doppler signal at the wrist that is different from the other hand and from personal experience may present with paroxysms of transient hand pain or paresthesias interspersed with asymptomatic intervals. Early observation is predicated on a purported theory of temporary arterial spasm, while series recom-

mending early surgery emphasize the high incidence of positive arterial findings at exploration weighted against the magnitude of devastating and permanent adverse outcomes should they befall a developing and otherwise healthy child. There is no role for angiography in a small child when the location of pathology is certain and the area of injury is so easily accessible. There is an increasing experience with duplex scanning whose low-cost, wide-availability, noninvasive, and portable nature makes it an attractive second level exam. However, modern consensus recommendations for diagnostic testing do not exist at this time and should not delay direct exploration when indicated and definitive treatment, when pathology is encountered (Fig. 9.5).

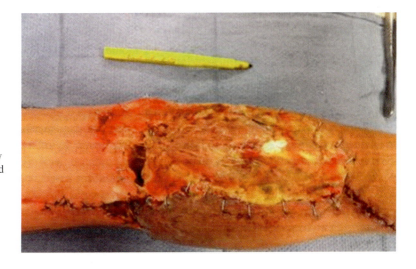

Fig. 9.5 Major crush injury with continued ischemia and infection of soft tissue coverage led to multiple bypass failures and ultimately limb loss (Courtesy of Dr. Jeff Kaufman)

Conclusion

The upper extremity is vulnerable to a variety of wounding mechanisms, both blunt and penetrating. Arterial injuries are relatively uncommon and presentation and prognosis can be separated by mechanism with penetrating injuries in general representing a lower-velocity wounding mechanism and a smaller zone of injury compared to blunt trauma which often presents a more proximal and wider zone of injury with higher associated injury severity scores. Regardless of mechanism, the success of arterial repair is outstanding. In addition, modern less invasive endovascular techniques offer some promise for both adjuvant care with balloon tamponade and definitive treatment by covered stent placement or branch embolization of difficult to expose proximal subclavian and axillary artery and branches. Rapid balloon occlusion is of particular benefit in the unstable or polytrauma patients with unmatched rapidity for control of bleeding and potential for definitive endovascular repair. In addition, the increased availability of rapidly acquired, noninvasive imaging by duplex and CTA has increased their role in triaging the multi-trauma patient by assisting simultaneously with both triage of multiple injuries and operative planning.

While modern trauma care combined with advances in vascular technique and endovascular care has resulted in outstanding success with limb salvage, it is the close proximity of additional structures and the coexisting orthopedic, neurologic, and soft tissue injuries that most likely determine the outcome. It is these associated nonvascular injuries that most likely and accurately determine disability and ultimately functional and from the standpoint of functional success override the rare incidence of failed vascular reconstruction. It is essential to have a multidisciplinary approach to these patients early in the presentation with open communication followed by early and aggressive rehabilitative services to optimize clinical outcomes which are more accurately and commonly defined by functional outcomes and disability scores than ischemic limb loss from a rare instance of failed arterial repair.

References

1. Zellweger R, Hess F, Nicol A, et al. An analysis of 124 surgically managed brachial artery injuries. Am J Surg. 2004;188(3):240–5.
2. Rich NM, Leppaniemi A. Vascular trauma: a 40-year experience with extremity vascular emphasis. Scand J Surg. 2002;91:109–26.
3. Franz RW, Skytta CK, Shah KJ, et al. A five-year review of management of upper-extremity arterial injuries at an urban level I trauma center. Ann Vasc Surg. 2012;26(5):655–64.
4. Tan TW, Joglar FL, Hamburg NM, et al. Limb outcomes and mortality in lower and upper extremity arterial injury: a comparison using the National Trauma Data Bank. Vasc Endovascular Surg. 2011;45(7):592–7.
5. Ergunes K, Yilik L, Ozsoyler I, et al. Traumatic brachial artery injuries. Tex Heart Inst J. 2006;33(1):31–4.
6. Klocker J, Falkensammer J, Pellegrini L, et al. Repair of arterial injury after blunt trauma in the upper extremity – immediate and long term outcome. Eur J Vasc Endovasc Surg. 2010;39(2):160–4.
7. Gill H, Jenkins W, Edu S, et al. Civilian penetrating axillary artery injuries. World J Surg. 2011;35(5):962–6.
8. Kiom JY, Buck 2nd DW, Forte A, et al. Risk factors for compartment syndrome in traumatic brachial artery injuries: an institutional experience in 139 patients. J Trauma. 2009;67(6):1339–44.
9. Griffin KJ, Walsh S, Markar S, et al. The pink pulseless hand: a review of the literature regarding management of vascular complications of supracondylar fractures in children. Eur J Vasc Endovasc Surg. 2008;36(6):697–702.
10. Brahmamdam P, Plummer M, Modrall JG, et al. Hand ischemia associated with elbow trauma in children. J Vasc Surg. 2011;54(3):773–8.

Radial, Ulnar, and Hand Injuries

10

Victor A. Moon and John B. Hijjawi

Contents

V.A. Moon, MD (✉)
Department of Surgery,
Hofstra North Shore – LIJ School of Medicine,
Hempstead, NY, USA

J.B. Hijjawi, MD
Departments of Plastic Surgery and General Surgery,
Medical College of Wisconsin, Milwaukee, WI, USA

10.1 Epidemiology

Traumatic injuries to the forearm and hand can be penetrating or blunt, which represent 4–36 % of upper extremity arterial trauma [1–3]. Because of the close proximity of the vessels and the nerves as they travel in the arm, injuries are rarely just vascular in nature, often complicating not only the presentation but also the long-term outcome. If not treated in a timely fashion and properly, such injuries can lead to loss of function, loss of limb, or even death [4, 5].

Patients with injuries to the forearm and hand can present in many different ways, from a seemingly clean laceration across the wrist or digit to a crush injury involving the hand and forearm (Fig. 10.1).

Injuries to the forearm and hand are often reported as part of upper extremity injuries, with brachial artery injuries accounting for 40–55 % and radial and ulnar arterial injuries 4–36 % of the injuries, with about 67 % resulting from penetrating trauma [2–4, 6]. Though it is associated with lower mortality, upper extremity injuries have a high amputation rate [7]. On the other hand, several studies have reported that vascular extremity trauma due to blunt mechanism leads to worse outcomes than penetrating injury [8]. This is likely due to the higher energy associated with crushing injuries and the higher potential for concomitant orthopedic trauma or soft tissue loss. The mortality rate of patients with upper extremity vascular injury is primarily related to

A. Dua et al. (eds.), *Clinical Review of Vascular Trauma*,
DOI 10.1007/978-3-642-39100-2_10, © Springer-Verlag Berlin Heidelberg 2014

Fig. 10.1 (**a**) Laceration across the wrist with transection of radial artery, median nerve, and flexor tendons. (**b**) Industrial crush injury with multisystem, segmental damage

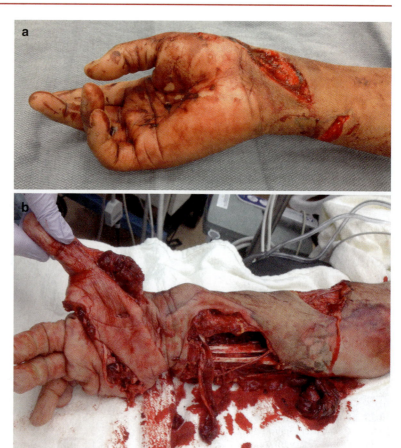

concomitant injuries such as head injury or abdominal trauma. Morbidity with upper extremity injuries, and especially with the forearm and hand, is closely associated with damage to the accompanying nerve, tendons, and associated bone fractures.

10.2 Etiology

The most common cause of forearm and hand vascular injury is penetrating trauma secondary to gunshot wounds and lacerations from stab wounds or glass. As mentioned previously, blunt trauma is not a common cause of vascular injury. As a result, vascular compromise can be easily missed during the initial assessment of a bluntly injured extremity. Therefore, a basic neurovascular exam is a critical component of any extremity exam, regardless of the

indication for the assessment or complaint. One consideration that should raise the index of suspicion is the amount of force associated with the blunt trauma. Closed bone fractures or dislocations can be associated with arterial injuries. These types of injuries result in intimal tears and subsequent thrombosis of the vessels without a frank of obvious vascular insult (Fig. 10.2) [9, 10]. An example is hypothenar hammer syndrome resulting from repetitive blunt trauma to the palm and subsequent injury to the ulnar artery via the same mechanism stated above [11].

Injuries involving the hand and fingers usually often require microsurgical skills because of the small and delicate nature of the vessels, and therefore a hand or reconstructive surgeon is often involved. A basic understanding of the anatomy and surgical principles is still valuable when managing polytrauma patients with vascular injuries to the upper extremity.

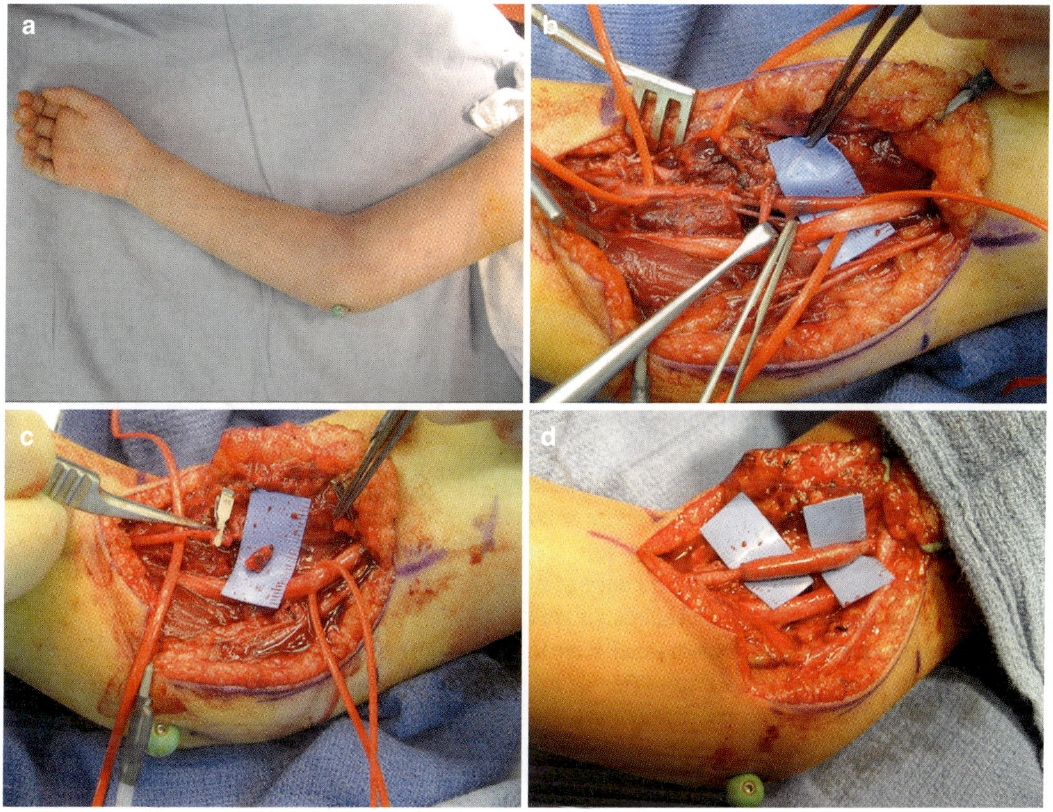

Fig. 10.2 (**a**) An 8-year-old girl treated for a closed supracondylar humerus fracture with closed reduction and percutaneous pin fixation. Postoperative examination revealed the extremity distal to the elbow to be ischemic. Urgent transfer was made. (**b**) The segment of brachial artery just proximal to the bifurcation is noted to have a thrombus within it. (**c**) The segment of brachial artery associated with the thrombus is presumed to have intimal damage given the blunt mechanism of injury and is resected. (**d**) A local vein graft is reversed and used to bypass the arterial gap created by debridement in a tension-free manner. Healing was uneventful

10.3 Anatomy/Physiology

The brachial artery, a continuation of the axillary artery, divides just distal to the elbow into the radial and ulnar arteries. Prior to its bifurcation, it gives off collateral branches around the elbow. In the distal aspect, the brachial artery is adjacent to the median nerve (Fig. 10.3).

Within the forearm, the radial artery begins near the neck of the radius and passes deep to the brachioradialis muscle, traveling distally on the anterior-radial part of the forearm. This serves as a landmark for the division between the anterior and posterior compartments of the forearm. As it approaches the wrist, it becomes more superficial and travels between the flexor carpi radialis and brachioradialis tendons and enters the wrist through the anatomical snuffbox and between the heads of the first dorsal interosseous muscle of the hand. It passes anteriorly between the heads of the adductor pollicis and becomes the deep palmar arch, which in turn will join with the deep branch of the ulnar artery.

As the radial artery travels down the forearm, it gives off several branches. In the forearm, the recurrent radial artery is the first branch, which will anastomose to the collateral arterial system around the elbow. Next, the palmar carpal branch arises near the lower border of the pronator quadratus and the superficial palmar branch just as it winds to the radial side of the wrist. At the wrist, the dorsal carpal branch and first dorsal metacarpal artery are

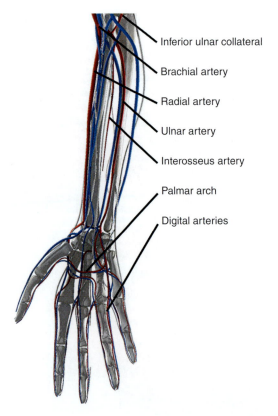

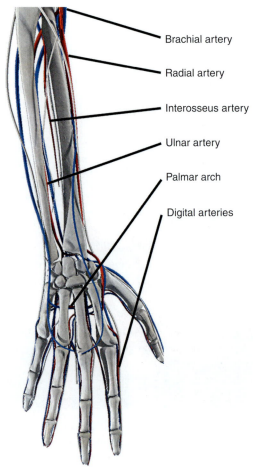

Fig. 10.3 Arterial anatomy of the ventral forearm and hand

noted and in the hand, the princeps pollicis artery, radialis indicis, and deep palmar arch.

The artery can be palpated on the radial aspect of the wrist, just radial to the flexor carpi radialis tendon, and in the anatomical snuffbox, and if during physical examination a pulse is present, it has been estimated to correlate with a systolic blood pressure of greater than 70 mmHg [12].

The ulnar artery is the larger branch of the two and runs under the pronator teres, flexor carpi radialis, palmaris longus, and flexor digitorum superficialis but over the brachialis and flexor digitorum profundus. As the brachialis bifurcation, it travels next to the median nerve on the medial side for about 2.5 cm and reaches the ulnar aspect of the forearm about midway between the elbow and wrist. It continues to travel distally on the ulnar border over the flexor digitorum profundus between the flexor carpi

Fig. 10.4 Arterial anatomy of the dorsal forearm and hand

ulnaris and flexor digitorum superficialis. About a third of the way down the forearm, the ulnar nerve travels on the medial side of the artery. At the wrist, it enters Guyon's canal, crossing the transverse carpal ligament on the radial side of the pisiform bone, and then divides into two branches: the superficial one which forms the superficial palmar arch and the deep branch that joins the deep palmar arch (Fig. 10.4).

The superficial palmar arch lies deep to the palmar fascia and gives rise to the volar common digital arteries and branches to the intrinsic muscles of the hand. Distally, the common digital arteries bifurcate into the proper digital arteries. Each digit has a radial and ulnar digital artery supplying it. The deep palmar arch lies at the base of the metacarpals, deep to the flexor tendons. It provides blood supply to the thumb and radial half of the index finger by the first metacarpal artery.

10.4 Clinical Assessment

Upon initial evaluation of a patient and following advanced trauma life support (ATLS) approach by the American College of Surgeons, during secondary survey, a thorough assessment of the extremity is undertaken [13, 14]. If persistent bleeding is present, direct pressure can be applied, or if hemorrhaging, then a tourniquet or blood pressure cuff should be placed proximal to the injury and inflated at least 50 mmHg above systolic pressure (usually 200–250 mmHg). Two issues surrounding tourniquet use are the proper location and associated tourniquet pain. The position of the tourniquet, whether on the forearm or upper arm, is equally effective in controlling bleeding and well tolerated [15, 16]. Under no circumstances should hemostats or any kind of clamp be used to control bleeding from the arm or forearm. The risk of iatrogenic injury to adjacent nerves is very high in this setting. A thorough history and physical examination, if able, should be obtained (Table 10.1).

The classic physical exam features of a vascular injury include diminished or absent distal pulses, a history of arterial bleeding, large or expanding hematoma, bruit at the site or injury, injury to anatomically related nerves, and injury in close proximity to a major artery [17]. These and other clinical signs have subsequently been stratified as "hard" and "soft" signs on their prediction of arterial injury in extremities, as shown in Table 10.2 [10]. The presence of a "hard" sign of vascular injury mandates immediate surgical intervention and repair, while "soft" signs are less specific and often need further studies to either confirm or exclude vascular injury [10].

The hand is perfused by the ulnar and radial arteries which terminate as the palmar arches, as previously described. In order to determine

Table 10.1 History and physical exam are the initial most important steps when assessing a patient with signs of vascular injury

History	Physical exam
Mechanism of injury	Radial and ulnar pulses – *Allen's test*
Time	Capillary refill
Handedness	Warmth
Occupation	Turgor
	Hand/wrist posture – tenodesis effect
	Sensation – radial, ulnar, median distribution
	Tendon exam

Table 10.2 Clinical signs for the prediction of arterial injuries in extremities

"Hard" signs	"Soft" signs
Active or pulsatile hemorrhage	Moderate hemorrhage occurring at the scene of injury
Pulsatile or expanding hematoma	Stable and nonpulsatile hematoma
Thrill or bruit (suggesting an AV fistula)	Proximity of wound to a major vessel
Evidence of ischemia (pallor, paresthesia, paralysis, pain, and poikilothermia)	Peripheral neurological deficit
Diminished or absent pulses	Asymmetric extremity blood pressures
	Presence of shock/hypoperfusion
	Associated fracture or dislocation

whether a patent palmar arch is present, an Allen's test should be performed (Fig. 10.5) [18]. This is done by applying firm pressure to both the ulnar and radial arteries just proximal to the wrist crease while the patient opens and closes his hand several times, until blanching is noted. The patient is asked to gently open his hand, in a position of rest, just short of full finger extension. The pressure over the ulnar artery is released while keeping pressure on the radial side, and perfusion of the hand is noted. This is then repeated but this time releasing the radial artery instead while holding pressure over the ulnar artery. Perfusion of the hand should take

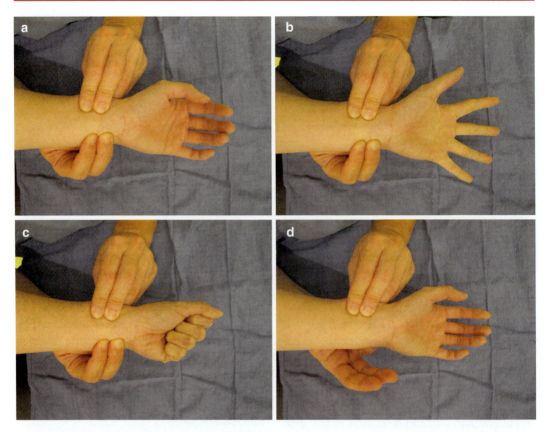

Fig. 10.5 Allen's test. (**a**) Firm pressure applied to both sides of the wrist over the ulnar and radial arteries while (**b**) opening and closing the hand. (**c**) Ulnar artery pressure is released and time for capillary refill of the hand is noted. (**d**) This is then repeated with the radial artery released while pressure is maintained in the ulnar side

5–10 s to suggest an intact palmar arch. Though it is an easy and simple exam to perform at the bedside, it is subjective and operator dependent, as shown by Benit et al. with up to 27 % of the population showing a discontinuous palmar arch based on this exam [19].

Evaluation of the vascular supply to the digits can be done in a similar fashion. Color, temperature, and turgor should be quickly assessed, while capillary refill can be used to assess adequate perfusion. It is generally brisk and less than 2 s. Another clinical test to assess blood flow to the digits is the pinprick test, usually done on an insensate finger or when the patient is anesthetized. Perfusion of the nail bed, which can be readily visualized through the nail plate, is helpful in darker-skinned patients. Allen's test, similar to the one used to evaluate for palmar arch patency, can be performed on the digits. The digit is exsanguinated by flexing it, and then the radial and ulnar digital arteries at the base of the digit are occluded. With release of either artery, it should result in brisk capillary refill to the digit. However, Allen's test is rarely required to determine if perfusion to a single digit is adequate.

10.5   Diagnostic Testing

10.5.1 Doppler Ultrasonography

Continuous wave Doppler or duplex ultrasound devices can be used to evaluate for vascular patency. A normal, triphasic signal should be heard over the radial, ulnar, and digital arteries. More complex or expensive techniques are rarely indicated in acute traumatic vascular injury to the forearm.

Fig. 10.6 Muscles of the forearm and digital arteries of the hand

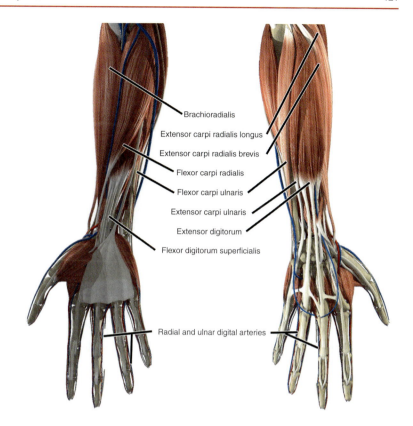

Brachioradialis

Extensor carpi radialis longus

Extensor carpi radialis brevis

Flexor carpi radialis

Flexor carpi ulnaris

Extensor carpi ulnaris

Extensor digitorum

Flexor digitorum superficialis

Radial and ulnar digital arteries

10.6 Operative Management

For forearm and hand arterial injuries, bony stabilization of associated fractures is performed first, before vascular repair, which will define the length of the defect and also avoid inadvertent injury to the repair if done in the reverse order. In cases where definitive vascular repair may need to be delayed because of severely comminuted fracture or need for extensive soft tissue debridement, a temporary intraluminal shunt can be placed until skeletal stabilization and debridement has been completed.

The primary vascular management strategy is primary repair. However, vascular bypass, with a reversed vein graft, is occasionally required [20]. In fact, in crush injuries vein grafts are very helpful in spanning gaps created by the proper debridement of devitalized vessels. If injury is in the forearm and there is absence of ischemic changes distal to either an isolated radial or ulnar artery injury, the options are ligation and repair of the vessel. One must confirm that there is

collateral blood supply if opting for ligation [20, 21]. Others opt for a repair of the vessel, even with no signs of ischemia, as they believe restoration of near-normal blood flow is optimal [22]. However, if both arteries are injured, repair of the ulnar artery is preferred because it is usually the dominant and larger vessel [23, 24]. The same algorithm can be used for finger injuries, as there is a dual blood supply to the digits, radial, and ulnar aspects of the fingers (Fig. 10.6).

If there is segmental loss, an interposition graft will be needed for repair of the arterial injury. Because the length of the defect is often short and the size of the lumen is usually measured in millimeters, a vein graft remains the "gold standard." Potential donor sites are the ipsilateral forearm and the dorsal foot. The contralateral forearm is often needed for vascular access. The more distal the injury in the forearm into the hand, the narrower the conduit that will be needed, and the veins on the dorsum of the foot are a good match (Fig. 10.7). Often injuries are in contaminated wounds, and although not an

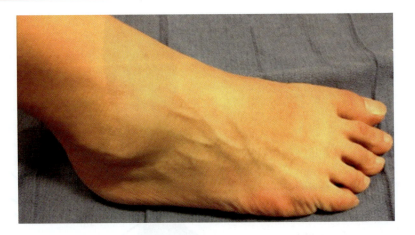

Fig. 10.7 Dorsal foot veins. A good donor site for vein grafts because of size match and minimal donor site morbidity

absolute contraindication to the use of prostheses for arterial repair, it is usually reserved for larger-caliber arteries, not extremity arteries [25].

10.6.1 Radial Artery Injury

As previously stated, the radial artery is not the dominant source of circulation to the hand, and if perfusion to the distal portion of the injured extremity is adequate, as evidenced by good capillary refill of the digits including the thumb, warmth, and a dopplerable signal over the palmar arch, the artery does not need to be repaired or reconstructed, unless the two ends are in close proximity. However, if the distal extremity shows any evidence of inadequate perfusion, the vessel should be repaired. If the mechanism of injury was a sharp transection of the artery, the ends can be repaired primarily. Additional length can be achieved by careful dissection of the vessel ends, allowing a tension-free repair of the artery. If there is segmental loss of the vessel, a graft will be needed to reconstruct it. A vein or arterial conduit can be used, with recent reports noting that arterial grafts might have higher patency [26]. It is likely however that the operative technique is a far more important factor in successful reconstruction.

10.6.2 Ulnar Artery Injury

The ulnar artery is the dominant artery to the hand. In most patients, however, it appears that

there is sufficient perfusion to the hand via the radial artery alone. Numerous studies of the ulnar artery forearm flap, which requires ligation of the ulnar artery, suggest that repair may not be essential to maintain adequate hand perfusion [27–29]. Regardless, the same operative principles as for radial artery injuries apply here.

10.6.3 Digital Artery Injury

There is normally an ulnar and a radial digital artery to each finger; thus, either can be sacrificed without consequence. After establishing that there is adequate perfusion of the digit from the contralateral neurovascular bundle, bleeding can be controlled usually by closing the skin laceration and applying pressure, after confirming that the digital nerve is intact. If the injury is circumferential to the digit, a repair or reconstruction of at least one digital artery will be required to establish perfusion to the distal finger. Repair requires the use of an operative microscope, and if there is segmental loss, a vein graft will be needed.

10.7 Endovascular Management

Over the past decade, there has been an increase in the use of endovascular techniques for management of trauma, from stenting traumatic dissections of the internal carotid to embolization techniques to stop hemorrhage from a pelvic fracture or solid organ injuries [30, 31]. There have been reports of the use of endovascular techniques in the management of brachial artery injuries of the upper arm with angioplasty and stenting for intimal disruptions and thrombosis and for transections [32, 33]. However, the utility of endovascular techniques remains limited for more distal injuries in the arm to endovascular embolization for transection, pseudoaneurysm, or arteriovenous fistula [11]. In the setting of acute trauma, injuries distal to the axillary artery are typically addressed surgically.

10.8   Fasciotomies

Prophylactic forearm fasciotomies should be performed in all extremities presenting with more than a few hours of ischemia due to the high risk of postoperative compartment syndrome secondary to reconstitution of arterial flow, leading to ischemia/reperfusion syndrome [34]. A very high index of suspicion should be maintained due to the profound morbidity associated with untreated compartment syndrome of the upper extremity.

Anatomically, the forearm can be divided into three compartments: dorsal, volar, and mobile wad compartments (Table 10.3). The dorsal or extensor compartment contains the finger, thumb, and ulnar wrist extensors. The volar or flexor

Table 10.3   Forearm compartments

Compartments	Muscles
Dorsal	*Superficial* – extensor digitorum communis, extensor carpi ulnaris, and extensor digiti minimi
	Deep – abductor pollicis longus, extensor pollicis brevis, extensor pollicis longus, extensor indicis, and supinator
Volar	*Superficial* – pronator teres, palmaris longus, flexor digitorum superficialis, flexor carpi radialis, and flexor carpi ulnaris
	Deep – flexor digitorum profundus, flexor pollicis longus, and pronator quadratus
Mobile wad	Brachioradialis, extensor carpi radialis longus, and extensor carpi radialis brevis

compartment contains the finger, thumb, and wrist flexors. The mobile wad or radial compartment of the forearm contains the brachioradialis, extensor carpi radialis longus, and extensor carpi radialis brevis. In the hand, there are ten compartments: four dorsal interosseous, three palmar interosseous, adductor pollicis, thenar, and hypothenar compartments.

10.8.1   Diagnostic Testing

In addition to the clinical findings associated with compartment syndrome, the pressure within the compartment in question can be measured. Although compartment syndrome is a clinical diagnosis, the measured pressure can aid when evaluating unconscious patients or when there is doubt in the diagnosis [35]. There are multiple methods, including the needle manometer, wick and slit catheters, and side-ported needle, with the latter technique appearing to be as accurate as the slit catheter [36–40]. The most commonly used cutoff pressure for the diagnosis of compartment syndrome is 30 mmHg [37, 41]. All three compartments of the forearm and ten compartments of the hand should be measured (Figs. 10.8 and 10.9). The clinical exam should always guide the surgeon in deciding whether or not to perform a fasciotomy. Seemingly normal compartment pressures in the setting of a concerning physical exam should not reduce the index of suspicion for compartment syndrome.

10.8.2   Operative Management of Compartment Syndromes of the Forearm and Hand

The three forearm compartments can be released usually via volar and dorsal incisions, as shown in Fig. 10.10. Through the volar incision, the lacertus fibrosus at the level of the elbow is released to decompress the median nerve, and the fascia of the forearm is opened from proximal to distal releasing the muscles of the volar compartment. The carpal tunnel should be released distally to ensure a full decompression (Fig. 10.11).

Fig. 10.8 Forearm compartments. At the junction of the proximal and middle third of the forearm, compartment measurements should be obtained. (**a**) Ulnar approach using ulna as guide to measure the deep volar compartment. (**b**) Dorsal approach to measure dorsal compartment

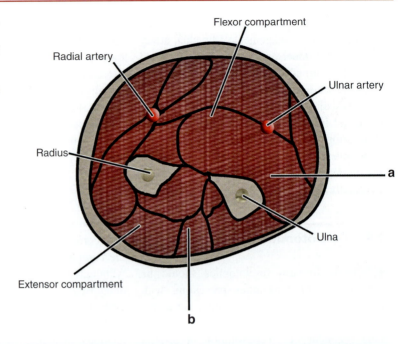

Fig. 10.9 Hand compartments – interosseous, thenar, hypothenar, and adductor compartments can be measured through these points

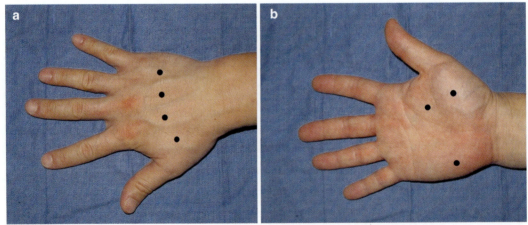

After releasing the volar compartment, one can either clinically or via direct compartment measurement determine if the other compartments of the forearm need to be released. Often time, by releasing the volar compartment, the remaining compartments do not need to be decompressed. If pressures remain elevated, a dorsal incision, as shown in Fig. 10.10, can be used to decompress the dorsal and mobile wad compartments.

Compartment syndrome of the hand is uncommon in acute penetrating trauma but can often be seen in patients with burns to the hand and high-pressure injection injuries [42]. Elevated compartment pressures are not well tolerated in the hand compartments, and so much lower values are considered indications for fasciotomy than in the forearm, with pressures greater than 15–20 mmHg being a relative indication for fasciotomy [43]. As shown in Fig. 10.12, the

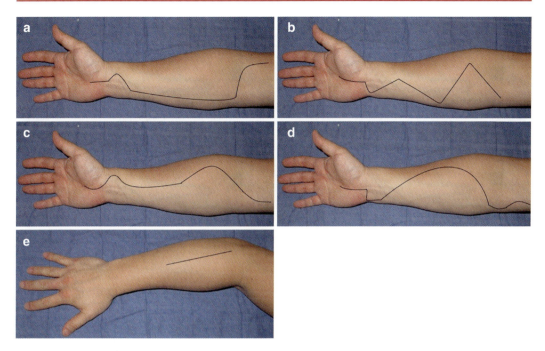

Fig. 10.10 Forearm fasciotomy. (**a-d**) Volar incision: several incisions have been used. (**e**) Dorsal incision: a line from lateral epicondyle to mid-wrist up to the junction of the middle and thirds of the forearm

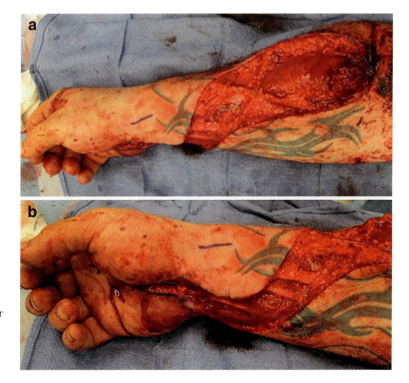

Fig. 10.11 (**a**) Forearm fasciotomy – a case of compartment syndrome after a brachial artery transection from a dog bite. (**b**) Volar incision extending through the carpal tunnel

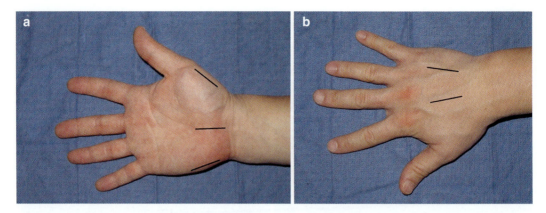

Fig. 10.12 (**a**) Ventral incision and (**b**) dorsal incision

dorsal and palmar interosseous compartments can be released via two dorsal incisions: the thenar and hypothenar compartments via incisions over the radial and ulnar aspect of the hand, respectively, and the adductor compartment via a carpal tunnel incision.

Once the compartments have been released, if skin closure is not possible, the arm/hand is immobilized in a non-compressive dressing and elevated. A delayed skin closure or skin grafting may need to be done once there is resolution of the edema. Ultimately, if the magnitude of injury to multiple systems in the hand and forearm is significant enough, then amputation may be the best option [44].

10.9　Complications

Early postoperative complications include vascular occlusion after either a primary repair or interposition graft and bleeding from disruption of the repair. These will require immediate reoperation. Iatrogenic injury to surrounding structures should be extremely limited if proper techniques are used and a detailed knowledge of upper extremity anatomy is employed.

10.10　Outcomes

Vascular trauma can cause a high degree of morbidity with severe consequences on function [45]. However, an approach that acknowledges

the upper extremity as a "multiorgan system" comprised of skin, blood vessels, musculotendinous structures, bones, and nerves will often result in excellent outcomes.

Conclusion

Vascular injuries to the forearm and hand have a wide variety of presentations. Although successful vascular reconstruction is the foundation for limb survival, appropriate management of injuries to concomitant structures, such as nerves, tendons, bone, and missing soft tissue, is mandatory for adequate limb function [6, 46]. A systematic and thorough approach combining history, physical exam, diagnostic studies, and coordination with other specialties will ensure the best possible outcomes.

References

1. Perry MO, Thal ER, Shires GT. Management of arterial injuries. Ann Surg. 1971;173(3):403–8.
2. Prichayudh S, Verananvattna A, Sriussadaporn S, Sriussadaporn S, Kritayakirana K, Pak-art R, et al. Management of upper extremity vascular injury: outcome related to the Mangled Extremity Severity Score. World J Surg. 2009;33(4):857–63.
3. Klocker J, Falkensammer J, Pellegrini L, Biebl M, Tauscher T, Fraedrich G. Repair of arterial injury after blunt trauma in the upper extremity – immediate and long-term outcome. Eur J Vasc Endovasc Surg. 2010; 39(2):160–4.
4. Joshi V, Harding GE, Bottoni DA, Lovell MB, Forbes TL. Determination of functional outcome following upper extremity arterial trauma. Vasc Endovascular Surg. 2007;41(2):111–4.

Overview of Chest Trauma

11

David J. Milia and Jasmeet S. Paul

Contents

D.J. Milia (✉) • J.S. Paul, MD
Division of Trauma and Critical Care,
Department of Surgery,
Medical College of Wisconsin,
Milwaukee, WI, USA
e-mail: dmilia@mcw.edu

11.1   Introduction

Injuries to the chest from both blunt and penetrating mechanisms account for approximately one-quarter of all traumatic deaths in the United States annually [1]. The majority of all chest injuries can be managed non-operatively with simple maneuvers such as securing a protected airway and performing a tube thoracostomy. To ensure the remaining patients receive the best chance at a meaningful survival, a firm understanding of the relevant anatomy, appropriate resuscitation techniques, surgical exposure, and operative management is of critical importance.

11.2   Anatomy

The anatomy of the thorax is complex and a detailed understanding of the relationship of surgically relevant structures is necessary for efficient exposure. Thorough overviews of the bony thorax, pleural cavities, and structures of the mediastinum can be found elsewhere in this text and in other resources. As an overview, this chapter serves to focus on the surface anatomy of the chest and how external landmarks relate to underlying anatomic structures.

11.3   Anatomic Definitions

11.3.1 Chest

The bony thorax consists of 12 paired ribs, 12 thoracic vertebrae, and the sternum. The fixation

A. Dua et al. (eds.), *Clinical Review of Vascular Trauma*,
DOI 10.1007/978-3-642-39100-2_11, © Springer-Verlag Berlin Heidelberg 2014

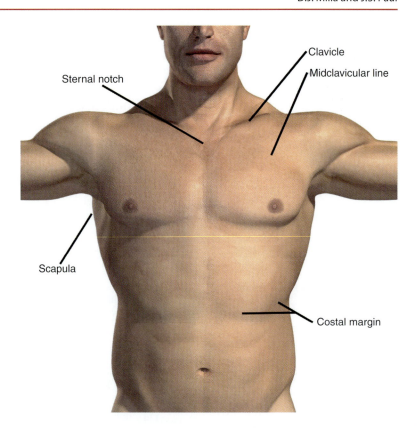

Fig. 11.1 Surface landmarks of the chest. The
craniocaudal border of the
chest is therefore defined as
the clavicle to the costal
margin. Posteriorly, the
inferior border lies at the
inferior margin of the
scapula

of the first through tenth ribs anteriorly (sternum)
and posteriorly (vertebrae) limits the deforma-
tions in the thoracic cage during the respiratory
cycle. The underlying diaphragm, however, can
be found as superior as the fourth thoracic vertebra or as inferiorly displaced as the costal margin
depending on where in the respiratory cycle the
patient is. The craniocaudal border of the chest is
therefore defined as the clavicle to the costal margin. Posteriorly, the inferior border lies at the
inferior margin of the scapula (Fig. 11.1). Injuries
within these borders are considered chest wounds
and require evaluation as outlined later in this
chapter.

There is crossover between the superior border of the abdomen and the inferior border of the
chest. Superiorly, the border of the abdomen is
defined as the nipple line. Wounds existing in the
area between the nipple (or inframammary fold
for females) and the costal margin are considered

thoracoabdominal and warrant both a thoracic
and abdominal evaluation.

11.3.2 The "Box"

The majority of stab wounds (approximately
80 %) causing injury to the heart enter through the
precordium. This area, often referred to as the
"box," is defined as an area bounded superiorly by
the clavicles, laterally by the nipples, and inferiorly by the xiphoid process (Fig. 11.2). This four-
sided area is extended posteriorly to the back.
Injuries to this area and missiles with trajectories
passing through this area mandate the proper cardiac evaluation as defined later in this section. It
should be noted that the majority of gunshot
wounds causing cardiac injury do not enter
through this anatomic area, so suspicion based on
presumed trajectory and clinical presentation is

Fig. 11.2 The box. The majority of stab wounds (around 80 %) causing injury to the heart enter through the precordium. This area, often referred to as the "box," is defined as an area bounded superiorly by the clavicles, laterally by the nipples, and inferiorly by the xiphoid process

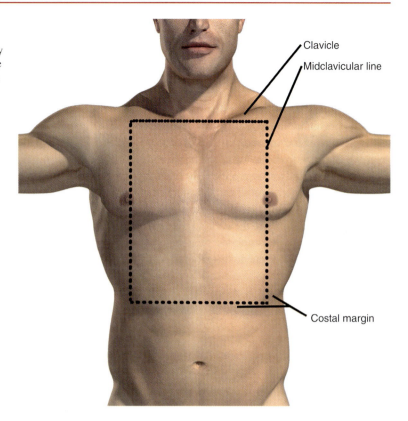

Clavicle

Midclavicular line

Costal margin

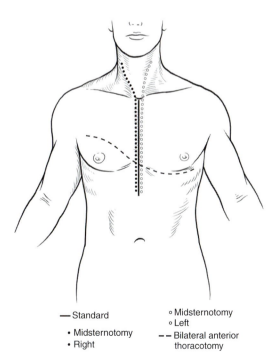

— Standard

• Midsternotomy
• Right

∘ Midsternotomy
∘ Left

– – Bilateral anterior
      thoracotomy

Fig. 11.3 Chest incisions

necessary for accurate and timely diagnosis [2]. The standard array of chest incisions are depicted in Fig. 11.3.

11.4   Anatomic Relationships

11.4.1 Heart

As stated above, the injuries to the precordium (especially stab wounds) are associated with a higher incidence of cardiac injury. Externally, the superior border of the heart lies approximately at the second intercostal space bordered laterally by points approximately 2 cm lateral to either side of the sternum. The inferior border, formed by the right ventricle, can be thought of as connecting the point of maximal impulse to the right sixth costal cartilage. Connecting the margins of the inferior and superior borders estimates the lateral borders of the heart. The left ventricle creates the left lateral border of the heart.

11.4.2 Arch Vessels

Arising from the aortic valve in the fibrous trigone of the heart, the short ascending aorta gives rise to the aortic arch. The arch is oriented primarily in the anterior-posterior plane with some leftward deviation beginning in the midline and ending up just to the left of the vertebral column. The three great vessels arise from the top of the aortic arch. Beginning proximally, they are the right brachiocephalic, left common carotid, and left subclavian arteries. The great vessels, in combination with the ligamentum arteriosum, fix the aorta to the chest. Over 90 % of aortic disruptions seen in blunt trauma occur in this area due to this fixation point.

11.4.3 Subclavian

The left subclavian artery arises reliably from the aortic arch. The right side typically arises from the brachiocephalic artery but may, rarely, arise directly from the aortic arch or from a common trunk shared by the right common carotid artery. Bilaterally, the arteries are divided into three parts by the anterior scalene muscles. The medial portion gives off the vertebral artery and thyrocervical trunk. The portion deep to the muscle gives rise to the costocervical artery. Laterally, the artery is without branches becoming the axillary artery as the artery crosses the medial portion of the clavicle.

11.5   Assessment and Initial Management

All patients with suspected injuries to the thorax should be evaluated and resuscitated according to the principles of the American College of Surgery-Committee On Trauma (ACS-COT) Advanced Trauma Life Support (ATLS) guidelines and protocols [3]. The primary survey will address immediate threats to life and will aid in the triage and further management of all injured patients. Prior to arrival, there should be communication with the transporting emergency services team in order to ascertain the hemodynamic status of the patient. Patients may be thought of as hemodynamically normal or abnormal or have

lost signs of life and are actively undergoing cardiopulmonary resuscitation, the latter potentially qualifying for a resuscitative (ED) thoracotomy.

Patients should undergo a standard airway assessment as outlined in ATLS. The decision to secure a patient's airway is multifactorial and takes into consideration the patient's physiologic presentation as well as other injuries. One pitfall is failure to recognize a tension pneumothorax in a patient presenting with respiratory distress. Patients presenting with respiratory distress with decreased breath sounds or a hyperinflated hemithorax along with hypotension (assessment of jugular venous distension may be compromised in the face of hypovolemia) should have their chest decompressed prior to attempting intubation. The reason is threefold: respiratory distress may resolve following appropriate chest decompression alleviating the need for intubation, intubation of a patient with tension physiology is difficult due to shifting anatomy, and induction agents may worsen the patient's shock state and hasten their cardiovascular collapse.

The importance of a properly inserted tube thoracostomy in the setting of thoracic trauma cannot be overstated. The majority of patients presenting with thoracic trauma will require only a thoracostomy tube in the management of their injuries. Findings of hemodynamic lability or respiratory distress should cue the treating physician to the potential need for a chest tube. Imaging studies are not necessary in this setting. Stable patients with abnormal physical exam findings (decreased breath sounds, crepitance, hyperinflation, etc.) can proceed with portable radiographic imaging prior to undergoing thoracostomy. The ideal location for a tube thoracostomy is in the mid-axillary line at approximately the level of the xiphoid (a consistent landmark which reduces the chances of placing the tube in the major fissure). While a 36 French or larger tube has been traditionally recommended, emerging data suggest a smaller tube may be as effective. For patients in extremis, however, a 36 French tube is still recommended [4, 5]. In the setting of acute trauma, a collection system with autotransfusion capability should always be considered. There is no indication to clamp a chest tube in the setting of trauma as this increases the potential for creating an iatrogenic tension pneumothorax. In the setting of a massive air leak leading to an inability to ventilate the patient, the tube may be placed to water seal en route to the operating room for definitive pulmonary repair.

If not addressed in the field, large-bore intravenous access should rapidly be obtained above the diaphragm in patients with thoracic trauma. If appropriate peripheral access cannot be obtained, there are many commercially available rapid infusion devices for placement into the subclavian, internal jugular, or femoral veins. Alternatively, interosseous access can rapidly be obtained in the humeral heads and/or tibias presuming the accessed extremities are uninjured. Patients with penetrating injuries are at increased risk for requiring a massive transfusion (MT, >10 units of blood in the first 24 h). Numerous clinical and laboratory predictors of MT exist and have been studied. One such model, referred to as the "ABC Score," examined non-weighted clinical parameters to determine the risk [6]. Patients with two of the following—penetrating mechanism, positive focused assessment sonography for trauma (FAST), initial $SBP \leq 90$ mmHg, and arrival $HR \geq 120$ bpm—are at significant increased risk for MT. As such, institutions treating unstable patients with penetrating thoracic wounds should have an MT protocol, which can be rapidly initiated.

Increased data have been reported targeting a lower systolic blood pressure in the resuscitation of patients sustaining penetrating trauma until vascular control is obtained. Following early preliminary work by Mattox, the landmark study by Bickell found patients (penetrating only) undergoing delayed resuscitation to have a survival benefit over those receiving a traditional resuscitation [7]. A large multicenter study is currently enrolling to examine if these findings are applicable to patients presenting to institutions with varying pre-hospital transport times and are inclusive of blunt injured patients.

Resuscitative thoracotomy (RT), originally described for medical cardiac arrest in the nineteenth century, gained acceptance in the trauma population soon after. The specific indications, however, have evolved since its first description and are still disputed today. There are those groups advocating a more restrictive approach and those purporting a liberal approach. Guidelines published by the American College of Surgery-Committee on Trauma (ACS-COT) discourage performing an RT on victims of blunt trauma presenting with cardiac arrest and sparingly in those that lose vital signs on presentation to the trauma center. They report the excessively low survival and low likelihood of neurological recovery. RT should be restricted to victims of penetrating trauma and in patients with witnessed physiologic parameters (vital signs, telemetric activity, pupillary reflexes, etc.) arriving to the trauma center within 15 min of EMS arrival [8]. This recommendation is supported in a recent retrospective study by Mollberg where after almost a decade of RTs at one institution, a strict adherence to the ACS-COT guidelines would account for all potential survivors while, at the same time, avoiding inappropriate resource utilization and operative hazards to healthcare providers [9]. The Western Trauma Association (WTA) has recently published guidelines promoting a more liberal approach to RT [10]. Their review, however, lacks appropriate evidence and is likely applicable to only a few trauma centers worldwide. Future evolution regarding RT is the concept of intravascular aortic occlusion. This is accomplished by inserting an inflatable balloon in the descending aorta through the femoral artery. Comparative data between this technique and the standard RT are currently time lacking.

11.6 Imaging

As in the case of all injured patients, the need for and choice of imaging studies will be dictated by the pattern of injury and clinical status. Patients presenting in extremis require few, if any, radiographs prior to proceeding to the operating room. Stable patients, conversely, may require more advanced imaging modalities depending on their injury pattern to further characterize their injuries prior to intervening.

In general, an AP chest film should be obtained sometime during the primary survey or soon thereafter. During the initial, primary survey, symptomatic, life-threatening airway and breathing problems can be addressed without imaging.

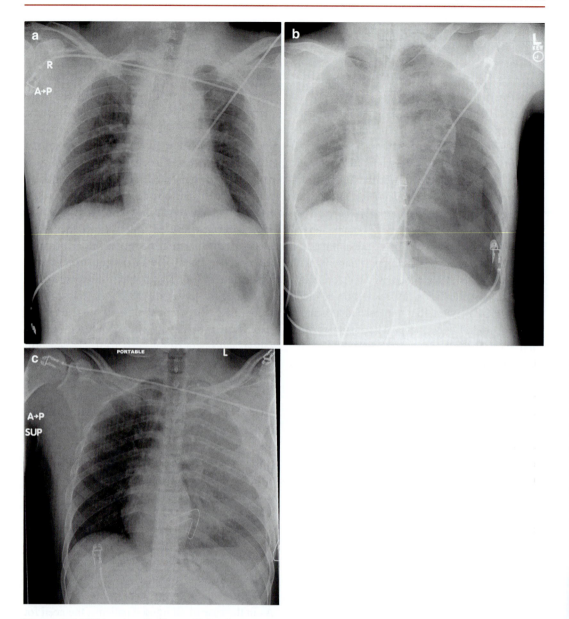

Fig. 11.4 (**a**) Widened mediastinum. (**b**) Tension pneumothorax. (**c**) Massive hemothorax

Concerns for symptomatic and tension pneumo-thoraces should be treated without delay. The chest film is regarded as a part of the circulatory assessment in order to evaluate for thoracic hem-orrhage. Hypotensive patients without signs of obstructive shock need to be evaluated for cavi-tary hemorrhage and a chest film is part of this assessment.

If not obtained during the primary survey, an x-ray of the chest should be performed as a resuscitative adjunct while the patient is undergo-ing a thorough secondary evaluation. Patients presenting with penetrating chest injuries should have radiographic markers placed over wound sites prior to imaging. If the clinical situation allows, a semierect film with the patient in the

Fig. 11.5 FAST view of pericardial window

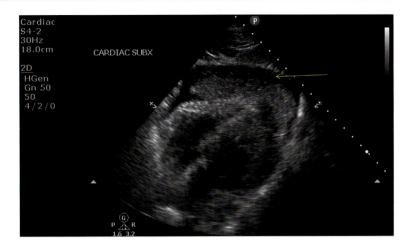

seated position is preferable. The XR is evaluated for tracheal position, parenchymal disease, hemopneumothorax, and mediastinal widening (Fig. 11.4a–c). Tube thoracostomy should be considered for all hemopneumothoraces seen on plain radiograph. Consideration should be given to connecting the chest tube to a collection system with autotransfusion capabilities. Stable patients with low-velocity penetrating injuries (i.e., stab wounds) presenting with normal radiographs may be safely discharged if a repeat film in 4–6 h fails to show the development of a pneumothorax [11]. Emerging data suggest patients may be safely discharged even earlier than the accepted 4–6 h [12]. Ultrasound has gained popularity for evaluation of blunt abdominal trauma and as such is being used with increasing frequency for the evaluation of thoracic injuries. Although operator dependent, the Focused Abdominal Sonogram for Trauma (FAST) exam carries a high specificity for the presence intraperitoneal fluid [13]. Part of the FAST exam includes a four-chamber subxiphoid view of the heart to evaluate for pericardial fluid (Fig. 11.5). In studies of patients with penetrating thoracic injuries, sensitivity and specificity have been noted as high as 97 % for cardiac injury [14]. The presence of a left hemo-/pneumothorax may reduce accuracy of ultrasound and further diagnostic workup may be necessary in this setting. Transesophageal echocardiography may have a

role in diagnosing cardiac and aortic injuries. This modality, however, is more invasive and operator dependent than traditional transthoracic echocardiography.

CT angiography has virtually replaced traditional aortography with regard to blunt chest trauma. This was evidenced in a comparison study between two similar AAST multicenter prospective studies separated by a decade (1997 and 2007) looking at blunt aortic injury [15]. The 2007 study noted a near-complete elimination of conventional angiography and TEE, with nearly all patients undergoing CT angiography [15]. Although limited prospective studies exist, stable patients presenting with transmediastinal gunshot wounds may be safely evaluated with axial imaging following appropriate primary and secondary surveys. The results of such an imaging study will determine the need for further diagnostic workup or operative interventions needed. The benefit of CTA is in its ability to delineate missile tract and vascular injury. Missile tracts remote from worrisome structures will help to limit further imaging studies. If concern for injury based on trajectory remains, further workup (e.g., endoscopy or fluoroscopy for esophageal evaluation) is warranted. Stable patients with periclavicular injuries should also have a CT angiogram to assess for vascular injury. Management of specific vascular injuries is addressed elsewhere in this text.

11.7   Overview of Operative Management

Figure 11.3 details the traditional incisional approaches to the chest cavity.

11.7.1 Resuscitative Thoracotomy

Resuscitative thoracotomy (RT), also known as emergency department thoracotomy, is an emergent procedure performed for a patient in extremis. Guidelines and indications for RT have been developed and proposed by several organizations including the ACS-COT as described above. The best results have been reported in patients with penetrating cardiac injuries as patients with penetrating non-cardiac thoracic injuries have a low survival rate.

The primary objectives of RT are release of pericardial tamponade, control of major vascular or cardiac bleeding, evacuation of bronchovenous air embolus, initiation of open cardiac massage, and control of the descending thoracic aorta [16]. Obviously, not every patient undergoing an RT will require all of these maneuvers, but this serves as a basic framework and a stepwise approach to the procedure.

Patients should be supine with their arms out to the side to allow for concurrent vascular access. This is the very definition of an emergency procedure and typical operation room practices need not be followed. If time allows, a stack of blankets is placed under the left hemithorax to elevate the chest. The chest is rapidly prepped with Betadine while the surgeon dons gloves and widely drapes out the entire chest with towels.

The incision is a left anterolateral thoracotomy made in the fourth or fifth intercostal space. In men this is the inferior border of the pectoralis muscle, and in women, the inframammary crease. The incision starts at the middle of the sternum and is continued laterally, curving upward towards the axilla to follow the curve of the rib, and terminates at the bed (Fig. 11.6). The underlying subcutaneous tissue and muscle are divided sharply until the chest wall is exposed. The chest is entered sharply on the superior aspect of the rib

to avoid the intercostal neurovascular bundle. Intercostal muscle and parietal pleura can then be divided with a scalpel or heavy scissors. A self-retaining rib spreader such as a Finochietto retractor is placed with the handle directed towards the bed in the axilla or towards the midline if the need for further exposure is anticipated. The sternum can be divided with a heavy scissors, trauma shears, or Lebsche knife to provide exposure to the heart and right chest if necessary. The internal mammary arteries will not bleed in the patient in extremis but will need to be ligated if the patient survives. The incision can be converted to a bilateral anterior thoracotomy (clamshell incision) by extending the incision across the sternum onto the right through the same intercostal space or going up one space. This incision provides exposure to the pulmonary artery, ascending aorta, aortic arch, innominate artery and vein, left common carotid artery, pulmonary hilum, and azygos vein.

Once the left chest has been entered and blood has been evacuated, the first maneuver is to evaluate the pericardium, relieve cardiac tamponade, and control cardiac injury. A normal-appearing pericardium does not rule out injury and a pericardiotomy should always be performed. The pericardium is grasped with Allis clamps anterior to the phrenic nerve and opened longitudinally, parallel to the phrenic nerve, with scissors (Fig. 11.7). If the pericardium is tense with underlying clot, it may be difficult to grasp, and the pericardium can be incised with a scalpel and then opened with scissors. All clots should be evacuated and bleeding sites should be controlled initially with digital pressure. Injuries to the atria may be controlled with side-biting vascular clamps prior to repair. Simple running suture or mattress sutures with 2-0 or 3-0 monofilament polypropylene suture should be used. A finer-gauge suture may be used; however, needle size is a consideration. Wounds in the ventricle can be controlled with digital pressure until definitive repair can be performed or temporally closed using a skin stapler. Attempting to control a ventricular wound with an inflated Foley catheter may inadvertently enlarge the wound and should be avoided.

Fig. 11.11 Trapdoor
incision

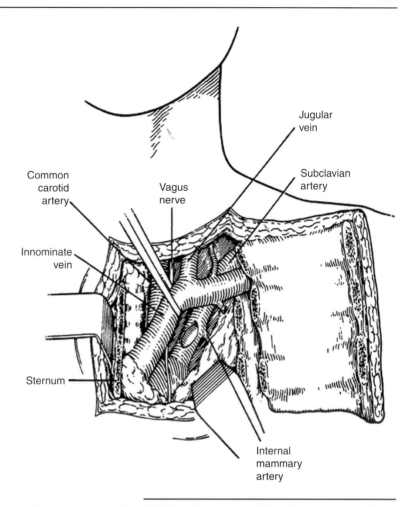

"trapdoor" is performed by making a standard left anterolateral thoracotomy in the fourth interspace (Fig. 11.11). A supraclavicular incision is then made 2 cm above the clavicle starting at the sternal notch extending laterally. The platysma is divided and the origins of the sternocleidomastoid and omohyoid muscles are exposed and divided. The carotid sheath is exposed and retracted medially exposing the anterior scalene muscle which is divided while preserving the phrenic nerve. The subclavian artery is then identified and controlled. A skin incision is made over the upper sternum to connect the medial borders of the supraclavicular and thoracotomy incisions. The sternum is divided with a sternal saw beginning at the suprasternal notch down to the fourth interspace. A sternal retractor is used to elevate the "trapdoor" and expose the entire artery for repair [4]. Most subclavian injuries can be repaired with primary repair or interposition grafts.

11.9   Postoperative Management

Specific post-op care of patients with chest injuries will be governed by the specific injuries and the exact procedure(s) performed. Patients having undergone a massive blood component resuscitation and prolonged operative course are at high risk for coagulopathy. These issues must be addressed immediately upon admission to the intensive care unit. Chest tubes should be placed to suction, and output should be followed closely as increased output despite correction of coagulopathy should prompt further workup and consideration for return to the operating room. Although numerous guidelines exist for determining when to remove chest tubes, they should remain in place until air leaks resolve, output has diminished (~100 cc/day), and the lung remains inflated with the collection system on water seal.

Patients suffering significant trauma, especially thoracic trauma, are at risk for developing acute respiratory distress syndrome (ARDS). This syndrome may develop indirectly following a large resuscitation or directly as a result of direct lung injury. Low-tidal-volume ventilation has been shown to decrease mortality in such patients, and thus patients should be screened daily for the presence of ARDS. Preliminary data have suggested that the benefits of a lung-protective ventilation strategy may extend to all patients, but strong evidence is lacking [22].

Other standard ICU practices should be followed. This includes, but is not limited to, appropriate venous thromboembolism (VTE) prophylaxis, enteric nutrition, and early removal of central lines and urinary catheters. A single perioperative dose of antibiotics is sufficient, and no data exist for subsequent doses unless needed to treat a specific infection.

References

1. Khandhar SJ, Johnson SB, Calhoon JH. Thoracic trauma overview of thoracic trauma in the United States. Thorac Surg Clin. 2007;17(1):1–9.
2. Buckman RF. Heart. In: Ivatury RR, Cayten CG, editors. The textbook of penetrating trauma. Baltimore: Williams & Wilkins; 1996. p. 500–1. Print.
3. Committee on Trauma, American College of Surgeons. ATLS: Advanced Trauma Life Support program for doctors. 8th ed. Chicago: American College of Surgeons; 2008.
4. Kulvatunyou N, Vijayasekaran A, Hansen A, Wynne JO, O'keefe T, Friese RS, Joseph B, Tang A, Rhee P. Two-year experience of using pigtail catheters to treat traumatic pneumothorax: a changing trend. J Trauma. 2011;71(5):1104–7.
5. Inaba K, Lustenberger T, Recinos G, Georgiou C, Velmahos GC, Brown C, Salim A, Demetriades D, Rhee P. Does size matter? A prospective analysis of 28–32 versus 36–40 French chest tube size in trauma. J Trauma Acute Care Surg. 2012;72(2):422–7.
6. Nunez TC, Voskresensky IV, Dossett LA, et al. Early prediction of massive transfusion in trauma: simple as ABC (assessment of blood consumption)? J Trauma. 2009;66(2):346–52.
7. Bickell WH, Wall Jr MJ, Pepe PE, Martin RR, et al. Immediate versus delayed fluid resuscitation for hypotensive patients with penetrating torso injuries. N Engl J Med. 1994;331(17):1105–9.
8. Working Group, Ad Hoc Subcommittee on Outcomes, American College of Surgeons. Committee on Trauma. Practice management guidelines for emergency department thoracotomy. Working Group, Ad Hoc Subcommittee on Outcomes, American College of Surgeons-Committee on Trauma. J Am Coll Surg. 2001;193(3):303–9.
9. Mollberg NM, Glenn C, John J, et al. Appropriate use of emergency department thoracotomy: implications for the thoracic surgeon. Ann Thorac Surg. 2011;92(2):455–61. Epub 2011 Jun 25.
10. Burlew CC, Moore EE, Moore FA, et al. Western trauma association critical decisions in trauma: resuscitative thoracotomy. J Trauma Acute Care Surg. 2012;73(6):1357–61.
11. Kerr TM, Sood R, Buckman Jr RF, Gelman J, Grosh J. Prospective trial of the six hour rule in stab wounds of the chest. Surg Gynecol Obstet. 1989;169(3): 223–5.
12. Berg RJ, Inaba K, Recinos G, Barmparas G, Teixeira PG, Georgiou C, Shatz D, Rhee P, Demetriades D. Prospective evaluation of early follow-up chest radiography after penetrating thoracic injury. World J Surg. 2013;37(6):1286–90.
13. Stengel D, Bauwens K, Sehouli J, Porzsolt F, Rademacher G, Mutze S, Ekkernkamp A. Systematic review and meta-analysis of emergency ultrasonography for blunt abdominal trauma. Br J Surg. 2001; 88(7):901–12.
14. Rozycki GS, Feliciano DV, Ochsner MG, et al. The role of ultrasound in patients with possible penetrating cardiac wounds: a prospective multicenter study. J Trauma. 1999;46(4):543–51; discussion 551–2.
15. Demetriades D, Velmahos GC, Scalea TM, et al. Diagnosis and treatment of blunt thoracic aortic injuries: changing perspectives. J Trauma. 2008;64(6): 1415–8; discussion 1418–9.
16. Mejia JC, Stewart RM, Cohn SM. Emergency department thoracotomy. Semin Thorac Cardiovasc Surg. 2008;20(1):13–8.
17. Ivatury RR. Resuscitative thoracotomy. In: Ivatury RR, Cayten CC, editors. The textbook of penetrating trauma. Philadelphia: Williams & Wilkins; 1996. p. 207–15.
18. Mattox KL. Thoracic great vessel injury. Surg Clin North Am. 1988;68(4):693–703.
19. Valentine RJ, Wind GG. Thoracic aorta. Anatomic exposures in vascular surgery. 2nd ed. Philadelphia: Lippincott, Williams & Wilkins; 2003.
20. Brewster SA, Thirlby RC, Snyder 3rd WH. Subxiphoid pericardial window and penetrating cardiac trauma. Archives of surgery. 1988;123(8): 937–41.
21. Hoyt DB, Coimbra R, Potenza BM, Rappold JF. Anatomic exposures for vascular injuries. Surg Clin North Am. 2001;81(6):1299–330, xii.
22. Serpa Neto A, Cardoso SO, Manetta JA, et al. Association between use of lung-protective ventilation with lower tidal volumes and clinical outcomes among patients without acute respiratory distress syndrome: a meta-analysis. JAMA. 2012;308(16): 1651–9.

Heart and Great Vessel Injuries

12

Martin A.S. Meyer, Jesper B. Ravn,
and Justin L. Regner

Contents

Jesper B. Ravn, MD and Justin L. Regner, MD contributed
equally as senior authors.

M.A.S. Meyer, BSc
Section for Transfusion Medicine,
Capital Region Blood Bank, Rigshospitalet,
Copenhagen University Hospital,
Copenhagen, Denmark

Department of Surgery,
Center for Translational Injury Research,
The University of Texas Health Science Center,
Houston, TX, USA

J.B. Ravn, MD
Department of Cardiothoracic Surgery,
Rigshospitalet, Copenhagen University Hospital,
Copenhagen, Denmark

J.L. Regner, MD (✉)
Trauma, Critical Care and Acute Care Surgery,
Scott and White Memorial Hospital,
Texas A&M University, Temple, TX, USA
e-mail: justin@yahoo.com

12.1   Introduction

Penetrating and blunt cardiac injuries are by their very nature extremely lethal, and consequently only a fraction of patients with a cardiac wound will be alive when reaching the hospital [1–4]. Patients that do arrive to the ED with penetrating thoracic trauma can be divided broadly into three hemodynamic categories on a continuum of physiologic derangements from "in extremis" or near death (5 %) to unstable (15 %) to stable (80 %), and for the former category immediate surgery and often a massive blood transfusion is the only treatment modality that offers possible survival [5]. For patients that arrive without any sign of life, only a select group is eligible for an emergency department thoracotomy [6, 7]. While the decision to operate is readily made for unstable patients, stable patients with a possible cardiac wound, i.e., patients with a penetrating injury or high-energy blunt force to the precordium but presenting without any apparent physiologic abnormalities, can be challenging to correctly diagnose and treat in a safe, timely, and minimally invasive fashion. Patients with suspected

A. Dua et al. (eds.), *Clinical Review of Vascular Trauma*,
DOI 10.1007/978-3-642-39100-2_12, © Springer-Verlag Berlin Heidelberg 2014

cardiac and great vessel injuries in extremis should receive the standard ED thoracotomy via a left anterolateral thoracotomy. Different imaging modalities, such as focused assessment with sonography in trauma (FAST), echocardiography, and computed tomographic arteriogram (CTA), can assist the diagnosis, but if equivocal a pericardial window may be the only way of ruling out intrapericardial bleeding [2, 3, 8–10].

The majority of blunt cardiac injuries (BCI) are contusions to the myocardium that can be treated conservatively with telemetry and expectant management; however, severe BCI may cause myocardial defects or valvular injuries which may require surgical repair with cardiopulmonary bypass. Historically the frequency of injury to the heart chambers in penetrating injuries has been reported to be predominantly and evenly affecting the ventricles, and less frequently the atria, with the left atrium being the least frequent [11]; this of course is highly dependent on the mechanism of injury and the trajectory of the wounding object. Accordingly, efforts should be made to establish the forces involved in the injuring process, e.g., bullet caliber, range, and for stab wounds the length of the object, as this will assist the diagnostic process.

Blunt cardiac injury (BCI) can be the result of a high-energy impact to the thorax, crushing, or a rapid deceleration [2, 3]. In cases of rapid deceleration, the heart may suffer injuries where fixed structures attach to the freely suspended heart, predominantly at the atria-vena cava junction and pulmonary vein [2, 3]. BCI can also result due to cardiac squeezing or sudden changes in intrathoracic or intra-abdominal pressure and may include cardiac rupture – often right atrium, septal injury, or valvular insufficiency [2]. In cases involving a blunt mechanism of injury, e.g., a motor vehicle accident, the injury to the heart itself may be of a penetrating nature, due to sharp fragments of bone from a rib, sternum, or spinal fracture, and therefore might not be readily observable during initial inspection.

12.2 Anatomy and Physiology

12.2.1 Anatomy

Salvaging trauma patients with cardiac and great vessel injuries requires intimate knowledge of both anatomy and physiology. The surgical anatomy includes the anterior, middle, posterior, and superior mediastinum, its vasculature and nerves. Physiology includes cardiac tamponade, hemorrhagic shock, and projectile path.

The mediastinum is defined by the diaphragm inferiorly, the pleura laterally, the sternum anteriorly, and the vertebral column posteriorly. Surgically, the mediastinum should be evaluated from the perspective of what is injured in the pericardium versus what could be injured outside the pericardium. The pericardium is a robust fibrous sac that completely contains and protects the heart. Its strength forms the basis of tamponade. The pericardium contains the heart, proximal ascending aorta, pulmonary artery, pulmonary veins, and inferior portion of the superior vena cava. In addition to these structures, the phrenic nerves reside in the lateral middle mediastinum bilaterally.

The remainder of the mediastinal structures resides outside the pericardium. The anterior mediastinum is mainly a potential space between the pericardium and sternum. Bleeding in this area is usually self-limited if from sternal fractures, but occasionally arises from internal mammary or proximal intercostal artery injuries. The posterior mediastinum contains the esophagus, descending thoracic aorta, thoracic duct, vagus nerves, and azygous and hemiazygous veins. These structures are discussed in preceding chapters. The superior mediastinum is divided from the middle mediastinum by the pericardium. This division may serve as a road map of safety to gain initial control of superior mediastinal hemorrhage since hematomas in this area are relatively uncontained making dissection difficult. The superior mediastinum includes the aortic arch, innominate, left carotid, and left subclavian arteries; innominate vein; superior portion of the superior vena cava; and vagus, recurrent laryngeal, and phrenic nerves.

The nerves of the mediastinum are easy to injure and difficult to locate in trauma. Bilateral phrenic nerves arise from cervical roots 3–5. The right runs inferiorly on the anterior border of the anterior scalene and enters the thoracic cavity anterior to the second portion of the subclavian artery but posterior to the subclavian vein. It then proceeds caudally to the inferior vena cava hiatus in the diaphragm by passing anterior to both the right atria and the right pulmonary hilum. The left phrenic nerve descends along the anterior scalene and passes into the thoracic cavity anterior to the first portion of the subclavian artery, posterior to the vein. It then passes anterior to the left pulmonary hilum and over the pericardium of the left ventricle to the left diaphragm. The left vagus nerve descends to the thoracic cavity in the carotid sheath. It passes anterior to the aortic arch between the left carotid and subclavian arteries. At the level of the aortic arch, it branches into the vagus and left recurrent laryngeal nerve. The left recurrent laryngeal nerve ascends superiorly to the larynx in the tracheoesophageal groove. The vagus descends into the abdomen posterior to the left pulmonary hilum to become the anterior vagus of the stomach as it exits the esophageal hiatus. The right vagus nerve descends in the carotid sheath and passes anterior to the right subclavian artery to divide into the recurrent laryngeal and the vagus. The right vagus then descends posterior to the pulmonary hilum to the esophageal hiatus to become the posterior vagus of the stomach.

12.2.2 Physiology

Cardiac and great vessel injuries create hemodynamic instability and death due to either cardiac tamponade or hemorrhagic shock. Cardiac tamponade is similar to the Monroe Doctrine of brain injury. The pericardium is a fairly fixed container divided into two separate spaces, intracardiac and extracardiac. Increases in one space force corresponding decreases in the other. With traumatic cardiac tamponade, the time to cardiac failure is based on the etiology of the blood source. If it is

an atrial injury or partial ventricular injury, it can be hours. Eventually the extracardiac pressure begins to approximate or exceed the atrial filling pressure with resultant hypotension and venous congestion. This hypotension can initially be overcome with increased preload, but is only a temporization. Cardiac tamponade left untreated will eventually result in cardiac failure with equalization of the extracardiac and intracardiac (both atrial and ventricular) pressures.

Hemorrhagic shock by its very nature requires blood loss; however, the source of shock may not be evident at first. Penetrating thoracic trauma to the heart and great vessels can hemorrhage directly from the entry and exit wounds or into an adjacent body cavity. However, these intrathoracic injuries may actually be tangential with the source of hemorrhage from another organ and body cavity. Historically the frequency of injury to the heart chambers with penetrating mechanisms has been reported predominantly affecting the ventricles, and less frequently the atria, with the left atrium being the least frequent [10]; this is highly dependent on the mechanism of injury and the trajectory of the wounding object. Accordingly, efforts should be made to establish the forces and vector involved in the injuring process, e.g., bullet caliber, range, and for stab wounds the length of the object, as this will assist in diagnosing. Cardiac injuries typically present with tamponade or direct bleeding. Great vessel injuries, on the other hand, can be more insidious. These superior mediastinal contents may suffer blast effect or contusion, tangential injuries, partial wall injury with pseudoaneurysm formation, or branch vessel injury. This difference in injury pattern accounts for the range of hemodynamic profiles present with this patient population.

12.3 Clinical Assessment and Diagnostic Testing

The aim of this section is to discuss the advantages and shortcomings of clinical signs, imaging modalities, and other diagnostic procedures in evaluating cardiac, great vessel, and hilar injuries. It must be emphasized again that emergent thoracotomy should not be delayed by diagnostic procedures in hemodynamically unstable patients and especially patients "in extremis." A simple and direct algorithm was developed by Mattox in 2000 and remains applicable today (Fig. 12.1).

Any patient with a penetrating mechanism, specifically a projectile, is at risk of a cardiac injury with subsequent cardiac tamponade or hemorrhage [2, 9, 12]. Traditionally, trauma surgeons have been taught to expect a cardiac injury when an exterior wound was located in "the box" (Fig. 12.2). However, with current military and civilian ballistics, cardiac injury can occur from any entry point into the body. The earliest signs of hemorrhage are due to sympathetic nervous system surge with increases in heart rate, respiratory rate, and peripheral vascular resistance, i.e., narrowed pulse pressure. On exam, these patients will have pallor, agitation, or anxiety [11–13]. If blood is collecting in the pericardium rather than being drained either externally or into the thoracic cavity, a cardiac tamponade can occur. Awake patients early in tamponade physiology will not be comfortable in the supine position as this compromises their venous return and right heart cardiac output. Many of the classical signs of tamponade or Beck's triad, i.e., muffled heart sounds, distension of jugular veins, and hypotension will often be absent or difficult to observe in the trauma bay [12]. Frequently trauma patients early in the tamponade physiology may not present with any symptoms of cardiac injury and yet later succumb to cardiac tamponade or exsanguinating wounds. In fact, an increased mortality from cardiac trauma has been reported in large case series when the exterior wound was located away rather than inside the precordium, possibly due to a lower-level of suspicion and attention from the clinical team [9].

Evaluation of the trauma patient and specifically the unstable patient occurs best with a regimented approach. Blunt injury to the pericardium can be evaluated in the same manner as penetrating. Portable chest radiographs remain the best initial film to assess the thorax for injury and ballistic vector. The FAST exam or ultrasound is the trauma surgeon's best friend in evaluating for internal bleeding [14]. All unstable blunt trauma patients once the initial ABC's of trauma are complete require a FAST exam [14, 15]. Patients with penetrating thoracic trauma require a focused cardiac ultrasound to evaluate for pericardial effusion [16, 17].

The FAST is specific and sensitive for intra-abdominal and cardiac injuries with a sensitivity for intra-abdominal fluid of 81–88 %, 99 %

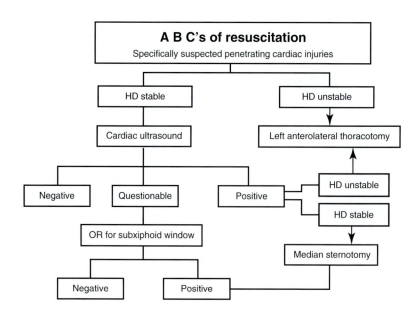

Fig. 12.1 Management of cardiac injuries (Adapted from Mattox et al. [31])

A B C's of resuscitation
Specifically suspected penetrating cardiac injuries

HD stable

HD unstable

Cardiac ultrasound

Left anterolateral thoracotomy

Negative

Questionable

Positive

HD unstable

HD stable

OR for subxiphoid window

Median sternotomy

Negative

Positive

Fig. 12.2 The mediastinum is defined by the diaphragm inferiorly, the pleura laterally, the sternum anteriorly, and the vertebral column posteriorly

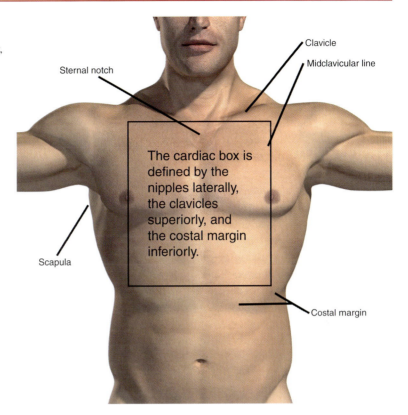

Sternal notch

Clavicle

Midclavicular line

The cardiac box is defined by the nipples laterally, the clavicles superiorly, and the costal margin inferiorly.

Scapula

Costal margin

specificity, and 97 % accuracy and sensitivity of pericardial fluid approaching 100 % [14–16]. The ultrasound can also evaluate pneumo- and hemothorax with excellent sensitivity assuming the patient does not have subcutaneous emphysema [16, 18]. If the patient is stable and the penetrating mechanism crosses the mediastinum without evidence of cardiac injury on ultrasound, then these patients require evaluation of their mediastinum for injuries. Multi-detector CTA of the chest provides excellent evaluation of the superior mediastinal vascular structures [19]. In addition, these images will assist with surgical planning, incision choice, and evaluation of other injuries. If concern remains regarding middle mediastinal injury, then the subxiphoid pericardial window should be considered the gold standard for detecting blood in the pericardium [8, 12]. For the most part penetrating cardiac and great vessel injuries will be diagnosed by either exsanguinating hemorrhage, ultrasound of the pericardium, CTA or angiography of the chest, or subxiphoid window.

Video-assisted thoracic surgery (VATS) is being introduced to evaluate hemodynamically stable patients for intrapericardial injuries [20]. We recommend a modified VATS approach, using only partial pulmonary deflation, and limiting the deflation to a few respiratory cycles, as well as reserving this diagnostic approach for the completely stable patients as not all patients will tolerate the periprocedural reduction in pulmonary capacity. This approach could be combined with an otherwise indicated chest tube placement. Unstable patients should be evaluated by TTE or TEE at the bedside or in the operating theater for the detection of complex cardiac injuries such as cardiac wall and septal defects, valvular insufficiency, or injuries to the pulmonary artery and vein [20]. For stable patients, a chest X-ray and 12-lead ECG should be obtained to screen patients suspected of myocardial ischemia or contusion, conduction abnormalities, or arrhythmias that may be present in BCI [2, 21]. Biomarkers of myocardial cell damage are generally not used to estimate the seriousness of injury as they can be either normal or elevated in the presence of significant cardiac injury [3]. However in blunt trauma, the combination of a normal ECG, normal chest X-ray, and normal levels of troponin I has a very high negative predictive value [22, 23].

12.4 Initial Management

Initial assessment and management of trauma patients should adhere to ATLS guidelines [11]. Specifically, unstable patients with suspected cardiac and great vessel injuries must have a secure airway, decompression or evaluation for tension pneumohemothorax, and adequate venous access as these patients are the highest-risk patients for receiving a massive blood transfusion [24]. Thoracotomy should not be delayed in the unstable patient. Every effort should be made to reuse the patient's blood via Cell Saver or autotransfusion from the Pleurovac.

Cardiac tamponade is the most typical presentation of a stable penetrating cardiac injury. Ironically, these patients generally remain stable as long as the tamponade persists. These patients require judicious boluses of intravenous fluids or blood products as the increased preload allows them to overcome the increased extrinsic forces of the tamponade on the thin-walled right atria and ventricle. This preloading is especially important while laying the patient flat to induce anesthesia.

12.5 Surgical Management

12.5.1 Choice of Incision and Supportive Care

Cardiac injury should be expected in all patients with mediastinal wound or when entry and/or exit wounds suggest a trans-mediastinal trajectory and in hemodynamically unstable patients with a relevant mechanism of injury and no other detected source of bleeding. Unstable patients should proceed with the most expedite incision, the left anterolateral thoracotomy. If injuries to

the great vessels, right hilum, or right heart need to be addressed then this incision can be extended across the sternum, i.e., the clam shell, for an excellent view of the entire anterior chest. For stable patients the median sternotomy should be considered as it offers good exposure of the heart, great vessels, and both pleural cavities [2, 8, 12]. In addition this incision can be extended up the neck or across the clavicles to address carotid and subclavian artery injuries as well.

For a subgroup of patients with acute cardiac failure due to their injuries, or when lung injuries cause a critically decreased ability to oxygenate, extracorporeal life support can offer a chance of survival [25–27]. As many trauma patients are already coagulopathic at admission, anticoagulation for extracorporeal life support should only be used with outmost caution. It can therefore be preferable to omit systemic anticoagulation and instead use extracorporeal membrane oxygenation (ECMO) tubing and filters coated with anticoagulation agents, e.g., heparin-like substances.

12.5.2 Specific Injuries and Repair

Upon entering the thorax, the pericardium should be evaluated for blood, and any clotted blood should be evacuated to allow cardiac filling and complete inspection.

12.5.2.1 Trauma Thoracotomy
The trauma patient should be prepped from the neck to the bilateral groins if time permits in preparation of emergent laparotomy for multi-cavity injuries, exposure and harvesting of the thigh veins, or extension into the neck for distal control. Both arms should be extended and abducted to allow anesthesia further venous or arterial access as required. Left anterolateral thoracotomy should begin on the sternum and extend along the fourth or fifthth intercostal space in the infra-pectoral or inframammary fold down to the intercostal muscles. Heavy Mayo scissors will divide the intercostal muscle insertion just above the inferior rib. Upon entering the thorax, open the chest with the rib spreader handle laterally to prevent impeding medial extension across the

sternum if required. The thorax should be evacuated of blood, and the inferior pulmonary ligament divided to just distal to the inferior pulmonary vein, which resides in the superior portion of the ligament. This maneuver will allow the lung to be mobilized or packed laterally away from the heart.

The pericardium should always be evaluated for blood. The only definitive mechanism to assess the pericardium for blood is to open it. The pericardium is usually tense and typically cannot be grasped with forceps. It should be pinched between fingers or grasped with an Allis clamp. Once the pericardium is lifted away from the heart, it should be incised and open with Metzenbaum scissors anterior and parallel to the phrenic nerve. Any clotted blood should be evacuated to allow cardiac filling and complete inspection. Cardiac tamponade, although lethal if allowed to progress, can be protective against exsanguination and is associated with an early survival advantage [7, 9]. Opening the tense pericardium can result in rapid exsanguinating bleeding, and blood products should be readily available to account for this. To insure early hemostasis digital pressure should be applied to the injured myocardium or vessels until a definitive repair can be accomplished.

If the cardiac chambers feel empty, the descending thoracic aorta should be occluded to maintain cardiac and cerebral perfusion. With the lung lifted anterior or superiorly, the aorta can be palpated to the left side of the vertebral column. If the aorta is flaccid due to the hemorrhagic shock, an orogastric tube can be passed to assist palpating the esophagus. Do not clamp this structure; the aorta should be left and lateral to the tube. The pleural overlying the aorta should be incised both anterior and posterior to the aorta. This incision can be performed with Metzenbaum scissors or fingers and should only be large enough to allow a straight or curved vascular clamp access. Too extensive dissection or spreading posterior to the aorta can injure the intercostal arteries and create more difficult to control bleeding.

The left anterolateral thoracotomy only allows adequate access to the left chest, left pulmonary hilum, left ventricle, and lateral right ventricle. If the patient's injuries involve the right chest, right heart, or great vessels, then the incision will need to extend across the sternum to the right third or fourth intercostal space. The sternum can be divided with a powered reciprocating bone saw, Gigli saw, or Lebsche knife. Once divided and the patient is stabilized, the internal mammary arteries must be ligated. The arteries receive dual blood supply; therefore, bilateral proximal and distal ends must be ligated.

12.5.2.2 Atrial

Atrial defects can be isolated by use of a vascular clamp (e.g., a Satinsky clamp) and repaired with nonabsorbable monofilament 2–0 or 3–0 suture (e.g., Prolene) by simple running or horizontal mattress suturing [7, 8]. Given the thin atrial wall and its consequent risk of tearing, a horizontal mattress can be advantageous [7, 8]. The suture bites should be full thickness to minimize atrial myocardial tear and maintain hemostasis. The most difficult part of suturing the myocardium (all chambers) is tying the knot with the appropriate tension. The tendency is for too much tension and subsequent tearing of the heart thereby creating a more severe injury.

12.5.2.3 Ventricular

Ventricular defects can be more challenging to suture than the atria due to the increased chamber pressures and vigorous contractions. Ventricular lacerations are repaired using 2–0 or 3–0 nonabsorbable monofilament sutures by simple, running, or horizontal mattress techniques, but should not be full-thickness bites to prevent injuring intraventricular structures. To avert having the sutures tear through the myocardium, the use of pledgets (0.5×1 cm), either Teflon or pieces of the pericardium, may be necessary [5, 8].

Injuries adjacent to the coronary arteries should be repaired utilizing horizontal mattress sutures, placed beyond or distal to the artery (Figs. 12.3 and 12.4) [7]. Lacerations of the coronary arteries can by managed by ligation if located in the distal third or small branches, while proximal injuries will likely require coronary artery bypass grafting (CABG) but are rarely survivable. If a penetrating object is retained in the

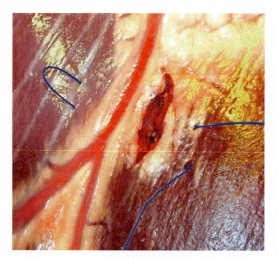

Fig. 12.3 Suture with no pledget. Injury adjacent to coronary artery. Use horizontal mattress technique and place the sutures deep and distant to the artery. Care should be taken not to restrict coronary blood flow when tightening the suture

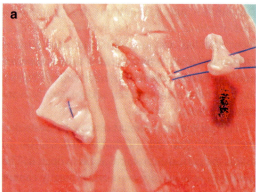

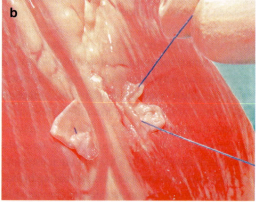

Fig. 12.4 Injury adjacent to coronary artery. Horizontal mattress technique as in Fig. 12.3. To avoid tearing the myocardium, pledgets can be utilized. Here shown with "pledgets" made impromptu from the pericardium. Shown before (**a**) and after (**b**) tightening the suture. Use same depth and distance to the coronary artery as without pledgets

wound, sutures must be placed prior to removing the object (Fig. 12.5).

Care should be given not to injure or restrict the flow of coronary arteries when suturing in their proximity. If ischemia occurs, the suture tension should be released or the entire suture should be replaced with the mattress stitch more distal to the artery.

Posterior cardiac injuries most commonly involve the left ventricle. These injuries are difficult to repair via a median sternotomy. A left anterolateral thoracotomy allows better access. Any upward traction of the heart can cause cardiac arrest due to outflow obstruction. Access to the posterior heart can be gained by sequential packing of gauze behind the heart to elevate.

12.5.3 Intracardiac Injuries

Intracardiac injuries can be difficult to diagnose initially if the patient is not evaluated with TTE or TEE, and some studies report a relatively high incidence of delayed diagnosis for these valvular injuries and septal defects [21, 22, 28]. Intracardiac injuries require cardiopulmonary bypass with systemic anticoagulation and cardiac

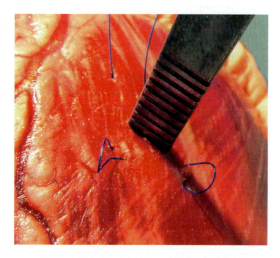

Fig. 12.5 Retained objects should be removed only when sutures have already been placed. Tighten the loop as the object is removed

arrest for repair. This might not be possible or even beneficial in the acute hemorrhagic setting. If the injuries are not threatening to strain the heart, which could otherwise result in cardiac failure, *and* adequate circulation with perfusion can be maintained, then it may be optimal to delay repair until the patient has stabilized. The repair of intracardiac injuries is a daunting task and should only be performed by a surgeon specialized in cardiac surgery.

12.5.4 Injuries to the Pulmonary Arteries and Veins

Hemorrhaging pulmonary hilar injuries have a high mortality rate due to rapid exsanguination and are very challenging to control or repair. The hilar structures are difficult to access, and proximal pulmonary artery or vein injuries often require extracorporeal circulation during repair. Hilar clamping requires complete mobilization of the inferior pulmonary ligament and often requires two hands to guide the Satinsky clamp around the hilum. This proximal control can facilitate bleeding cessation and alleviate the passage of air emboli from the injured lung, but will increase cardiac afterload considerably and might not be tolerated by the already strained right heart.

The lung twist technique described by Mattox is for peripheral pulmonary injuries and should not be used in cases of hilar injuries. If attempted with hilar injuries, it may create further tearing of the vessels and should be used only as a last resort. If en bloc pneumonectomy is considered, then proceed quickly with a vascular load TA stapler as a compromised heart will not survive this increased afterload. Survival from this can be as high as 42 %, but postoperative care may require extracorporeal membrane oxygenation (ECMO) [29].

12.5.5 Injuries to the Great Vessels

First rule of great vessel injuries is to keep it simple and call for help. Second rule is to consider shunting all complex injuries initially, especially the carotid artery.

Patients with injuries to the great vessels present in two manners: relatively stable after blunt or penetrating mechanisms or unstable after penetrating mechanisms. Stable patients with trauma to the great vessels are typically diagnosed on CTA of the chest. These patients allow for time to plan operative approach and seek specialists' assistance. Advancements in endovascular techniques have made open repair of great vessel injuries less frequent and have greatly improved at least short-term outcomes [30].

Penetrating injury to the great vessels creates unstable patients; therefore, the trauma surgeon frequently is forced to explore these injuries emergently via a clam shell incision. If, however, these patients arrive reasonably stable and best projectile mapping suggests injuries to the superior mediastinum, then a median sternotomy will allow increased access and versatility to approach the great vessels. The incision should be started 2 cm superior to the manubrium and extend 2 cm beneath the xiphoid process. Blunt dissection along the posterior aspect of the sternum will create a safe plane for placement of a sternal saw or Lebsche blade. While dividing the sternum always lift away from the patient and heart to protect the mediastinal structures. At completion of the sternotomy, bone bleeding can be controlled with cautery, bone wax, or lap pads behind the sternal retractors.

Once the chest is open, two scenes evolve: either a large expanding hematoma or pulsatile bleeding. Pulsatile bleeding should be controlled by finger compression, usually the assistant's. To gain access to the great vessels, the thymus should be divided first. The next structure to be identified and encountered is the innominate vein. If it is the only injury and less than ½ the circumference is involved, simple repair with 4–0 or 5–0 nonabsorbable monofilament suture via lateral wall venorrhaphy is sufficient. If it is completely transected or deeper mediastinal access is required, the innominate vein should be divided and ligated.

Once the left innominate vein is controlled, mobilization of the aortic arch and great vessels is required to explore the mediastinum, control bleeding, and repair injuries. The easiest method to define the anatomy and facilitate exploration is to open the pericardium in the midline and extend this incision superiorly along the ascending aorta. The pericardial reflection should be divided along the patient's right side of the ascending aorta, thereby completely freeing anterior mobilization of the aortic arch.

At this point with the innominate vein divided and the pericardium open, the heart, ascending aorta, aortic arch, and great vessels (specifically innominate artery and left carotid) should be completely exposed. Before further dissection continues, the vagus nerve anatomy should be verified. Both vagus nerves descend from the neck in the carotid sheath between the carotid artery and jugular vein. The right vagus nerve will pass anterior to the right subclavian artery and then dive deep to the pulmonary hilum after the right recurrent laryngeal wraps around the subclavian artery to ascend superiorly in the tracheoesophageal groove. The left vagus nerve will descend lateral to the carotid artery, and it will pass anterior to the aortic arch between the carotid artery and subclavian artery ostia where the left recurrent laryngeal nerve wraps around the arch.

With the mediastinum exposed and the bleeding controlled, reconstruction with the assistance of intraoperative consults to cardiovascular surgery should be considered. Regarding specific injuries, simple aortic injuries can be repaired with side-biting clamps and interrupted suture of 3–0 monofilament. The great vessels may be shunted or occluded with balloon catheters while proximal and distal exposure and control is attained. Distal control may require extending the median sternotomy incision in the direction of the vessel injured. The proximal great vessel injuries may require bypass from the aorta with Dacron or ePTFE interposition grafts prior to exposure of the injury or as definitive repair. Distal injuries will be repaired with interposition grafts if simple repair is not possible.

12.5.6 Special Considerations

The use of Foley catheters to occlude and control bleeding from myocardial defects facilitates temporary hemostasis; however, there is risk of enlarging the defect when inflating the catheter, and their use should be limited [8]. The Foley catheter technique should use saline to inflate the balloon to just large enough to control the bleeding (usually <10 mL). Skin staplers may allow rapid repair of myocardial injuries and could possibly reduce the risk for needlestick injuries; however, this technique may not provide adequate hemorrhage control and the long-term effects of skin staplers in the myocardium are largely unknown [7]. Sternal closure may be omitted initially in patients that remain unstable after initial repair and resuscitation or when return to the OR for re-exploration after stabilization in the ICU is expected; instead a vacuum closure such as Vacuum-assisted closure (VAC) can be used. Acutely, the surgeon can "pack" the patient with gauze or hemostatic dressing if bleeding persists and cover with a dressing.

12.5.7 Equipment

Most cardiac injuries can be repaired with a minimum of equipment; however, due to the very acute nature of cardiac bleeding, preparations should be made to ensure immediate availability of the following (Fig. 12.6):

- Disinfectant fluid for rapidly prepping the patient
- Scalpel, scissors, needle holder, and forceps
- Rib retractor
- Vascular clamps, e.g., a Satinsky clamp, and two long curved clamps
- 2–0 and 3–0 monofilament nonabsorbable sutures and skin staplers for temporary repairs
- Internal defibrillator paddles

12.6 Postoperative Management

Postoperatively patients should be monitored and evaluated for the development of tamponade, arrhythmias, conduction abnormalities, or heart failure after admission to the surgical ICU. Temporary pacing may be necessary especially in patients with septal injuries, and these temporary epicardial electrodes should optimally be placed during surgery. If a TEE has not been performed

Fig. 12.6 An example of a "kit" for emergency thoracotomy. Disinfectant fluid, sutures, and internal defibrillator paddles not shown

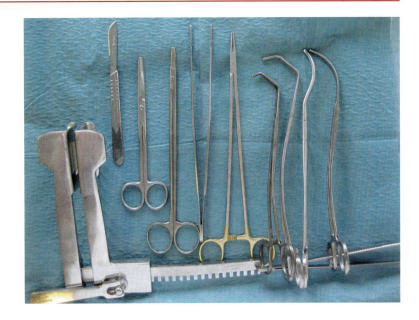

intraoperatively, all patients with cardiac injury should postoperatively receive a TEE to assess for injuries to the septum or valves and/or decreased wall motion. If myocardial ischemia is evident, coronary angiography (CAG) and percutaneous coronary intervention (PCI) with balloon dilation or stenting can be performed if the patient's condition allows. This also includes ischemia secondary to surgical repair of cardiac wounds, with sutures inadvertently causing strictures of coronary arteries.

12.7 Outcomes

For cardiac injuries the reported mortality rates are highly variable; however, early predictors of poor outcome includes prehospital loss of vital signs, asystole, and fixed dilated pupils at admission, and the perioperative observation of global myocardial stunning, collapsed coronary arteries, and the presence of air emboli in the coronary veins [7, 12]. Stab wounds rather than gunshot wounds are reported to have more favorable outcomes [7, 12]. In blunt cardiac injury there are often associated injuries in other organ systems including the central nervous system which accordingly will influence the outcomes in a negative direction [3].

Conclusion

The management of the trauma patient is often dictated by local guidelines and influenced by available diagnostic capabilities and surgical expertise. Cardiac and great vessel injuries come with a high level of morbidity and mortality, requiring prompt diagnosis and often surgical repair. A high level of suspicion is necessary as symptoms might not be present at admission though the patient may have a potentially mortal cardiac wound. We recommend that a cardiovascular surgeon be consulted early if cardiac or great vessel injury is suspected as complex injuries will require cardiopulmonary bypass and complex surgical repair.

References

1. Campbell NC, Thomson SR, Muckart DJ, Meumann CM, Van Middelkoop I, Botha JB. Review of 1198 cases of penetrating cardiac trauma. Br J Surg. 1997; 84:1737–40.
2. El-Menyar A, Al TH, Zarour A, Latifi R. Understanding traumatic blunt cardiac injury. Ann Card Anaesth. 2012;15:287–95.
3. Nan YY, Lu MS, Liu KS, et al. Blunt traumatic cardiac rupture: therapeutic options and outcomes. Injury. 2009;40:938–45.

4. von Oppell UO, Bautz P, De GM. Penetrating thoracic injuries: what we have learnt. Thorac Cardiovasc Surg. 2000;48:55–61.

5. Lenworth MJ, Gross R, Luk S. Advanced trauma operative management. Woodbury, CT: American College of Surgeons, Cine-Med, Inc; 2004.

6. Moore EE, Knudson MM, Burlew CC, et al. Defining the limits of resuscitative emergency department thoracotomy: a contemporary Western Trauma Association perspective. J Trauma. 2011;70:334–9.

7. Asensio JA, Soto SN, Forno W, et al. Penetrating cardiac injuries: a complex challenge. Injury. 2001;32:533–43.

8. O'Connor J, Ditillo M, Scalea T. Penetrating cardiac injury. J R Army Med Corps. 2009;155:185–90.

9. Degiannis E, Loogna P, Doll D, Bonanno F, Bowley DM, Smith MD. Penetrating cardiac injuries: recent experience in South Africa. World J Surg. 2006;30:1258–64.

10. Wall Jr MJ, Mattox KL, Chen CD, Baldwin JC. Acute management of complex cardiac injuries. J Trauma. 1997;42:905–12.

11. American College of Surgeons. Advanced trauma life support for doctors. 8th ed. Chicago: American College of Surgeons; 2008.

12. Kang N, Hsee L, Rizoli S, Alison P. Penetrating cardiac injury: overcoming the limits set by nature. Injury. 2009;40:919–27.

13. Casos SR, Richardson JD. Role of thoracoscopy in acute management of chest injury. Curr Opin Crit Care. 2006;12:584–9.

14. Rozycki GS, Ochsner MD, Schmidt JA, et al. A prospective study of surgeon-performed ultrasound as the primary adjuvant modality for injured patient assessment. J Trauma. 1995;39:492–500.

15. McKenney MG, Martin L, Lentz K, et al. 1,000 Consecutive ultrasounds for blunt abdominal trauma. J Trauma. 1996;40:607–12.

16. Rozycki GS, Feliciano DV, Ochsner MG, et al. The role of ultrasound in patients with possible penetrating cardiac wounds: a prospective multicenter study. J Trauma. 1999;46:543–52.

17. Alrajhi K, Woo MY, Vaillancourt C. Test characteristics of ultrasonography for the detection of pneumothorax: a systematic review and meta-analysis. Chest. 2012;141(3):703–8.

18. Sisley AC, Rozycki GS. Rapid detection of traumatic effusion on using surgeon-performed ultrasonography. J Trauma. 1998;44:291.

19. O'Connor JV, Scalea TM. Penetrating thoracic great vessel injury: impact of admission hemodynamics and preoperative imaging. J Trauma. 2010;68:834–7.

20. Wall Jr MJ, Soltero ER. Trauma to cardiac valves. Curr Opin Cardiol. 2002;17:188–92.

21. Cha EK, Mittal V, Allaben RD. Delayed sequelae of penetrating cardiac injury. Arch Surg. 1993;128:836–9.

22. Velmahos GC, Karaiskakis M, Salim A, et al. Normal electrocardiography and serum troponin I levels preclude the presence of clinically significant blunt cardiac injury. J Trauma. 2003;54:45–50.

23. Cook CC, Gleason TG. Great vessel and cardiac trauma. Surg Clin North Am. 2009;89:797–820.

24. Cotton BA, Dossett LA, Haut ER, et al. Multicenter validation of a simplified score to predict massive transfusion in trauma. J Trauma. 2010;69:S33–9.

25. Evans BJ, Hornick P. Use of a skin stapler to repair penetrating cardiac injury. Ann R Coll Surg Engl. 2006;88:413–4.

26. Reade MC. Temporary epicardial pacing after cardiac surgery: a practical review. Part 2: selection of epicardial pacing modes and troubleshooting. Anaesthesia. 2007;62:364–73.

27. Reade MC. Temporary epicardial pacing after cardiac surgery: a practical review: part 1: general considerations in the management of epicardial pacing. Anaesthesia. 2007;62:264–71.

28. Demetriades D, Charalambides C, Sareli P, Pantanowitz D. Late sequelae of penetrating cardiac injuries. Br J Surg. 1990;77:813–4.

29. Halonen-Watras J, O'Connor J, Scalea M. Traumatic pneumonectomy: a viable option for patients in extremis. Am Surg. 2011;77(4):493–7.

30. Hershberger RC, Aulivola D, Murphy M, Luchette FA. Endovascular grafts for treatment of traumatic injury to the aortic arch and great vessels. J Trauma. 2009;67(3):660–71.

31. Mattox et al. Trauma. 4th ed. 2000.

Thoracic Aortic Injuries

13

Ahmed Al-Adhami, Sapan S. Desai,
and Ali Azizzadeh

Contents

A. Al-Adhami, MBChB (Hons), MSc
Department of Cardiothoracic Surgery,
Golden Jubilee National Hospital, Glasgow, UK

S.S. Desai, MD, PhD, MBA
Department of Surgery,
Duke University, Durham, NC, USA

Department of Cardiothoracic and Vascular Surgery,
University of Texas Medical School,
Houston, TX, USA

A. Azizzadeh, MD (✉)
Department of Cardiothoracic and Vascular Surgery,
University of Texas Houston Medical School,
Houston, TX, USA

Memorial Hermann Heart & Vascular Institute,
Texas Medical Center, Houston, TX, USA
e-mail: ali.azizzadeh@uth.tmc.edu

13.1   Introduction

Injury to the aorta and the arch vessels can occur following blunt and penetrating trauma. While penetrating trauma commonly occurs secondary to gunshot and stab wounds, blunt trauma is often secondary to motor vehicle accidents. Traumatic aortic injury (TAI) is the second most common cause of death after blunt trauma [1, 2]. In recent autopsy series involving traffic accidents, 33 % of the victims had associated TAI, with 80 % dying prior to hospital arrival [2]. TAI is a significant modern health problem. Considering that 37,661 motor vehicular deaths occurred in 2010, an estimated 12,553 (33 %) may have involved TAI [3]. In comparison, aortic aneurysms and dissections were responsible for 10,397 deaths in the same year. Significant advancements have been made in the diagnosis and treatment of aortic injuries over the past two decades. These include the widespread use of CTA for diagnosis, medical management of minimal aortic injuries, delayed repair (>24 h) for stable patients, and broad implementation of endovascular repair. This chapter describes the anatomy, pathophysiology, diagnosis, management, and outcomes of TAI.

A. Dua et al. (eds.), *Clinical Review of Vascular Trauma*,
DOI 10.1007/978-3-642-39100-2_13, © Springer-Verlag Berlin Heidelberg 2014

13.2 Anatomy

13.2.1 Ascending Aorta

The ascending aorta begins within the pericardial sac, gives off the right and left coronary arteries at the root of the aorta, and travels approximately 5 cm before giving off the branches of the aortic arch.

13.2.2 Aortic Arch

The brachiocephalic, left common carotid, and left subclavian arteries (LSAs) are the three major branches of the arch in most patients. The brachiocephalic artery bifurcates to form the right common carotid and right subclavian arteries (Fig. 13.1). The ligamentum arteriosum is the remnant of the patent ductus arteriosum, which shunts blood from the pulmonary artery to the aorta during development.

13.2.3 Descending Aorta

The descending aorta begins after the ligamentum arteriosum and travels to the aortic hiatus at the level of the diaphragm near the T12 vertebra, where it becomes the abdominal aorta. The thoracoabdominal aorta lies posterior to the esophagus at this level, near which it gives off bronchial arteries, esophageal arteries that travel to the middle third of the esophagus, several mediastinal arteries that travel to the posterior mediastinum, pericardial arteries, nine pairs of posterior intercostal arteries that supply the 3rd–11th intercostal spaces, two subcostal arteries, superior phrenic arteries that supply the diaphragm, and a number of lumbar branches that travel to the spinal cord.

13.2.4 Variant Anatomy

A variety of congenital alterations to the aortic arch exist, such as the true bovine arch and so-called bovine arch. The true bovine arch is a rare

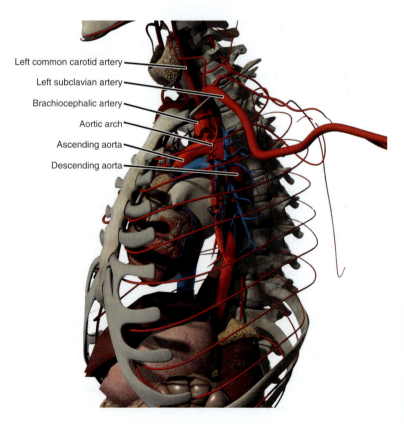

Left common carotid artery
Left subclavian artery
Brachiocephalic artery
Aortic arch
Ascending aorta
Descending aorta

Fig. 13.1 Lateral view of the great vessels of the aorta

variant in which a single, large common brachio-cephalic trunk comes off the arch and separates into the right and LSAs and the bicarotid trunk. This bicarotid trunk then bifurcates to form the right and left common carotid arteries. A more common variant is the so-called bovine arch, present in as many as 20 % of patients [4]. The so-called bovine arch includes a brachiocephalic trunk that splits into the right subclavian, right common carotid, and left common carotid arteries. The LSA comes off separately from the arch of the aorta. Other variants include the left vertebral artery coming off directly from the arch in 2.5 % of patients and the existence of a right-sided aortic arch in patients with dextrocardia or situs inversus.

Anatomic variants with the aorta can masquerade as traumatic injury. For example, a ductus diverticulum may be present along the anterior surface near the ligamentum arteriosum, which may be confused with pseudoaneurysm formation. Ductus diverticula appear as a smooth outline within the aortic lumen and do not have intimal flaps. In contrast, true pseudoaneurysm formation typically presents as an irregular out-pouching with an irregular base and intimal flaps. An aortic spindle may present as circumferential dilatation between the LSA and ligamentum arteriosum.

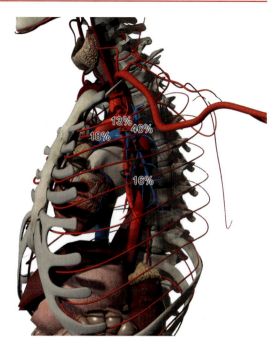

Fig. 13.2 The incidence of injury to the thoracic aorta ranges from 18 % at the ascending aorta, 13 % at the arch, 46 % at the ligamentum arteriosum, to 16 % at the descending aorta

the thoracic aorta, the rate of injury is 18 % at the ascending aorta, 13 % at the arch, and 16 % at the descending aorta (Fig. 13.2) [5, 8–12].

13.3   Pathophysiology

More than 85 % of patients with blunt TAI die prior to hospital arrival. The majority of patients who survive to undergo imaging and intervention have an injury at the aortic isthmus that is limited to the intima and media [5]. Survival of more advanced injuries (free rupture of the aorta) is rare [6, 7]. Nearly 99 % of patients who survive to make it to the hospital will die without surgical intervention: 15 % will die within the first hour, 30 % within 6 hours, nearly 50 % within 1 day, nearly 75 % within 1 week, and 90 % within 4 months [5]. The most common site of blunt TAI is at the proximal descending aorta, near the location of the ligamentum arteriosum, occurring at a rate of approximately 46 %. Elsewhere within

13.3.1 Mechanism of Injury

The cause of blunt TAI is multifactorial and includes high-shearing forces, torsion, and extreme stretch at fixed points of the aorta, such as the ligamentum arteriosum, aortic root, and sites of major branches, such as the arch [7]. Differential relative motion at different points of fixation further contributes to trauma, especially at the isthmus [13, 14]. Penetrating injuries to the thoracic aorta are uncommon. When present, they are likely to lead to rapid exsanguination, and many of these patients do not survive transport to the hospital. For those rare survivors, open repair is indicated for unstable patients. Endovascular repair may be attempted in a stable patient who is an anatomically suitable candidate based on preoperative imaging.

13.3.2 Classification of Injury

Based on CTA imaging, TAI is classified by severity: grade 1 injuries have an intimal tear (*without* external contour abnormality); grade 2 injuries involve the media and develop an intramural hematoma (*with* external contour abnormality); grade 3 extend to the adventitia and lead to pseudoaneurysm formation; and grade 4 have a free rupture of the aorta (Figs. 13.3 and 13.4) [15]. Management of grade 1 injuries can be conservative, with strict blood pressure control and follow-up CTA in 6 weeks to verify resolution. Grade 2 and 3 injuries should be urgently repaired, while grade 4 injuries require emergent intervention.

13.4 Clinical Presentation

The most common causes of blunt TAI include motor vehicle collision (MVC) (78 %), motorcycle accident (9 %), pedestrian (7 %), fall (5 %), and bicycle (1 %) [9]. The use of a seat belt decreases the risk of TAI by fourfold [16].

Concurrent injuries in patients with blunt TAI include major abdominal injury (57 %), closed head injury (50 %), major peripheral vascular injury (46 %), multiple rib fractures (46 %), pulmonary contusion (38 %), pelvic trauma (31 %), upper extremity trauma (20 %), flail chest (12 %), and spine injury (12 %) [8, 17].

Up to one-third of patients with blunt TAI have minimal signs of chest wall injury, which may contribute to missed injuries in favor of more obvious orthopedic or peripheral vascular trauma. Physical exam findings are nonspecific and are not sensitive for the diagnosis of blunt TAI (Table 13.1). Penetrating TAI typically presents with evidence of chest wall trauma, and physical findings include distended neck veins, muffled heart sounds, and hypotension secondary to tamponade physiology.

13.5 Diagnosis

The diagnosis of TAI in patients with blunt trauma can be suspected on plain chest x-ray (Table 13.2). A widened mediastinum may be seen on plain chest x-ray in more than 90 % of patients with TAI

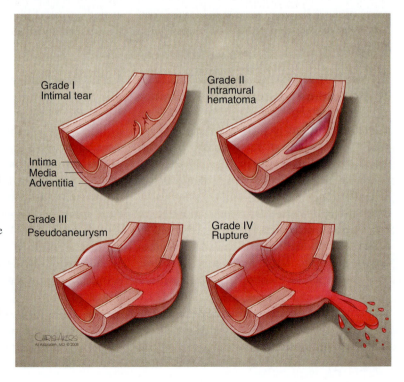

Fig. 13.3 Classification of traumatic aortic injury. Grade I injuries present with an intimal tear and can often be managed with anti-impulse control. Grade II injuries have an intramural hematoma and are often managed with endovascular stent graft placement. Grade III injuries develop a pseudoaneurysm and should be covered with a stent graft to avoid rupture. Grade IV injuries have frank rupture of the aorta and require emergency surgery

Grade I	Grade II	Grade III	Grade IV

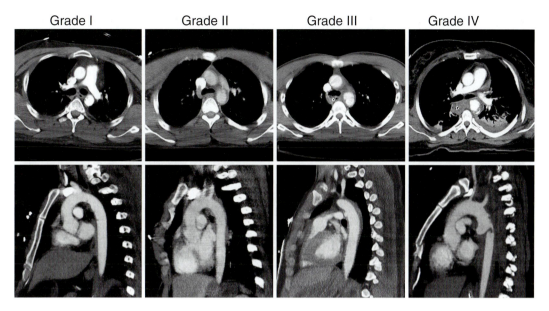

Fig. 13.4 CTA images of patients with grade I–IV traumatic aortic injuries

Table 13.1 Stigmata of aortic injury on clinical examination

Symptoms	Signs
Chest pain[a]	Unexplained hypotension
Dyspnea	Upper limb hypertension[b]
Cough	Decreased lower limb pulses[c]
Dysphagia	Systolic murmur[d]
Hoarseness[e]	Anterior chest wall contusion
Hemoptysis[f]	Sternal or thoracic spine fractures
	Expanding hematoma at the thoracic outlet

[a]Most commonly recorded symptom [38]
[b]Acute coarctation syndrome
[c]With normal upper limb pulses and differences in pulse amplitude (Acute coarctation syndrome)
[d]Audible over base of heart or between the scapulae
[e]Hoarseness results from compression of the left recurrent laryngeal nerve by an aneurysm
[f]Impending aneurysm rupture into a bronchus may be preceded by hemoptysis with or without associated hemothorax

Table 13.2 Stigmata of aortic injury on plain chest radiography

Widened mediastinum
Abnormal aortic outline
Loss of the aortopulmonary window
Depression of the left mainstem bronchus (more than 140° from trachea)
Lateral deviation of trachea to the right of midline
Lateral deviation of nasogastric tube to the right of midline
Widened right paratracheal stripe
First and second rib fractures
Sternal fracture
Multiple rib fractures with a crushed chest
Large hemothorax
Left apical cap (hematoma)
Clavicular fracture[a]
Anterior displacement of trachea (lateral radiograph)

[a]In the context of a high energy injury or multisystem trauma

[18, 19]. CTA is highly sensitive (95–100 %) with a negative predictive value approaching 100 % for TAI [18, 20–22]. False-positive studies, however, are possible [23, 24]. While CTA is the diagnostic modality of choice, patients with equivocal studies can undergo traditional angiogram and intravascular ultrasound (IVUS). If additional imaging is required after an equivocal CTA, we have found that IVUS is more sensitive than angiography. Therefore, we advocate the use of IVUS in suspected TAI patients for whom angiography is being considered (Fig. 13.5) [25].

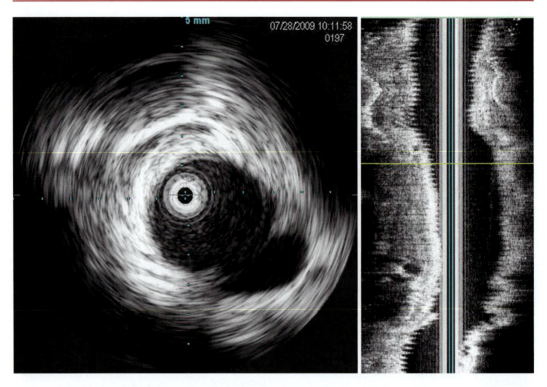

Fig. 13.5 Intravascular ultrasound in a patient with a grade III traumatic aortic injury. The pseudoaneurysm can be seen in the 4 o'clock position

13.6 Management

The initial management of patients with TAI should be to initiate the advanced trauma life support (ATLS) guidelines, including an assessment of the airway, breathing, circulation, disability, and exposure. Immediate management of life-threatening injuries should be the focus. Permissive hypotension should be the norm to avoid exacerbating major vascular injuries, and elevations in blood pressure should be avoided to minimize the risk of vascular rupture. Specifically, a mean arterial pressure below 80 mmHg should be the target [26]. There should be an appropriate balance between permissive hypotension and maintaining a satisfactory cerebral perfusion pressure. The patient's overall hemodynamic status dictates the management strategy. Hemodynamically unstable patients should be managed in the operating room, especially those with major concurrent trauma. Patients with high-volume chest tube drainage (i.e., more than 1,500 mL or a rate greater than 250 mL/h for 4 h) should also be managed in the operating room [27].

13.6.1 Medical Management

Patients with grade I TAI can be treated medically. Decreasing the intra-aortic shear force by decreasing blood pressure can be achieved using beta-blockers and other antihypertensive agents. Use of a nicardipine and esmolol drip should be initiated in patients who do not promptly respond to oral or intermittent intravenous therapy to decrease their heart rate below 100 beats per minute and blood pressure below 100 mmHg. Replacement of the drips with an oral regimen should be instituted over a period of days. New symptoms, continuing pain, or progression of injury on a CT scan are indications for operative intervention [28].

13.6.2 Delayed Surgical Management

Delayed repair (>24 h) may be suitable for selected patients with grade 2 or 3 injuries who have concurrent severe trauma [29, 30]. For example, patients with severe closed head injuries, severe sepsis, or major multisystem trauma may require more immediate management of life-threatening injuries prior to treatment of TAI. Strict blood pressure control is necessary, and some delay in operative management may improve physiologic optimization without compromising overall care [27, 31].

13.6.3 Operative Management

13.6.3.1 Open Repair

Open repair commences following general anesthesia via a double-lumen endotracheal tube. Aortic perfusion distal to the arch is achieved using a Bio-Medicus (Minneapolis, MN) pump with an inline heat exchanger. This is used with outflow cannulation from the left inferior pulmonary vein to either the distal descending aorta or left common femoral artery. An alternative strategy includes cannulating the left atrium or superior pulmonary vein, depending on what structure is most accessible. The patient is therapeutically heparinized and the aorta cross-clamped proximal to the LSA in cases of TAI to the isthmus. An alternative approach to therapeutic heparinization is to use a Carmeda®-coated circuit, in which only 5,000 units of heparin need to be administered. A longitudinal incision is made to visualize the tear, and hemostasis achieved. Transverse incisions can also be utilized to divide the aorta, which permits inspection and debridement of the ends of the aorta. The site of injury is bypassed using a woven Dacron tube graft, which is sewn in place with a running 4–0 pledgeted polypropylene suture at both the proximal and distal anastomosis. Protamine is given to reverse the heparin and the patient transported to the intensive care unit (ICU) [15].

Table 13.3 Types of endoleaks

I. Incomplete seal at either side of the stent graft
II. Blood accumulation in the excluded segment as a result of back bleeding from branches covered by the stent graft
III. Blood leakage between overlapping stent grafts
IV. Blood leakage due porosity of graft material leads to leakage. This was seen mainly in early stent grafts and rarely seen nowadays

13.6.3.2 Endovascular Repair

Following induction of general anesthesia, endovascular repair is performed in an operating room equipped with imaging technology. The abdomen and bilateral groins are prepped. A diagnostic arch aortogram is performed through percutaneous femoral artery access. The cerebrovascular anatomy is evaluated, especially if LSA coverage is required. The patient is anticoagulated with intravenous heparin, but at a lower dose (0.5 mg/kg) than the weight-based protocol. A thoracic stent graft is selected according to the manufacturer's instructions for use and based on cross-sectional measurements of the aorta. The device is delivered via open or percutaneous femoral artery access. Once deployed, a completion aortogram is performed to ensure satisfactory placement and ensure that there are no endoleaks (Table 13.3). Selective balloon angioplasty can be performed as necessary if there is concern about graft apposition. The heparin is reversed with protamine. The patient is then transferred to the trauma ICU.

13.6.3.3 Subclavian Artery Coverage

The LSA can be covered with the stent graft if necessary to achieve a proximal seal. LSA revascularization using a left carotid to subclavian bypass or subclavian transposition can be performed selectively. Indications for LSA revascularization are listed in Table 13.4. Posterior cerebral and cerebellar ischemia can occur in patients with a posterior inferior cerebellar artery (PICA) syndrome in which an aberrant vertebral artery terminates directly into the PICA instead of the basilar artery. Coverage of a left internal mammary artery that was used as part of a coronary artery bypass graft (CABG) should also be

Table 13.4 Indications for left subclavian artery revascularization

Preoperative
Left internal mammary artery bypass graft
Left vertebral arising from the arch
Dominant left vertebral in comparison to the right
Left vertebral terminating in the posterior inferior cerebellar artery
Stenotic or occluded right vertebral artery
Spinal protection (in patients who are at high risk for paraplegia)
Left upper extremity hemodialysis access
Postoperative
Left upper extremity claudication
Vertebrobasilar insufficiency

avoided. In emergent situations, LSA revascularization can be delayed unless an absolute indication for revascularization is present.

13.7 Postoperative Management

Close monitoring of the patient following the procedure and appropriate management of their concomitant injuries is necessary. Most patients with TEVAR can be discharged within 3–7 days, assuming their other injuries do not require further management. As long-term data (i.e., greater than 10 years) is unavailable, our midterm results indicate that endovascular repair remains durable up to 7 years. Follow-up surveillance should be completed by clinical examination and CT imaging at 1 month, 6 months, and then annually.

13.8 Complications

In comparison to open repair, TEVAR is associated with a lower rate of death, paraplegia, renal failure, transfusion requirement, reoperation, myocardial infarction, respiratory failure, and overall length of stay when controlled for ISS and age [32]. Specific risks associated with endovascular repair include device malfunction, migration of the stent graft, endoleak, aortic dissection, and trauma to the access vessels. Device collapse has been reported in TAI patients who undergo

TEVAR. According to a recent study, 65 % of patients who experienced device collapse had undergone TEVAR for TAI [31]. A tight aortic curvature and excessive device oversizing were among the most commonly reported risk factors.

13.9 Outcomes

In a recent systematic review of the literature involving 7,768 patients from 139 studies, Murad et al. reported a significantly higher mortality rate for nonoperative management and open repair compared to TEVAR (nonoperative 46 %, odds ratio [OR] 19 %, and TEVAR 9 %; $P<0.01$) [33]. TEVAR was associated with a lower mortality (RR 0.61; 95 % CI 0.46–0.80), spinal cord ischemia (RR 0.34; 95 % CI 0.16–0.74), end-stage renal disease, and systemic and graft infections as compared to open repair. However, there were increased secondary interventions for device-related complications in the TEVAR group.

In a review of our 15-year experience with 338 patients with TAI, we found that the in-hospital mortality for all patients arriving with TAI was 41 % (139/338) [9]. Early mortality for those who underwent aortic intervention was 17 % (27/175). Hospital mortality for patients with TAI who did not undergo aortic intervention was 69 % (112/163). TEVAR was associated with a 4 % (3/69) mortality, which was significantly less than open repair with clamp-and-sew technique (31 %, 9/29) ($P=0.002$). In comparison, the mortality for patients who underwent open repair using distal aortic perfusion was 14 % (11/77). In the patients who underwent operative intervention, a mortality reduction of 3.0 % per year ($P<0.001$) over the course of the study was observed. Mean follow-up for patients undergoing TEVAR was 2.5 years with 1- and 5-year survival of 92 and 87 %, respectively.

We have also investigated the cost of TEVAR compared to open repair for TAI [15]. The adjusted mean fixed, variable, and total costs of the two treatment modalities were compared. We found that while the variable costs were significantly higher for TEVAR compared to open repair, the fixed and total costs were not significantly different.

13.9.1 Special Cases

13.9.1.1 Ascending Aorta and Arch

Trauma affecting the ascending aorta and arch is uncommon, and the vast majority of afflicted patients die at the scene. Repair progresses via a median sternotomy and cardiopulmonary bypass with deep hypothermic circulatory arrest, followed by placement of an interposition graft. Replacement of the root may be required in rare circumstances (Table 13.5) [9, 34–36].

13.9.1.2 Innominate Artery

Trauma to the innominate artery can be repaired following median sternotomy with right cervical extension to obtain satisfactory proximal and distal control. As trauma commonly affects the base of the innominate artery, repair is best completed through placement of a woven Dacron graft bypass from the ascending aorta to the bifurcation of the innominate [37, 38].

13.9.1.3 Left Common Carotid Artery

Trauma to the left common carotid artery can be approached via a median sternotomy with left cervical extension, with a bypass graft from the arch or subclavian artery to a location distal to the site of injury on the carotid artery [27, 39]. However, endovascular techniques are increasingly utilized with placement of a covered stent to avoid the morbidity associated with a median sternotomy [40–42]. Routine surveillance and use of antiplatelet agents (i.e., aspirin and clopidogrel) is recommended to reduce the risk of in-stent thrombosis [43, 44].

13.9.1.4 Subclavian Arteries

Trauma to the subclavian arteries is typically secondary to penetrating trauma, and management should be dictated by preoperative imaging whenever possible to help optimize surgical planning. Injury to the right subclavian artery may require a "mini" median sternotomy with right cervical extension, or simply an infraclavicular incision. A left anterior thoracotomy or left infraclavicular incision may be completed to isolate the LSA. A supraclavicular incision can also be made to achieve distal exposure.

Table 13.5 Recommended incisions for suspected aortic and branch vessel injury

Injured segment	Recommended incision
Uncertain injury (hemodynamically unstable)	Left anterolateral thoracotomy ± Transverse sternotomy ± Right anterolateral thoracotomy (clamshell)
Ascending aorta	Median sternotomy
Transverse aortic arch	Median sternotomy ± Neck extension
Descending thoracic aorta	Left posterolateral thoracotomy (fourth intercostal space)
Innominate artery	Median sternotomy with right cervical extension
Left common carotid artery	Median sternotomy with left cervical extension
Left subclavian artery	Left anterolateral thoracotomy (third or fourth intercostal space) with separate left supraclavicular incision ± connecting vertical sternotomy ("book" thoracotomy)

Adapted from Mattox [27]

Endovascular management of subclavian artery trauma can be completed, even with transection of these vessels [40, 45, 46]. Placement of a covered stent graft can be accomplished in most patients using a variety of endovascular techniques. In cases of complete transection and nonunion, the use of a snare technique and extra-anatomic endovascular coverage can be completed.

13.9.1.5 Contaminated Fields

Penetrating or blunt trauma may occasionally lead to concomitant esophageal injury or gross contamination from the environment. Management of these injuries follows the same principles of damage control laparotomy: stabilization of the patient is the first priority. The preferred option is to achieve hemostasis, repair any esophageal or tracheal injuries, and decontaminate the surrounding region with infection control strategies, such as aggressive debridement and wide drainage. Emergency prosthetic graft placement may be necessary even in contaminated fields. If the patient survives the trauma, excision of the graft and autogenous or extra-anatomic bypass can be completed electively. Morbidity and mortality remain very high.

13.10 Controversies

There are several controversies associated with TAI. While stable patients should undergo urgent repair due to the risk of rupture, delayed management (>24 hours) is acceptable in patients with more severe injuries who require more immediate attention. Medical management with strict blood pressure control and follow up imaging in 6 weeks is suitable for patients with grade I injuries. TEVAR is the treatment of choice for all anatomically suitable candidates for TAI, regardless of age. Long-term results on the durability of endovascular repair remain to be determined. Selective revascularization of the LSA is recommended unless absolute indications exist. Systemic heparinization, albeit at a lower dose compared to open repair, is permissible for TEVAR. Routine spinal drainage is not routinely necessary following open repair of an aortic disruption, as only a limited portion of the aorta is replaced. Routine spinal drainage may be necessary if extensive stent grafting is expected [9].

Conclusion

Considerable progress has been made over the last two decades in the diagnosis and management of TAI. The current body of evidence supports the preferential use of endovascular repair compared to open surgery for all anatomically suitable candidates. Meticulous preoperative planning can help avoid many of the reported complications. The short- and midterm outcomes of TEVAR appear very favorable, but the long-term durability of the current devices is unknown. Continued improvements in imaging and device technology will expand the treatment options available. Adherence to the follow-up imaging is necessary to detect long-term complications.

References

1. Arajarvi E, Santavirta S, Tolonen J. Aortic ruptures in seat belt wearers. J Thorac Cardiovasc Surg. 1989; |98(3):355–61.
2. Teixeira PG, Inaba K, Barmparas G, Georgiou C, Toms C, Noguchi TT, Rogers C, Sathyavagiswaran L, Demetriades D. Blunt thoracic aortic injuries: an autopsy study. J Trauma. 2011;70(1):197–202.
3. Murphy SL, Xu J, Kochanek KD. Deaths: preliminary data for 2010. Natl Vital Stat Rep. 2012;60(4):7.
4. Desai SS, Lidsky M, Pascarella L, Shortell CK. Principles of vascular surgery in clinical review of vascular surgery. In: Desai SS, Shortell CK, editors. Clinical Review of Vascular Surgery. Surgisphere Corporation; 2010.
5. Parmley LF, Mattingly TW, Manion WC, Jahnke Jr EJ. Nonpenetrating traumatic injury of the aorta. Circulation. 1958;17(6):1086–101.
6. Richens D, Field M, Neale M, Oakley C. The mechanism of injury in blunt traumatic rupture of the aorta. Eur J Cardiothorac Surg. 2002;21(2):288–93.
7. Riesenman PJ, Brooks JD, Farber MA. Acute blunt traumatic injury to the descending thoracic aorta. J Vasc Surg. 2012;56(5):1274–80.
8. Fabian TC, Richardson JD, Croce MA, Smith Jr JS, Rodman Jr G, Kearney PA, et al. Prospective study of blunt aortic injury: multicenter trial of the American Association for the Surgery of Trauma. J Trauma. 1997;42(3):374–80.
9. Estrera AL, Miller CC, Salinas-Guajardo G, Coogan SM, Charlton-Ouw KM, Safi HJ, Azizzadeh A. Update on blunt thoracic aortic injury: 15-year single-institution experience. J Thorac CV Surg. 2013;145(3 Suppl):S154–8.
10. Feczko JD, Lynch L, Pless JE, Clark MA, McClain J, Hawley DA. An autopsy case review of 142 nonpenetrating (blunt) injuries of the aorta. J Trauma. 1992; 33(6):846–9.
11. Brundage SI, Harruff R, Jurkovich GJ, Maier RV. The epidemiology of thoracic aortic injuries in pedestrians. J Trauma. 1998;45(6):1010–4.
12. Burkhart HM, Gomez GA, Jacobson LE, Pless JE, Broadie TA. Fatal blunt aortic injuries: a review of 242 autopsy cases. J Trauma. 2001;50(1):113–5.
13. Pearson R, Philips N, Hancock R, et al. Regional wall mechanics and blunt traumatic aortic rupture at the isthmus. Eur J Cardiothorac Surg. 2008;34(3):616–22.
14. Schmoker JD, Lee CH, Taylor RG, et al. A novel model of blunt thoracic aortic injury: a mechanism confirmed? J Trauma. 2008;64(4):923–31.
15. Azizzadeh A, Keyhani K, Miller 3rd CC, Coogan SM, Safi HJ, Estrera AL. Blunt traumatic aortic injury: initial experience with endovascular repair. J Vasc Surg. 2009;49(6):1403–8.
16. Greendyke RM. Traumatic rupture of aorta; special reference to automobile accidents. JAMA. 1966;195(7): 527–30.
17. Downing SW, Sperling JS, Mirvis SE, et al. Experience with spiral computed tomography as the

sole diagnostic method for traumatic aortic rupture. Ann Thorac Surg. 2001;72:495–501.

18. O'Conor CE. Diagnosing traumatic rupture of the thoracic aorta in the emergency department. Emerg Med J. 2004;21:414–9.

19. Woodring JH. The normal mediastinum in blunt traumatic rupture of the thoracic aorta and brachiocephalic arteries. J Emerg Med. 1990;8:467–76.

20. Gavant ML, Menke PG, Fabian T, Flick PA, Graney MJ, Gold RE. Blunt traumatic aortic rupture: detection with helical CT of the chest. Radiology. 1995;197:125–33.

21. Mirvis SE, Bidwell JK, Buddemeyer EU, Diaconis JN, Pais SO, Whitley JE, et al. Value of chest radiography in excluding traumatic aortic rupture. Radiology. 1987;163:487–93.

22. Wicky S, Capasso P, Meuli R, Fischer A, Segesser L, Schnyder P. Spiral aortography: an efficient technique for the diagnosis of traumatic aortic injury. Eur Radiol. 1998;8:828–33.

23. Bruckner BA, DiBardino DJ, Cumbie TC, Trinh C, Blackmon SH, Fisher RG, et al. Critical evaluation of chest computed tomography scans for blunt descending thoracic aortic injury. Ann Thorac Surg. 2006;81:1339–46.

24. Patel NH, Hahn D, Comess KA. Blunt chest trauma victims: role of intravascular ultrasound and transesophageal echocardiography in cases of abnormal thoracic aortogram. J Trauma. 2003;55:330–7.

25. Azizzadeh A, Valdes J, Miller 3rd CC, Nguyen LL, Estrera AL, Charlton-Ouw K, Coogan SM, Holcomb JB, Safi HJ. The utility of intravascular ultrasound compared to angiography in the diagnosis of blunt traumatic aortic injury. J Vasc Surg. 2011;53(3):608–14.

26. Bickell WH, Wall Jr MJ, Pepe PE, Martin RR, Ginger VF, Allen MK, Mattox KL. Immediate versus delayed fluid resuscitation for hypotensive patients with penetrating torso injuries. N Engl J Med. 1994;331:1105–9.

27. Mattox KL. Approaches to trauma involving the major vessels of the thorax. Surg Clin North Am. 1989;69(1):77–91.

28. Azizzadeh A, Charlton-Ouw KM, Chen Z, Estrera AL, Rahbar MH, Amer H, Coogan SM, Holcomb JB, Safi HJ. An outcome analysis of endovascular vs. open repair of blunt traumatic aortic injuries. J Vasc Surg. 201357(1):108–14.

29. Demetriades D, Velmahos GC, Scalea TM, Jurkovich GJ, Karmy-Jones R, Teixeira PG, Hemmila MR, O'Connor JV, McKenney MO, Moore FO, London J, Singh MJ, Spaniolas K, Keel M, Sugrue M, Wahl WL, Hill J, Wall MJ, Moore EE, Lineen E, Margulies D, Malka V, Chan LS. Blunt traumatic thoracic aortic injuries: early or delayed repair–results of an American Association for the Surgery of Trauma prospective study. J Trauma. 2009;66(4):967–73.

30. Nagy K, Fabian T, Rodman G, Fulda G, Rodriguez A, Mirvis S. Guidelines for the diagnosis and management of blunt aortic injury: an EAST Practice Management Guidelines Work Group. J Trauma. 2000; 48(6):1128–43.

31. Jonker FH, Giacovelli JK, Muhs BE, Sosa JA, Indes JE. Trends and outcomes of endovascular and open treatment for traumatic thoracic aortic injury. J Vasc Surg. 2010;51(3):565–71.

32. Cheng D, Martin J, Shennib H, et al. Endovascular aortic repair versus open surgical repair for descending thoracic aortic disease a systematic review and meta-analysis of comparative studies. J Am Coll Cardiol. 2010;55:986–1001.

33. Murad MH, Rizvi AZ, Malgor R, Carey J, Alkatib AA, Erwin PJ, Lee WA, Fairman RM. Comparative effectiveness of the treatments for thoracic aortic transection. J Vasc Surg. 2011;53(1):193-199. e1–21.

34. Samanidis G, Dimitriou S, Sakorafas A, Khoury M. Repair of a penetrating aortic arch injury using deep hypothermic circulatory arrest and retrograde cerebral perfusion. Interact Cardiovasc Thorac Surg. 2012;14(3):356–8.

35. Serna DL, Miller JS, Chen EP. Aortic reconstruction after complex injury of the mid-transverse arch. Ann Thorac Surg. 2006;81(3):1112–4.

36. Symbas P. Cardiothoracic traumas. London: WB Saunders; 1989.

37. Graham JM, Feliciano DV, Mattox KL, Beall Jr AC. Innominate vascular injury. J Trauma. 1982;22(8): 647–55.

38. Symbas PN. Great vessels injury. Am Heart J. 1977; 93(4):518–22.

39. Brown MF, Graham JM, Feliciano DV, Mattox KL, Beall Jr AC, DeBakey ME. Carotid artery injuries. Am J Surg. 1982;144(6):748–53.

40. DuBose J, Recinos G, Teixeira PG, Inaba K, Demetriades D. Endovascular stenting for the treatment of traumatic internal carotid injuries: expanding experience. J Trauma. 2008;65(6):1561–6.

41. Gomez CR, May AK, Terry JB, Tulyapronchote R. Endovascular therapy of traumatic injuries of the extracranial cerebral arteries. Crit Care Clin. 1999;15(4):789–809.

42. Cox MW, Whittaker DR, Martinez C, Fox CJ, Feuerstein IM, Gillespie DL. Traumatic pseudoaneurysms of the head and neck: early endovascular intervention. J Vasc Surg. 2007;46(6):1227–33.

43. Bhatt DL, Kapadia SR, Bajzer CT, Chew DP, Ziada KM, Mukherjee D, et al. Dual antiplatelet therapy with clopidogrel and aspirin after carotid artery stenting. J Invasive Cardiol. 2001;13(12):767–71.

44. Liu AY, Paulsen RD, Marcellus ML, Steinberg GK, Marks MP. Long-term outcomes after carotid stent placement treatment of carotid artery dissection. Neurosurgery. 1999;45(6):1368–73.

45. Carrick MM, Morrison CA, Pham HQ, Norman MA, Marvin B, Lee J, et al. Modern management of traumatic subclavian artery injuries: a single institution's experience in the evolution of endovascular repair. Am J Surg. 2010;199(1):28–34.

46. Shalhub S, Starnes BW, Hatsukami TS, Karmy-Jones R, Tran NT. Repair of blunt thoracic outlet arterial injuries: an evolution from open to endovascular approach. J Trauma. 2011;71(5):E114–21.

Subclavian Artery and Vein Injuries

14

K. Shad Pharaon and Martin A. Schreiber

Contents

14.1 Introduction

Injuries to the subclavian artery and vein occur infrequently. These vessels are well protected by an extensive bony skeleton. When these injuries do occur, they have a high mortality due to their difficult surgical exposure. Most surgeons see only a small number of such injuries in their career. Limited clinical experience combined with difficult exposure makes these injuries challenging. A surgeon must have a thorough understanding of the surrounding anatomy and a well-thought-out plan for exposure to give the patient the best chance at survival. A surgeon familiar with endovascular techniques, imaging, and how to combine open and catheter-based options is better prepared to manage these cases.

14.2 Epidemiology

Men in their 20s are the most common group of patients to suffer subclavian vessel injury. Most subclavian artery and vein injuries are caused by penetrating trauma. The top three mechanisms of penetrating injury are gunshots, stabs, and shotgun wounds. Most of these victims will die before reaching the hospital. While gunshot wounds are most common, shotgun injuries have the highest mortality. Most of the patients that arrive alive with these injuries will have an isolated subclavian artery or vein injury, but there is injury to both vessels in 25 % of cases [1–3]. Brachial plexus injuries are found in about one-third of

K.S. Pharaon, MD
Division of Trauma,
Critical Care and Acute Care Surgery,
Oregon Health and Science University,
Portland, OR, USA
e-mail: pharaon@ohsu.edu

M.A. Schreiber, MD (✉)
Department of Surgery,
Oregon Health and Science University,
Portland, OR, USA
e-mail: schreibm@ohsu.edu

A. Dua et al. (eds.), *Clinical Review of Vascular Trauma*,
DOI 10.1007/978-3-642-39100-2_14, © Springer-Verlag Berlin Heidelberg 2014

patients with penetrating trauma to the subclavian vessels. A few patients will have a simultaneous intra-abdominal source of hemorrhage requiring an exploratory laparotomy. Blunt trauma to the subclavian vessels is less common. When it occurs, it is usually from a clavicle fracture or a stretch injury such as falling from a motorcycle or great height [1–3].

14.3   Anatomy

The subclavian artery is divided into three individual segments based on its relation to the anterior scalene muscle (Fig. 14.1). The first segment of the subclavian artery is medial to the anterior scalene muscle and typically gives rise to three significant vessels: the vertebral artery, the internal mammary artery, and the thyrocervical trunk. The second segment lies deep to the anterior scalene and typically gives rise to the costocervical trunk. The third segment is lateral to the anterior

scalene muscle and gives origin to the dorsal scapular artery. The subclavian artery becomes the axillary artery at the medial border of the pectoralis minor muscle. From a surgical standpoint, the right and left subclavian arteries are exposed differently depending on the location of injury with respect to the vertebral artery. The arch of the aorta does not curve from right to left as depicted in many texts. Instead, the arch curves from anterior to posterior (Fig. 14.2). This is important when a surgeon needs to access the distal left subclavian artery. Its posterior location makes it most accessible through a thoracotomy and very difficult to expose or control via median sternotomy.

The subclavian vein is the continuation of the axillary vein that arises from the cephalic, brachial, and basilic veins of the arm (Fig. 14.3). The cephalic vein traverses the lateral side of the arm from the hand to the shoulder. The basilic vein traverses the medial side of the arm. The brachial or deep vein of

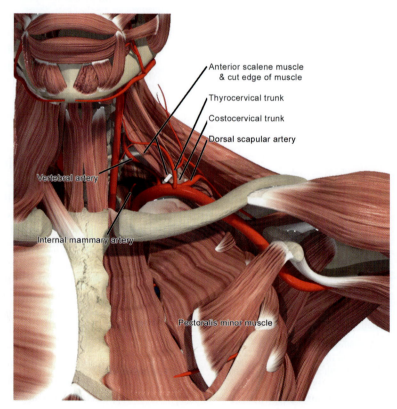

Fig. 14.1 Divisions of the subclavian artery and its key branches. The first segment of the subclavian artery is medial to the anterior scalene muscle and typically gives rise to three significant vessels: the vertebral artery, the internal mammary artery, and the thyrocervical trunk. The second segment lies deep to the anterior scalene and typically gives rise to the costocervical trunk. The third segment is lateral to the anterior scalene muscle and gives origin to the dorsal scapular artery. The subclavian artery becomes the axillary artery at the medial border of the pectoralis minor muscle

Fig. 14.2 Lateral view of
the aorta. The arch of the
aorta does not curve from
right to left as depicted in
many texts. Instead, the arch
curves from anterior to
posterior

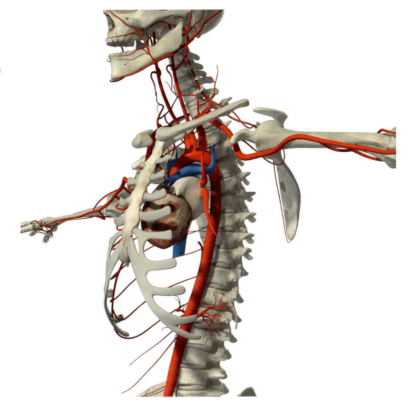

Fig. 14.3 Major veins of the
head, neck, and upper
extremity

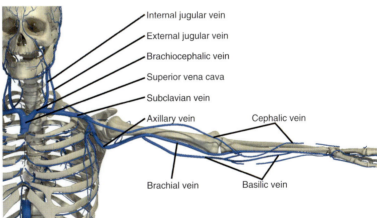

Internal jugular vein
External jugular vein
Brachiocephalic vein
Superior vena cava
Subclavian vein
Axillary vein   Cephalic vein

Brachial vein   Basilic vein

the arm joins the basilic vein to become the
axillary vein. In the shoulder, the cephalic vein
pierces the deltopectoral fascia and empties
into the axillary vein. After the cephalic vein
joins the axillary vein, it becomes the subclavian vein. The subclavian vein extends from
the outer border of the first rib to the medial
border of the anterior scalene muscle. Here, the
internal jugular vein joins the subclavian vein,
and it is now referred to as the brachiocephalic
vein. Once the brachiocephalic vein joins its
counterpart from the other side, it becomes the
superior vena cava. The subclavian vein lies
anterior to the anterior scalene muscle. The
subclavian artery lies posterior to the anterior
scalene muscle. Hence, the anterior scalene
muscle is sandwiched between the subclavian
vein and artery.

14.4 Clinical Assessment

The initial assessment and management should follow standard Advanced Trauma Life Support (ATLS) protocols. After determining that the patient has an adequate airway, the next priority is assessment of labored breathing and adequate breath sounds. Air bubbling through a wound and subcutaneous emphysema may indicate a pneumothorax. A thorough pulse exam should be performed to assess circulation. The absence of a pulse does not necessarily mean that there is an arterial injury, and the presence of a pulse does not necessarily mean that there is no injury. Nonetheless, the presence or absence of a pulse upon admission should be documented.

A focused neurologic exam should be obtained, with particular attention to neurologic compromise of the ipsilateral upper extremity. Because of the close anatomical relationship of the neurovascular structures, the brachial plexus is injured in about one-third of patients with subclavian vessel injury. Therefore the axillary, median, radial, ulnar, and musculocutaneous nerve exams should be documented. Plexus injuries can be caused by penetrating injuries that directly transect nerve roots or by blunt injuries that result in shear or traction forces [1–3].

14.5 Initial Management

Once the exam is complete, the critical decision point in a patient with a suspected subclavian vessel injury is determining if the patient is stable or unstable. Hemodynamically unstable patients are transported to the operating room without delay, and those in extremis require an immediate anterolateral ED thoracotomy.

The second most important management decision is to ensure adequate intravenous access. Intravenous (IV) lines should be inserted on the contralateral side of the injury; as infused fluids via an ipsilateral IV will extravasate from the wound. These patients are at high risk of a massive transfusion, and the blood bank should be notified of such.

The most common physical finding indicative of vascular injury is hematoma formation. Direct pressure should be applied to help control

bleeding. Some injuries behind the clavicle will not benefit from direct pressure. A commonly described technique of balloon tamponade with a Foley catheter inserted into the missile tract is often ineffective. Remember the pulse exam is an insensitive sign of subclavian artery injury. Collateral circulation around the shoulder may result in a normal pulse when in fact there is an injury to the artery.

14.6 Diagnostic Testing

Bilateral upper extremity blood pressures should be recorded in all patients with suspected upper extremity vascular injury. A difference of more than 5–10 mmHg should prompt a more thorough evaluation of possible injury sites. A chest x-ray should be obtained. Stable patients with suspected upper extremity vascular injury should undergo computed tomographic angiography (CTA) of the neck, chest, and upper extremity. CTA can be invaluable for identifying the location of injury as well as evaluating the mediastinal vascular and nonvascular structures.

14.7 Endovascular and Operative Management

After a diagnostic work-up on a stable patient, the next step is a therapeutic intervention. This can be pursued in an open or endovascular fashion. Many hospitals are building hybrid operating rooms that allow open or endoluminal management, thus allowing the surgeon to bring a trauma patient directly to the operating theater for diagnostic work-up, endovascular repair, endovascular adjunctive care, or an open operation.

Endovascular options, including balloon tamponade and stent grafting via percutaneous access or in conjunction with open surgical repair, can be life and limb saving. Arterial access is commonly approached percutaneously through the femoral artery, though percutaneous or open brachial approaches can also be utilized and are sometimes necessary in conjunction with the femoral access. Once guide wire traversal through the area of injury has been achieved, a covered

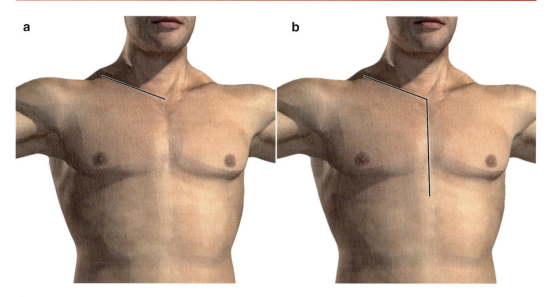

Fig. 14.4 (**a**) Clavicular incision for accessing the innominate, common carotid, and subclavian arteries. (**b**) Median sternotomy extension for more proximal access.

This incision starts at the sternoclavicular junction and extends over the length of the clavicle

stent graft upsized by roughly 10 % of the diameter of adjacent healthy vessel is deployed. Lesions that appear difficult to traverse are sometimes accessed through the brachial vessels because this provides a direct, shorter, less tortuous approach. Pseudoaneurysm, arteriovenous fistula, arterial intimal flap, and lacerations of subclavian vessels have all been treated with endovascular repairs. Endovascular covered stent placement in the appropriate patient eliminates the acute need for surgical dissection, anterolateral thoracotomy, decreasing the risk for injuring structures such as the vagus nerve, recurrent laryngeal nerve, phrenic nerve, and innominate vein. Careful patient selection is necessary, and only focal lesions that can safely be traversed with a guide wire can be approached in this fashion. Contraindications to endovascular repair include a hemodynamically unstable patient, long segmental arterial injury, and insufficient proximal or distal fixation points. Some patients will have an arteriogram that demonstrates a contraindication to an endovascular repair and will require an open operation, in which case proximal balloon occlusion can be useful [4–7].

For patients that do require an open surgical approach, the surgeon should be able to respond quickly with a systematic approach in mind for exposure. The right and left subclavian arteries are exposed via different incisions and patient positioning depending on the location of injury with respect to the vertebral artery. For right-sided injury distal to the vertebral artery, the preferred method is to start with a right supraclavicular incision. This incision starts at the sternoclavicular junction and extends over the length of the clavicle (Fig. 14.4). Should additional exposure be needed, such as those with injury proximal to the vertebral, median sternotomy is performed utilizing a Lebsche knife or sternal saw (Fig. 14.5). The dissection and exposure of the right subclavian artery begins first by dissecting and removing the underlying scalene fat pad. Once it is removed, the phrenic nerve must be identified. This is a key anatomical landmark that must be preserved. The nerve courses lateral to medial along the anterior scalene muscle. The nerve can be isolated with a vessel loop and gently retracted out of the way. The anterior scalene muscle should be cut as low as possible, and the subclavian artery will be found behind it.

The choice of surgical incision for left-sided injury is more difficult due to the orientation of the aorta and the very posterior origin of the left subclavian artery. There are three ways to expose the left subclavian artery – a supraclavicular

Fig. 14.5 Lebsche knife used for completing a median sternotomy

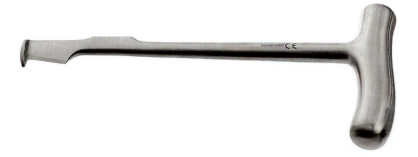

Fig. 14.6 Supraclavicular incision used for accessing the left subclavian artery. The supraclavicular incision is made one fingerbreadth above and parallel to the clavicle extending from the sternal notch to the lateral end of the clavicle

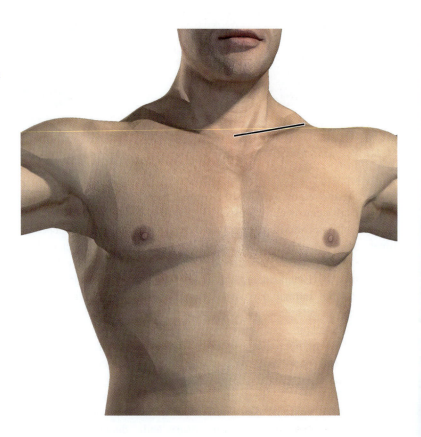

incision with clavicle resection, a left antero-lateral thoracotomy, and a sternoclavicular flap (trapdoor). The supraclavicular incision is made one fingerbreadth above and parallel to the clavicle extending from the sternal notch to the lateral end of the clavicle (Fig. 14.6). Cautery is used to score the clavicle, a periosteal elevator is used to peel the periosteum off the clavicle in a circumferential fashion, and the clavicle is divided in the middle with bone cutters. Once the clavicle is cut, it can be grabbed with a towel clip and removed from its bed. The clavicle is then removed from the sternum. The clavicle can be resected with surprisingly little disability and deformity. The clavicle does not need reconstruction with orthopedic plating. Dissection of the left subclavian artery commences similar to as described above for the right. A supraclavicular incision is adequate if the injury is distal to the vertebral [8–10].

When a supraclavicular incision is inadequate, such as those with injury of the left subclavian

Fig. 14.7 Clavicular incision and anterior left thoracotomy incision. The preferred sequence of steps to obtain control of the left subclavian artery in an injury that has not been preoperatively identified is to begin with a supraclavicular incision and quickly move to a thoracotomy if the necessary exposure is not obtained

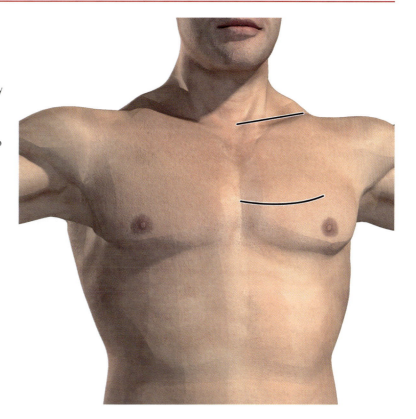

artery proximal to the vertebral, an anterolateral thoracotomy is used. An anterolateral thoracotomy through the third intercostal space will provide access to the origin of the subclavian. Technically speaking, the incision that gives the best ability to obtain proximal and distal control of the left subclavian artery is through the chest using a posterolateral thoracotomy with the patient in the right lateral decubitus position. However, given that the patient will be supine on the operation room table to allow access to any possible injury, an anterolateral thoracotomy is a more practical approach. The preferred sequence of steps to obtain control of the left subclavian artery in an injury that has not been preoperatively identified is to begin with a supraclavicular incision and quickly move to a thoracotomy if the necessary exposure is not obtained. If exposure is still inadequate, as a last resort, the supraclavicular and thoracotomy incisions can be connected with a median sternotomy, completing the trapdoor (Figs. 14.7 and 14.8) [8–12].

Once the vessel is exposed and the injury defined, proximal and distal control of the vessel is required. A small laceration in the artery may be repaired primarily, but usually the injury requires an interposition graft. Attempting to mobilize the soft and friable subclavian artery to gain enough length for an end-to-end repair is rarely successful. Therefore the majority of subclavian artery injuries and especially for extensive injuries, an interposition graft should be performed using vein or polytetrafluoroethylene (PTFE). Vein is preferred, particularly in an infected field, but if the patient is unstable and time does not permit vein harvest, then PTFE is acceptable. A proximal and distal Fogarty balloon thrombectomy is performed, and the artery is repaired with the interposition conduit using 4 or 5-0 monofilament suture. A completion angiogram should be performed.

For subclavian vein injuries, thrombosis often results due to the low-pressure venous system. Venous injuries are only repaired if the patient

a

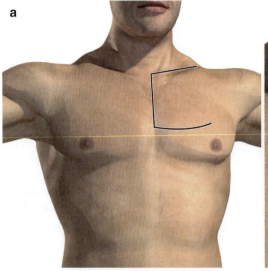

b

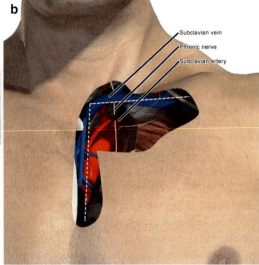

Fig. 14.8 (**a**) Clavicular incision, median sternotomy, and thoracotomy incision. (**b**) Contents of the mediastinum once trapdoor flap is pulled back. Once the vessel is exposed and the injury defined, proximal and distal control of the vessel is required. A small laceration in the artery may be repaired primarily, but usually the injury requires an interposition graft

remains stable, and the repair can be performed without producing stenosis or requiring an interposition graft. If this is not possible, the vein should be ligated. Besides transient edema, no significant long-term complications result from venous ligation.

Although subclavian artery injuries should ideally be repaired if possible, some patients will be too unstable and require damage control surgery for life salvage. For these patients in extremis, the subclavian artery can be ligated. This can be tolerated if ligation occurs proximal to the vertebral artery ostia because of retrograde flow to the extremity through the vertebral and collateral circulation of the shoulder. If the subclavian artery is ligated distal to the vertebral artery, the viability of the extremity becomes questionable. If any portion of the subclavian artery is ligated, a fasciotomy should be considered. The role, however, of prophylactic fasciotomy remains controversial. Routine prophylactic fasciotomy is generally not preferred, as it may be not necessary in many patients and can be associated with significant morbidity and prolonged hospital stay. Close observation and fasciotomy when needed is the preferred approach. Another option in the unstable patient is to place a temporary arterial shunt and defer definitive repair until the patient has been stabilized.

14.8 Postoperative Management

Patients status post-subclavian artery repair and especially with concomitant vein ligation should be managed postoperatively in an intensive care setting. The patient should have frequent (every 1–2 h) neurovascular checks for the first 24 h. Pulmonary toilet with use of incentive spirometry and chest physiotherapy is started on the first postoperative day. Pain control is often given by use of patient controlled analgesia. Early thromboembolic events can occur, and duplex or CTA of the chest and upper extremity should be performed aggressively for any acute change in exam. A high index of suspicion should be maintained for the development of compartment syndrome in the first 24–48 h. Physical and occupational therapy are started in the immediate postoperative period for the injured extremity. All of these patients are started on low-dose aspirin. However, there is currently no data for lifelong use in these patients as studies supporting lifelong use were conducted in coronary artery disease (CAD) patient populations.

14.9   Complications and Pitfalls

The presence of a large hematoma in zone I of the neck after a gunshot wound increases the risk of laryngotracheal trauma or airway compromise from soft tissue edema. This type of injury may make endotracheal intubation difficult and dangerous. Inability to secure the airway in such a patient can lead to severe respiratory compromise and, ultimately, cardiac arrest. Thus, the most qualified person should make the first attempt at intubation, and a surgeon should be ready to perform a cricothyroidotomy. Cervical spinal immobilization with a neck collar remains a common practice in the prehospital setting. Spinal immobilization may complicate the evaluation and diagnostic work-up. Its application in the presence of a large or expanding hematoma may increase the risk of respiratory obstruction. For this reason, spinal immobilization is not recommended for penetrating trauma to the neck and chest. The risks outweigh the benefits unless the patient has neurologic evidence of spinal cord injury or radiographic evidence of potentially unstable bony injury.

A normal heart rate and blood pressure does not assure the absence of shock, as early shock may not be associated with abnormalities in vital signs. All potential subclavian vessel injuries should be treated as surgical emergencies. Bleeding from vessels behind the clavicle is difficult to control with direct pressure. Digital compression through the hole with a gloved finger can be attempted, but balloon tamponade using a Foley into the missile tract and blind clamping of bleeding vessels should be avoided. The risk of further vascular or nerve damage is very high.

Failure to accurately document the patient's neurologic exam on admission and postoperatively will compromise the surgeon's ability to detect and/or correct potential compartment syndrome. The patient's neurologic exam should be accurately documented on initial presentation and serially checked after interventions. Many patients will present to the hospital manifesting a permanent neurologic deficit from a brachial plexus injury, while others may develop deficits from the surgical intervention or onset of compartment syndrome.

Covered stents placed in the subclavian artery near the thoracic outlet maybe subject to compression between the first rib and the clavicle and thus need close follow-up for possible stenosis or thrombosis. Other potential disadvantages of endovascular repair are early thromboembolic events, late stenosis, and infected grafts, which is why many times these techniques are considered a bridging therapy. Vascular reconstruction at a later point with carotid-subclavian bypass may be performed in a more elective fashion as necessary for increased patency and durability. Long-term follow-up is necessary to identify those patients that develop stenosis; however, patient compliance with respect to follow-up is generally poor.

For those that undergo an open operation, exposure of the subclavian artery and vein allows assessment of associated injuries but also places uninjured anatomy at risk. If during an operation a transected trunk of the brachial plexus is discovered, the nerve should be repaired by a consulting hand or plastic surgery team versus tagged with a suture for subsequent repair at reexploration. Phrenic nerve injury may be repaired but usually leads to ipsilateral hemidiaphragm paralysis. An injured thoracic duct should be ligated.

Ligation of the subclavian vein will lead to transient edema of the arm, but often there are no long-term complications. Resection of the medial half of the clavicle does not result in functional disability. Reconstruction is an option for cosmesis as opposed to function. There is the rare patient with a subclavian artery injury who presents in extremis with a poor anastomotic network of collaterals around the shoulder that may be at risk for amputation. Criticisms of the trapdoor approach are prolonged time to make the incision, division of thick muscles which often leads to bleeding, severe postoperative pain due to iatrogenic rib fractures, high incidence of postoperative respiratory complications, and difficulty in wound closure. Sternal wound infection is rare but can be a devastating complication after sternotomy. Infection can lead to sternal dehiscence. Early detection and treatment are fundamental to successful treatment of sternal wound infections. Pectoralis major muscle flaps are often used for coverage and have decreased the hospital stay and mortality associated with sternal wound infections, but these procedures generally require a plastic surgery consult for assistance.

14.10 Outcomes

The most frequent cause of subclavian vessel injury is penetrating trauma. Blunt trauma accounts for only 2–3 % of all subclavian artery injuries in the largest published series [1–3]. Mortality rate of surgical series ranged from 5 to 30 %. Fifty percent of subclavian vessel injuries are amendable to an endovascular approach [13]. Different stents were used in published series: balloon expandable, self-expanding, covered with a Dacron graft, or with PTFE. To date, no significant differences in patency and outcome have been reported. Short-term and midterm results of endovascular repair are encouraging with low restenosis and low occlusion rates. Long-term durability has not been established. Subclavian vessel injuries occur infrequently, and it is unlikely that a prospective randomized trial with a sufficient number of patients will be conducted comparing the endovascular and open approaches.

Conclusion

Injury to the subclavian vessels is a rare occurrence but one that a surgeon must be prepared for before the patient arrives in the emergency department. Detailed knowledge of the anatomy is critical for the complex surgical exposure of the subclavian vessels. It is important to follow ATLS protocols. Specifically, secure an airway, establish appropriate IV access in the contralateral extremity, and control hemorrhage. Initially, the surgeon must completely assess and attempt to account for all other potential sources of blood loss prior to committing the entire focus on the vascular injury as the cause of shock.

The critical decision is determining if the patient can afford a more thorough diagnostic work-up to plan repair versus emergent open exploration. Traumatic vascular injuries have traditionally been managed with conventional open surgery but are now evolving to include more endovascular therapies. The subclavian artery may be most amendable and best managed with these evolving techniques. Treatment will depend on available resources and expertise of IR, trauma and vascular surgeons. In stable patients, endografts have led to significant advances in the care of the injured patient and, with a few caveats, are the treatment of choice. In the unstable patient, repair of the subclavian artery can usually be performed with PTFE or autologous vein. Subclavian vein injury is usually treated with ligation. Exposure of these vessels will depend on the site of injury. For right-sided injury, a supraclavicular incision with possible median sternotomy is usually sufficient. For left-sided injury, a supraclavicular incision may be adequate. The anterolateral thoracotomy provides more exposure, and only rarely is a trapdoor needed. Postoperatively, these patients may develop respiratory complications, inadequate pain control, and acute thromboembolic events and should be initially monitored in an intensive care setting. Physical and occupational therapy are beneficial. A multidisciplinary effort is necessary for the successful management of these rare vascular injuries.

References

1. Lin PH, Koffron AJ, Guske PJ, Lujan HJ, Heilizer TJ, Yario RF, Tatooles CJ. Penetrating injuries of the subclavian artery. Am J Surg. 2003;185(6):580–4.
2. Demetriades D, Chahwan S, Gomez H, Peng R, Velmahos G, Murray J, Asensio J, Bongard F. Penetrating injuries to the subclavian and axillary vessels. J Am Coll Surg. 1999;188(3):290–5.

3. Demetriades D, Asensio JA. Subclavian and axillary vascular injuries. Surg Clin North Am. 2001;81(6):1357–73.

4. Arthurs ZM, Sohn VY, Starnes BW. Vascular trauma: endovascular management and techniques. Surg Clin North Am. 2007;87(5):1179–92.

5. du Toit DF, Strauss DC, Blaszczyk M, de Villiers R, Warren BL. Endovascular treatment of penetrating thoracic outlet arterial injuries. Eur J Vasc Endovasc Surg. 2000;19(5):489–95.

6. Patel AV, Marin ML, Veith FJ, Kerr A, Sanchez LA. Endovascular graft repair of penetrating subclavian artery injuries. J Endovasc Surg. 1996;3(4):382–8.

7. Parodi JC, Schonholz C, Ferreira LM, Bergan J. Endovascular stent-graft treatment of traumatic arterial lesions. Ann Vasc Surg. 1999;13(2):121–9.

8. Hoyt DB, Coimbra R, Potenza BM, Rappold JF. Anatomic exposures for vascular injuries. Surg Clin North Am. 2001;81(6):1299–330.

9. Old W, Oswaks R. Clavicular excision in management of vascular trauma. Am Surg. 1984;50:286–9.

10. Schaff HV, Brawley RK. Operative management of penetrating vascular injuries of the thoracic outlet. Surgery. 1977;82:182–91.

11. Buscaglia LC, Walsh JC, Wilson JD, Matolo NM. Surgical management of subclavian artery injury. Am J Surg. 1987;154(1):88–92.

12. Graham JM, Feliciano DV, Mattox KL, Beall Jr AC, DeBakey ME. Management of subclavian vascular injuries. J Trauma. 1980;20(7):537–44.

13. White R, Krajcer Z, Johnson M, Williams D, Bacharach M, O'Malley E. Results of a multicenter trial for the treatment of traumatic vascular injury with a covered stent. J Trauma. 2006;60(6): 1189–95.

Thoracic Duct Injuries

15

Leslie M. Kobayashi

Contents

15.1   Anatomy/Physiology

Lymph tissue can be found in dermis, subdermal tissues, and fascia. The vessels created by lymphatic endothelium lack a basement membrane, and the highly permeable lymphatic system collects protein and lipid-rich fluid, as well as red blood cells, lymphocytes, and bacteria from the extravascular space and returns it to the venous system via the thoracic duct [1]. The thoracic duct also carries chyle from the abdomen and viscera back to the venous circulation. Chyle is rich in chylomicrons, cholesterol, triglycerides, and fat soluble vitamins A, D, E, and K [2] The anatomy of the thoracic duct varies but the most common variant, occurring in 50–65 % of the population, has the duct arising from the cisterna chyli near the second and third lumbar vertebrae (Fig. 15.1) [2, 3]. The duct enters the chest via the aortic hiatus on the right side where it travels cephalad between the aorta and the azygos vein, before coursing behind the aortic arch to the left chest at the fifth thoracic vertebra. As the duct exits the thoracic outlet, it passes behind the carotid sheath before draining into the junction of the left subclavian and jugular veins in the neck (Fig. 15.2) [3, 4].

15.2   Background/Incidence/ Epidemiology

Lymphatic vessels are thin and easily damaged; however, clinical manifestations are generally only seen when disruption of the major ducts

L.M. Kobayashi, MD
Division of Trauma, Surgical Critical Care
and Burns, University of California-San Diego,
San Diego, CA, USA
e-mail: lkobayashi@ucsd.edu

A. Dua et al. (eds.), *Clinical Review of Vascular Trauma*,
DOI 10.1007/978-3-642-39100-2_15, © Springer-Verlag Berlin Heidelberg 2014

Fig. 15.1 Anatomical illustration of the origin, course, and termination of the thoracic duct (Reproduced with permission from Stranding et al. [20])

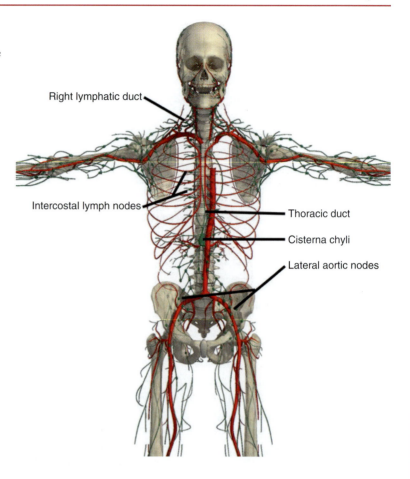

Right lymphatic duct

Intercostal lymph nodes

Thoracic duct

Cisterna chyli

Lateral aortic nodes

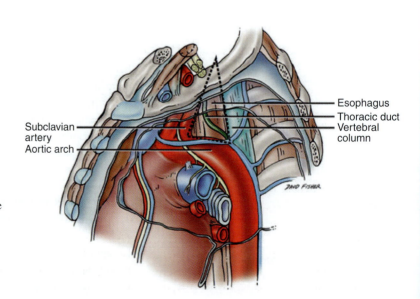

Subclavian artery

Aortic arch

Esophagus

Thoracic duct

Vertebral column

DAVID FISHER

Fig. 15.2 Poirier's triangle (*dotted line*) bounded by the left subclavian artery, vertebral column, and arch of the aorta (Reproduced with permission from Tubbs et al. [21])

occurs resulting in chylous pseudocysts, fistulae, or chylous effusions of the thoracic cavity (chylothorax), pericardium, or peritoneum (chylous ascites). Loss of the protein and immune cell rich fluid caused by large volume of chyle leaks can result in malnutrition and immunosuppression. Without proper management, this loss of chyle can also cause dehydration, severe electrolyte abnormalities, and pulmonary insufficiency. Prior to the development of total parenteral nutrition (TPN) and surgical treatment of thoracic duct injuries mortality rates for thoracic duct leaks could approach 50 % [2, 5, 6].

Because of its location, protected by the spine, aorta, and mediastinum, injury to the thoracic duct is rare. When it does occur the most common causes of injury are iatrogenic during surgical procedures or, less commonly, due to traumatic injury [1, 7]. Iatrogenic injury to the thoracic duct occurs most commonly with neck or thoracic procedures, including central venous line placement, complicating between 0.37 and 2 % of thoracic procedures and up to 1–5 % of esophagectomies [2, 7–9]. Traumatic thoracic duct injury is rare, accounting for only 3 % of chylothoraces, and occurring in only 0.9 % of cases following penetrating neck trauma [9–11]. When due to penetrating trauma, it is often found in conjunction with visceral or vascular injuries. Isolated thoracic duct injuries occur in only 0.06 % of all penetrating neck and chest trauma [6]. Injury to the thoracic duct following blunt trauma is also very rare and is thought to be due most commonly to overstretching and rupture of the duct across the thoracic spine during hyperextension or by direct laceration by broken bones or osteophytes [2, 7, 12–14].

15.3 Clinical Assessment

As with all traumas, patients suspected of having a thoracic duct injury following blunt or penetrating trauma should be evaluated in a systematic fashion. Problems of airway, breathing, and circulation, as well as neurological deficits, should be identified and treated according to Advanced Trauma Life Support Protocols. Those with hard signs of vascular or aerodigestive injury such as pulsatile hemorrhage, lack of distal pulses, expanding hematoma, or air or saliva bubbling through open wounds should be taken to the operating room immediately for appropriate surgical exploration. Patients with effusions, pneumothoraces, or tension physiology should have tube thoracostomies placed. Once associated life-threatening injuries have been identified and addressed, thoracic duct injuries primarily present in one of two ways, either through manifestation of a chylothorax or during operative exploration. Less commonly, chyle fistula via the wound tract or chyle pseudocyst formation can be seen following penetrating trauma to the neck or chest.

The location of the thoracic duct injury will have a great deal of influence on how the injury manifests (Fig. 15.2). Injuries located high in the neck are often found with associated injuries and are commonly diagnosed when chyle is seen in the surgical field during neck exploration. When injured in the chest, thoracic duct injuries primarily manifest with chylothorax formation. Chylothorax presents most commonly with asymptomatic opacity found on chest x-ray, when symptoms are present they can include shortness of breath, chest pain, or cough. When injured high in the chest, most commonly within Poirier's triangle, the space bounded by the left subclavian artery, vertebral column, and arch of the aorta, the injury presents with a left sided chylothorax [6]. Whereas injuries lower in the duct, below the cross over at the fifth thoracic vertebra, will result in right sided chylous effusions. Initial chest tube drainage may demonstrate the classical milky white drainage; however, fluid may initially be serous, serosanguinous, or bloody. There are several reasons for delay in obvious chylothorax: blood from associated injuries may mask the chyle leak, the duct injury may be small and chyle leakage may be slow requiring time to manifest clinically, and patients may be in a fasting state causing the chyle to be more serous in appearance. Typically chylothorax will manifest within 1–7 days of the initial injury [2, 6].

15.4 Diagnostic Testing

If there is concern for thoracic duct injury due to milky drainage from a thoracostomy tube, there are several options to confirm the presence of chyle. First, the fluid can be sent for triglyceride levels, if levels are greater than 110 mg/dL this is diagnostic for chyle leak, if less than 50 mg/dL the chances of chyle leak are less than 5 % and thoracic duct injury can effectively be ruled out [3]. For patients with triglyceride levels between 50 and 110 mg/dL, lipoprotein analysis or light microscopy can be used to detect chylomicrons confirming the presence of chyle, alternatively Sudan III stain can be used to confirm the presence of fat globules [2]. Additionally, the clinician can perform a cell count, chyle will demonstrate a predominance of lymphocytes (>90 %) or if the patient is on a diet cream can be administered and the drainage observed for change in character. Administration of milk or cream is also useful preoperatively for identification of the injury and localization for duct ligation.

More invasive methods of identifying and, more importantly, localizing thoracic duct injury include lymphangiography where diffusible blue dye is injected into the interdigital web spaces and lymphoscintigraphy with similar injection of a radiotracer and serial scanning (Fig. 15.3) [1, 2]. However, both of these methods are invasive and can be painful and poorly tolerated by patients and either technique may not be available in all hospitals.

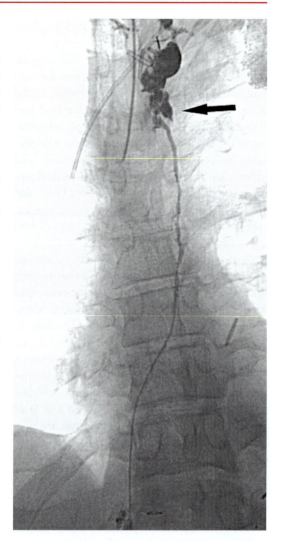

Fig. 15.3 Radiographic image showing extravasation of the contrast in the upper part of the thoracic duct (*arrow*), following injection of the duct with iodinated contrast through the microcatheter (Reproduced with permission from Itkin et al. [8])

15.5 Initial Management and Outcomes

Initial management of thoracic duct injury depends upon presentation and volume of the leak. In patients in whom the injury has been identified intraoperatively, maneuvers should be taken to localize the injury, such as the administration of cream or absorbable dye. Once the injury is localized, the duct should be ligated proximal and distal to the injury. Attempts at surgical repair are unlikely to be successful and are

impractical to perform due to the delicate nature of the lymphatic vessels [6, 11]. In those patients presenting with chylothorax, initial management consists of adequate pleural drainage with placement of tube thoracostomies, with or without image guidance. Drainage must be adequate to evacuate all fluid and allow the collapsed lung to fully re-expand. Maneuvers to reduce the volume of chyle should then be undertaken. The patient may be made nothing per os (NPO) and placed on TPN.

Alternatively, the patient may be allowed a fat free diet enriched in medium-chain triglycerides. Use of octreotide or somatostatin, which reduces gastrointestinal secretion and absorption and subsequently may reduce chyle production, has also been reported [2–4, 13, 15]. Electrolytes, fluids, and fat-soluble vitamins should be monitored closely and aggressively replaced intravenously. Low and moderately low output chylothoraces, those with <500 and <1,000 mL/day, respectively, generally respond well to dietary manipulation and drainage without requiring invasive interventions. The overall success rate of conservative management has been reported to be as high as 88 % [2, 9, 10]. Once the fluid draining has cleared from milky to serous, and the output has decreased to less than 250 mL/day, a high-fat meal challenge should be given, if no increase in output or change in character of the drainage is noted, the chest tubes can be removed [15].

It is unclear how long patients should be trialed on medical management before it should be considered unsuccessful and surgical management performed. Studies vary from 1 to 4 weeks; however, most advocate for intervention if the chyle leak has failed to resolve within 2 weeks, particularly as sufficient T cell loss to place the patient at severe risk for sepsis can occur within 8 days [2, 3, 6, 16].

In those patients with high-output chylothoraces, in whom leaks exceed 1,000–1,500 mL/day for adults or 100 mL/kg/day in children, conservative management is unlikely to be successful [2, 6, 16]. In these patients, intervention should be performed early in their hospital course to reduce the risk of morbidity, particularly infectious, and mortality. With early intervention and adequate nutritional support mortality can be reduced to 0–10 % [2, 4–6, 14]. Early intervention may also reduce hospital length of stay [6].

15.6   Operative and Interventional Management and Outcomes

Treatment options for high-output chylothoraces or for those of low to moderate output who fail to resolve with conservative management include percutaneous thoracic duct embolization and ligation of the thoracic duct by either open or video-assisted thoracoscopic surgical (VATS) approaches. Surgical ligation of the thoracic duct has been the gold standard treatment with a success rate of 90–95 % and associated mortality of 0–16 % and morbidity of 0–16.7 % [2, 6, 8–11]. Associated injuries and comorbidities likely contribute to mortality; however, deaths occur primarily because of malnutrition, sepsis, and respiratory failure due to the persistent chylous fistula. Early ligation, optimal management of fluids, nutrition and electrolytes, and use of minimally invasive VATS techniques have decreased mortality and morbidity rates, and may result in shorter lengths of stay. Surgical approach will be dictated by cause and location of the chylothorax.

Iatrogenic injuries are best approached via the initial surgical incision. The patient can be given cream, milk, or dye preoperatively to help localize the site of the injury. Once the injury has been localized, it should be suture ligated proximal and distal to the site of injury. This can be augmented with the use of pledgets in the suture ligation, clips, and placement of fibrin or artificial glue sealants. Thought can also be given to buttressing the site of ligation with a pleural flap. For traumatic chylothoraces without prior surgery, open thoracotomy or VATS can be used to explore the affected hemithorax, and the site of injury should be localized and ligated proximal and distal to the site of injury. If there is concern regarding the ability to localize the injury, again the patient can be given a lipid heavy food bolus or absorbable dye approximately 4 h prior to exploration or lymphangiography can be utilized to locate the source of the injury. Alternatively, if these methods have not successfully located the injury or are not available the thoracic duct can be ligated within the preaortic tissues at the diaphragmatic hiatus. This technique has the advantage of stopping potential flow from accessory lymphatic ducts, and may be performed in conjunction with or without talc pleurodesis.

In some cases, patients may not tolerate thoracic procedures due to poor reserve, associated lung injury, or pneumonia; or it may be unfeasible due to prior surgeries. In these cases the thoracic duct can be ligated via a transabdominal approach. Exposure of the abdominal portion of the thoracic duct can be performed by mobilizing the left lobe of the liver and dividing the gastrohepatic ligament. The stomach and esophagus are retracted laterally to the left, and the retroperitoneum and median arcuate ligament are divided as are the interdigitating fibers of the diaphragmatic crura. This exposes the origin of the celiac trunk and the supraceliac aorta. The proximal thoracic duct can be found at this level to the right of the aorta and ligated. This technique has been reported to be successful at resolving chylothorax with both open and laparoscopic approaches [17–19].

A new alternative to surgical ligation of the thoracic duct is percutaneous embolization. This technique requires pedal lymphangiography to localize the cisterna chyli, the cisterna is then accessed percutaneously by transabdominal catheterization. The thoracic duct can then be interrogated radiographically to localize the source of injury and can then be embolized with coils, chemical coagulants, or a combination of the two agents. A review of the existing literature regarding thoracic duct embolization up to 2004, including 91 patients, found a technical success rate of 79 % and a clinical success rate (complete resolution of chylothorax) of 69 %. This was associated with no mortalities and a 2 % morbidity rate, with most complications being minor and self limited [10]. Subsequently, a large series of 109 patients treated with thoracic duct embolization had a similar success rate of 71 %, with a complication rate of only 3 %. This series included 20 patients who had already failed surgical ligation of the thoracic duct; within this subgroup success of thoracic duct embolization was 88 % [8].

15.7 Postoperative Management and Complications

Patients undergoing open or VATS thoracic duct ligation or embolization should have thoracostomy tubes left in place post procedure to asses

for change in character and quantity of drainage. Once drainage has ceased being chylous and output has diminished, patients should undergo oral challenge with a fatty meal. If quantity and character of the drainage does not change with the challenge, the drains can be removed.

Recurrent chylothorax can occur in 5–10 % of patients following surgical ligation and in 29–31 % of patients following embolization [9–11]. If there is continued or recurrent chylous drainage following either surgical ligation or embolization, continued medical management can be continued with bowel rest, TPN, and fluid and electrolyte replacement with or without octreotide. If the leak does not respond to conservative management following embolization, surgical ligation should be performed. Strong consideration should be given to ligation at the level of the diaphragmatic hiatus to ligate possible collateral lymphatic vessels. If the chyle leak occurs after surgical ligation, there is some evidence to suggest success with embolization in a high percentage of these patients, up to 88 % [8]. Alternatively, patients who fail surgical ligation can undergo talc pleurodesis which generally has a good success rate or less commonly pleuroperitoneal shunt placement [3, 9].

Conclusion

Thoracic duct injury is a rare consequence of both blunt and penetrating trauma; it is most commonly due to iatrogenic injury following neck or chest surgery, particularly esophagectomy. It can be associated with significant morbidity including sepsis, malnutrition, dehydration, and electrolyte abnormalities, these complications can result in death if not appropriately treated in a timely fashion. If suspected intraoperatively, provocative maneuvers such as enteral administration of cream can be performed to localize the site of injury for ligation. In patients who present postoperatively or post-injury with chylothorax, conservative management with drainage, bowel rest, intravenous fluids and nutrition, with or without octreotide, is quite successful if output is low or moderate. In those patients with high volume output or in those who do not respond to conservative management within 2 weeks, percutaneous embolization or surgical ligation should be performed expeditiously in order to minimize morbidity and mortality. Recurrent chylothorax is an uncommon complication following surgical ligation and embolization, and can be treated with conservative management or if high volume or unresponsive with talc pleurodesis with good results.

References

1. Greenfield LJ. Lymphatic system disorders. In: Greenfield L, Mulholland M, Oldham K, Zelenock G, Lillemore K, editors. Surgery: scientific principles and practice. Philadelphia: Lippincott Williams and Wilkins; 2001. p. 1897–900.
2. Seitelman E, Arellano JJ, Takabe K, Barrett L, Faust G, Angus LD. Chylothorax after blunt trauma. J Thorac Dis. 2012;4(3):327–30.
3. Sugarbaker DJ, Zellos L, Davis BD. Chest wall, pleura, mediastinum, and nonneoplastic lung disease. In: Greenfield L, Mulholland MW, Oldham KT, Zelenock GB, Lillemore KD, editors. Surgery: scientific principles and practice. Philadelphia: Lippincott Williams and Wilkins; 2001. p. 1417–9.
4. Maddaus MA, Luketich JD. Chest wall, lung, mediastinum, and pleura. In: Brunicardi FC, Andersen DK, Biliar TR, Dunn DL, Hunter JG, Pollock RE, editors. Schwartz's manual of surgery. New York: McGraw-Hill; 2006. p. 434.
5. Sachs PB, Zelch MG, Rice TW, Geisinger MA, Risius B, Lammert GK. Diagnosis and localization of laceration of the thoracic duct: usefulness of lymphangiography and CT. AJR Am J Roentgenol. 1991;157(4).
6. Worthington MG, de Groot M, Gunning AJ, von Oppell UO. Isolated thoracic duct injury after penetrating chest trauma. Ann Thorac Surg. 1995;60(2): 272–4.
7. Apostolakis E, Akinosoglou K, Koletsis E, Dougenis D. Traumatic chylothorax following blunt thoracic trauma: two conservatively treated cases. J Card Surg. 2009;24(2).
8. Itkin M, Kucharczuk JC, Kwak A, Trerotola SO, Kaiser LR. Nonoperative thoracic duct embolization for traumatic thoracic duct leak: experience in 109 patients. J Thorac Cardiovasc Surg. 2010;139(3): 584–9.
9. Paul S, Altorki NK, Port JL, Stiles BM, Lee PC. Surgical management of chylothorax. Thorac Cardiovasc Surg. 2009;57(4):226–8.
10. Marcon F, Irani K, Aquino T, Saunders JK, Gouge TH, Melis M. Percutaneous treatment of thoracic duct injuries. Surg Endosc. 2011;25(9):2844–8.
11. Whiteford MH, Abdullah F, Vernick JJ, Rabinovici R. Thoracic duct injury in penetrating neck trauma. Am Surg. 1995;61(12):1072–5.
12. Silen ML, Weber TR. Management of thoracic duct injury associated with fracture-dislocation of the spine following blunt trauma. J Trauma. 1995;39(6): 1185–7.
13. Pakula AM, Phillips W, Skinner RA. A case of a traumatic chyle leak following an acute thoracic spine injury: successful resolution with strict dietary manipulation. World J Emerg Surg. 2011;6:10.
14. Gartside R, Hebert JC. Chylothorax following fracture of the thoracolumbar spine. Injury. 1988;19(5): 363–4.
15. DeCamp MM, Sodha NR. Applied anatomy of the chest wall and mediastinum. In: Fischer JE, editor. Mastery of surgery. Philadelphia: Wolters Kluwer/ Lippincott Williams and Wilkins; 2007. p. 566–8.
16. Selle JG, Snyder 3rd WH, Schreiber JT. Chylothorax: indications for surgery. Ann Surg. 1973;177(2): 245–9.
17. Schumacher G, Weidemann H, Langrehr JM, Jonas S, Mittier J, Jacob D, Schmidt SC, Spinelli A, Pratschke J, Pfitzmann R, Alekseev D, Neuhaus P. Transabdominal ligation of the thoracic duct as treatment of choice for postoperative chylothorax after esophagectomy. Dis Esophagus. 2007;20(1):19–23.
18. Tsubokawa N, Hamai Y, Hihara J, Emi M, Miyata Y, Okada M. Laparoscopic thoracic duct clipping for persistent chylothorax after extrapleural pneumonectomy. Ann Thorac Surg. 2012;93(5):e131–2.
19. Vassallo BC, Cavadas D, Beveraggi E, Sivori E. Treatment of postoperative chylothorax through laparoscopic thoracic duct ligation. Eur J Cardiothorac Surg. 2002;21(3):556–7.
20. Stranding S, Healy J, Johnson D, Williams A. The mediastinum. In: Ellis H, editor. Gray's anatomy: the anatomical basis of clinical practice. Edinburgh: Elsevier/Churchill Livingstone; 2004. p. 985.
21. Shane Tubbs R, Noordeh N, Parmar A, Comert A, Loukas M, Shoja MM, Cohen-Gadol AA. Reliability of Poirier's triangle in localizing the thoracic duct in the thorax. Surg Radiol Anat. 2010;32:757–60.

Part IV

Abdomen

John A. Weigelt and Sherene Shalhub

Abdominal Aorta Injuries

16

Sherene Shalhub and Benjamin W. Starnes

Contents

16.1   Introduction

Traumatic abdominal aortic injury is uncommon but remains one of the most challenging injuries to successfully manage. Many patients die of hemorrhage prior to arrival to the hospital and those who survive to the hospital are hypotensive due to massive blood loss and associated injuries [1, 2]. Penetrating injuries account for 70–95 % of abdominal vascular trauma with gunshot wounds exceeding stab wounds and affecting men primarily [1–4]. Blunt abdominal aortic injury (BAAI) occurs with less than 1 % incidence [5]. In an autopsy series, 5 % of aortic lacerations occurred in the abdominal aorta [6]. Since 1996, 100 cases of blunt abdominal aortic injury were reported as case reports or case series with motor vehicle crashes being the predominant mechanism and affecting men primarily [5, 7–54]. The most common associated injuries include abdominal visceral injuries and lumbar spine fracture [5]. Table 16.1 summarizes the demographics and type of aortic injury of these cases.

16.2   Anatomy/Physiology

Abdominal aortic mechanism of injury relates to the biomechanical direct and indirect forces incurred while it is tethered between the spinal column, the peritoneum, and abdominal viscera [5, 6]. The most frequent force causing

S. Shalhub, MD, MPH (✉) • B.W. Starnes, MD
Division of Vascular Surgery,
University of Washington,
Seattle, WA, USA
e-mail: shalhub@uw.edu

A. Dua et al. (eds.), *Clinical Review of Vascular Trauma*,
DOI 10.1007/978-3-642-39100-2_16, © Springer-Verlag Berlin Heidelberg 2014

Table 16.1 Summary of BAAI literature review of clinical presentation, associated injuries, and location of abdominal aortic injury

	$N = 100$ (values are also %)
Age median (range)	30 years (1–89)
Male	70
Hypotensive on admission (<90 mmHg)	34
Cardiac arrest in route, ED or OR	14
Associated injuries	
Traumatic brain injury	11
Rib fractures	10
Pneumothorax/hemothorax	13
Abdominal wall ecchymosis	34
Abdominal wall degloving	9
Solid organ injury	25
Mesenteric hematoma/laceration	26
Small bowel injury	38
Colon injury	22
Spine fracture	32
Pelvic fracture	16
IVC injury	8
Retroperitoneal hematoma	50
Lower extremity ischemia	17
Location on aorta	
Zone I: superior to SMA	8
Zone II: SMA to RA	6
Zone III: infrarenal	86

SMA superior mesenteric artery, *RA* renal artery

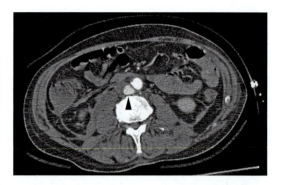

Fig. 16.1 Blunt abdominal aortic pseudoaneurysm (*arrowhead*) as seen on axial view with CT angiography

an abdominal aorta injury is compressive, associated with deceleration [55]. Indirect forces occur when the aortic wall is directly stretched and compressed against a high-pressure column of blood leading to intimal tears, pseudoaneurysm, rupture, or thrombosis [56, 57]. Atherosclerotic changes of the aorta are associated with a weakening of the intima in addition to loss of elasticity and compliance and thus thought to increase the risk of aortic injury [58, 59]. These forces can occur during motor vehicle collisions when the aorta is compressed by the seat belt, thus termed "seat belt aorta" [60]. Other mechanisms include long-distance falls, direct compression of the aorta, and penetrating injuries.

The underlying pathologic lesion of BAAI is the disruption of the intima. Depending on the magnitude of the traumatic forces, BAAI presents as a spectrum of disease ranging from a minimal aortic injury (MAI) to free rupture of the aorta [61]. The increasing use of CT scanning with angiography to evaluate patients with blunt trauma has resulted in increasing numbers of MAI diagnosed [61]. These traumatic intimal tears can manifest as intimal flaps or dissection which can be uncomplicated or progress to thrombosis or acute arterial insufficiency [21, 22, 29, 56]. Injuries involving the adventitia lead to pseudoaneurysm formation (Fig. 16.1) or even rupture of the aortic wall. Rupture of the aortic wall can also be due to branch vessel avulsion [2].

The majority of the injuries occur inferior to the renal arteries. Aortic injuries are classified based on presence of aortic contour abnormality and presence of free rupture [5]. This classification is based on experience with blunt thoracic aortic injury [62]. Intimal tears/flaps are not associated with external aortic contour abnormality. A pseudoaneurysm presents as a contained rupture and is clearly associated with an aortic contour abnormality. The most common associated injuries are small bowel injuries (38 %) and thoracolumbar spine injuries (25 %). The most common anatomic findings since 1996 were intimal tears/flaps (41 %) followed by reports of pseudoaneurysms (29 %) [8, 10, 11, 15–47].

16.2.1 Clinical Assessment and Diagnostic Testing

The initial presentation is dependent on presence or absence of free rupture of the abdominal aorta, branch vessel avulsion, or concomitant inferior vena cava injury [2]. Those with rupture typically present with hypotension due to hemorrhagic shock. Emergency room anterolateral thoracotomy is used to provide cross clamping the aorta in the distal thorax. In our recent BAAI series, all patients with rupture were hypotensive, and 75 % had cardiac arrest in the emergency department with 38 % requiring an emergency department thoracotomy [5]. Tamponade is usually associated with a retroperitoneal hematoma which improves survival [2, 3]. Abdominal wall ecchymosis is seen in one third of BAAI cases and should raise the index of suspicion for aortic and associated hollow viscus injuries [5].

16.2.2 Diagnostic Testing

Diagnostic testing is dependent on the initial presentation. In the hypotensive patient, the focused assessment with sonography for trauma (FAST) scan or a diagnostic peritoneal lavage (DPL) is the first step. If significant hemoperitoneum is present, then operative exploration is warranted. In the temodynamically stable patient an abdominal and pelvic CT scan with contrast is done allowing the evaluation of the aortic anatomy and concomitant injuries [63].

16.3 Initial Management

Management of aortic injury varies and risk of mortality rises with the severity of the pathologic lesion. In a recent review of the National Trauma Data Bank of 436 patients with BAAI from 180 centers from 2007 to 2009, 90 % were managed nonoperatively. Of those who underwent operative repair, 69 % underwent endovascular repair, with the remainder undergoing open aortic repair and two extra-anatomic bypasses [64]. In general,

cases of BAAI with uncomplicated intimal flaps are managed nonoperatively with anti-impulse (β-blockers) and antiplatelet (aspirin) therapy and close follow-up. The natural history of intimal flaps is a decrease in size and complete resolution [9]. Cases of aortic pseudoaneurysms require operative repair to prevent rupture, but these can be managed on a semi-elective basis during the initial hospitalization. Cases complicated by thrombosis, acute arterial insufficiency, and free rupture require an operative or endovascular repair.

The timing of repair also depends on the patient's associated injuries. Patients with pulse and neurologic deficits, an expanding hematoma and concomitant intra-abdominal injuries, require emergent exploration and immediate repair. Otherwise, treatment can be individualized in the hemodynamically normal trauma patient.

16.4 Open Repair

Initial management is determined by the hemodynamic state of the patient. Hypotensive patients are managed with an exploratory laparotomy. A midline laparotomy incision allows exposure of all zones of the abdomen. Initial inspection identifies areas of ongoing hemorrhage, contained hematoma, or evidence of bowel ischemia [3]. Operative management of aortic injury is guided by its associated Zone 1 hematoma which may be supramesocolic or inframesocolic. Common pitfalls and pearls regarding management of the patient with an aortic injury are discussed below.

16.4.1 Exposure and Control of the Aorta

Exposure is guided by the location of the retroperitoneal hematoma. In the case of a supramesocolic hematoma, proximal control of the aorta can be obtained at the diaphragm. The supraceliac aorta is exposed by opening the gastrohepatic ligament, lateral retraction of the left lobe of the liver, and caudal retraction of the stomach. The esophagus is mobilized laterally, its location

Fig. 16.2 Manual clamping of the supraceliac aorta, followed by placement of an atraumatic vascular clamp over the fingers

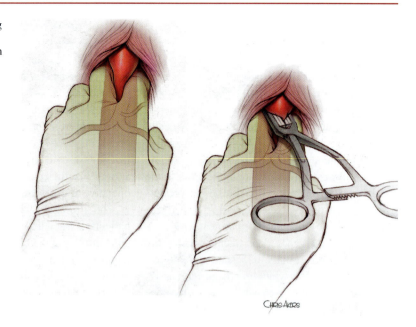

facilitated by the presence of a nasogastric or orogastric tube. This allows identification of the abdominal aorta at the diaphragmatic hiatus. Control is achieved manually with compression or by vascular clamp placement (Fig. 16.2). Full exposure of the supraceliac aorta and its branches is achieved with left medial visceral rotation (the Mattox maneuver). For an inframesocolic hematoma, the exposure is obtained in a transperitoneal fashion similar to that for an infrarenal aneurysm. This is achieved with caudal retraction of the transverse colon, retraction of the small intestine to the right, and cephalad mobilization of the third and fourth portions of the duodenum. The proximal extent of this exposure is the left renal vein which can be divided if necessary between clamps for more cephalad access to the aorta. Proximal control of the aorta is obtained immediately below the renal arteries or at the diaphragm [65].

16.4.2 Repair of the Aorta

Repair of the aorta is determined by extent of injury and on presence of gross contamination from hollow viscus injury. In cases of aortic tears, multiple injuries can be connected and closed in linear fashion using polypropylene suture,

Dacron patch aortoplasty, or Dacron graft interposition depending on the size of the tear [65]. In cases of intimal flaps complicated by thrombosis and acute arterial insufficiency, repair is accomplished with thrombectomy and tacking sutures of the intimal flap or Dacron graft interposition if the damage to the intima is substantial (Fig. 16.3). Pseudoaneurysms usually require excision with primary end-to-end anastomosis or interposition grafting.

Gross contamination from hollow viscus injury can jeopardize aortic grafts due to risk of infection. Thus ligation of the injured aorta with extra-anatomic bypass, such as axillobifemoral bypass, may be required. In cases in which damage control laparotomy is needed, shunts such as chest tubes, endotracheal tubes, or carotid shunts can be used to establish temporary control, in a damage control fashion until hypothermia, coagulopathy, and acidosis are corrected.

16.5 Endovascular Management of Aortic Injuries

Reports of endovascular stent placement in cases of aortic injuries have recently increased in frequency because these techniques are less invasive

Fig. 16.3 Blunt abdominal aortic injury associated with thrombosis of the infrarenal aorta (*arrow*) and bilateral proximal iliac arteries (**a**). Complete intimal disruption seen (**b**)

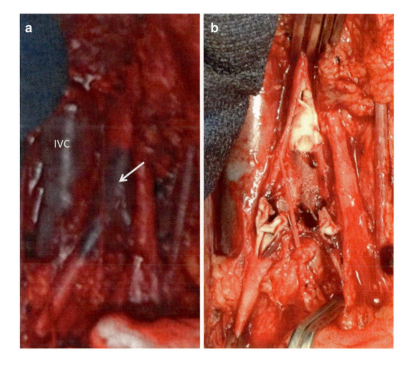

and an attractive alternative for patients with both isolated aortic injuries and multisystem injuries in a manner similar to that of blunt thoracic aortic injury (Fig. 16.4). The use of stent grafts is not widely adopted, and most of the literature is limited to case reports and small case series where endovascular stents, aortic extension cuffs, and limb extensions have all been used in cases of blunt and penetrating trauma [23, 24, 29, 31, 34, 35, 44, 66–69]. Indications include cases with associated gross contamination from hollow viscus injury that can jeopardize aortic grafts due to risk of infection or management of injuries difficult to expose by conventional means. Endovascular interventions can be used as a stabilizing measure for critically ill patients and a bridge to open definitive repair. From an endovascular perspective as it relates to trauma, abdominal aorta zones of injury can be classified [5] based on feasibility of endovascular approach as follows: *Zone I injuries* occur from diaphragmatic hiatus to the superior mesenteric artery (SMA). *Zone II injuries* include the SMA to renal arteries. *Zone III injuries* are inferior to the renal arteries to the aortic bifurcation (Fig. 16.5). Zone I and III injuries are amenable to endovascular

repair, whereas Zone II lesions are not amenable to endovascular stenting without fenestration for the SMA and renal arteries. The timing of the repair is dependent on the patient's hemodynamic status and the presence of acute limb ischemia. Endovascular repair can be used for injuries from the diaphragmatic hiatus to the superior mesenteric artery or for injuries below the renal arteries to the aortic bifurcation. Injuries that involve the aorta in the vicinity of the SMA and renal arteries are not easy to manage by an endovascular technique as this would require graft fenestration for the SMA and renal arteries

16.5.1 Intra-Aortic Occlusion Balloon (IAOB)

The most common cause of death from aortic trauma remains hemorrhagic shock compounded by ongoing coagulopathy; thus early proximal control of the aorta is a key maneuver [2, 5, 6, 10]. The use of transfemoral IAOB to obtain proximal control at the level of the diaphragm prior to entering the abdomen may have a role in early control of hemorrhage from the

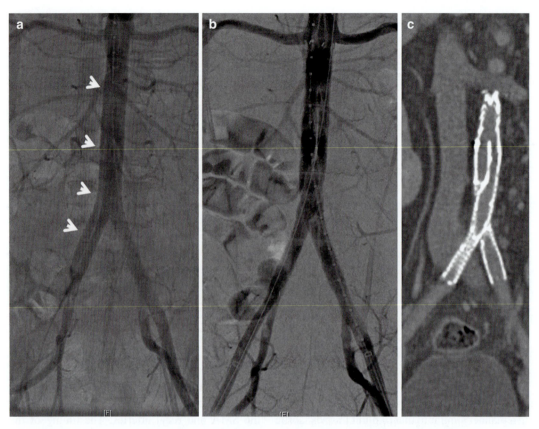

Fig. 16.4 Blunt abdominal aortic dissection. (**a**) An intraoperative arteriogram showing the dissection flap (*arrows*) in the infrarenal aorta and extending to the right common iliac artery. (**b**) Arteriogram post endovascular stent graft placement. (**c**) Coronal view of CT angiography 6 weeks post repair

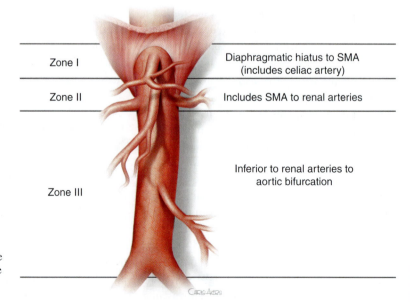

Fig. 16.5 Zone I injuries occur from diaphragmatic hiatus to the superior mesenteric artery (*SMA*). Zone II injuries include the SMA to Renal arteries. Zone III injuries are inferior to the renal arteries to the aortic bifurcation

Zone I — Diaphragmatic hiatus to SMA (includes celiac artery)

Zone II — Includes SMA to renal arteries

Zone III — Inferior to renal arteries to aortic bifurcation

injured aorta [70]. Placement of the IAOB can be done expeditiously and would not delay the laparotomy as demonstrated in proximal control of the aorta in cases of ruptured abdominal aortic aneurysms [71]. Current studies are evaluating the use of this modality in animal models [72, 73].

16.6 Pearls, Complications, and Pitfalls

- Patient preparation includes a warmed room to minimize patient hypothermia.
- Placement of the patient on a radiolucent table allows the option for endovascular intervention. Prior to incision, a nasogastric or orogastric tube is placed to decompress the stomach and facilitate identification of the esophagus during supraceliac aortic clamping. A Foley catheter is inserted to decompress the bladder and avoid injury during laparotomy as well as for urine output monitoring.
- Concomitant limb ischemia may be present due to intimal flaps complicated by thrombosis and acute arterial insufficiency; thus it is imperative to assess the peripheral vasculature for involvement of limb ischemia prior to the start of the case and at the conclusion of the procedure.
- The patient is prepped from sternal notch to upper anterior thigh. This allows access to the anterior thorax should a thoracic injury be identified or if vascular control via the thorax is needed. Distally preparing the upper anterior thighs allows for saphenous vein harvest should vascular reconstruction be deemed necessary.
- Broad spectrum antibiotic is administered prior to incision.

16.7 Outcomes

Injury to the abdominal aorta is highly lethal. Among those who survive the transport to the hospital mortality rates range from 32 to 78 % with hemorrhagic shock being the most common cause of associated mortality [2, 4–6, 10]. Outcomes in cases requiring a resuscitative thoracotomy remain poor [74, 75]. In BAAI, mortality varies by the type of aortic injury. When minimal aortic injuries, dissections of the aorta, and pseudoaneurysms are included, aggregate mortality is 11 % [5]. In cases treated by endovascular repair, the long-term durability of aortic endografts for abdominal aortic trauma is not well described. Clearly long-term follow-up will be required in these cases.

Conclusion
Abdominal aortic injury is rare and remains associated with high morbidity and mortality. High index of suspicion with expeditious diagnosis and repair is lifesaving. Temporizing measures such as shunts or endovascular repair used in a damage control manner my increase survival though this remains to be seen. Using newer adjuncts for obtaining proximal aortic control such as IAOB or the move to a hybrid suite is on the horizon in the management of this population.

References

1. Asensio JA, Chahwan S, Hanpeter D, Demetriades D, Forno W, Gambaro E, et al. Operative management and outcome of 302 abdominal vascular injuries. Am J Surg. 2000;180(6):528–33.
2. Deree J, Shenvi E, Fortlage D, Stout P, Potenza B, Hoyt DB, et al. Patient factors and operating room resuscitation predict mortality in traumatic abdominal aortic injury: a 20-year analysis. J Vasc Surg. 2007;45(3):493–7.
3. Goaley TJ, Dente CJ, Feliciano DV. Torso vascular trauma at an urban level I trauma center. Perspect Vasc Surg Endovasc Ther. 2006;18(2):102–12.
4. Paul JS, Webb TP, Aprahamian C, Weigelt JA. Intraabdominal vascular injury: are we getting any better? J Trauma. 2010;69(6):1393–7.
5. Shalhub S, Starnes BW, Tran NT, Hatsukami TS, Lundgren RS, Davis CW, et al. Blunt abdominal aortic injury. J Vasc Surg. 2012;55(5):1277–85.
6. Burkhart HM, Gomez GA, Jacobson LE, Pless JE, Broadie TA. Fatal blunt aortic injuries: a review of 242 autopsy cases. J Trauma. 2001;50(1):113–5.
7. Tracy Jr TF, Silen ML, Graham MA. Delayed rupture of the abdominal aorta in a child after a suspected handlebar injury. J Trauma. 1996;40(1):119–20.

8. Borioni R, Garofalo M, Seddio F, Colagrande L, Marino B, Albano P. Posttraumatic infrarenal abdominal aortic pseudoaneurysm. Tex Heart Inst J. 1999; 26(4):312–4.

9. Aladham F, Sundaram B, Williams DM, Quint LE. Traumatic aortic injury: computerized tomographic findings at presentation and after conservative therapy. J Comput Assist Tomogr. 2010;34(3):388–94.

10. Roth SM, Wheeler JR, Gregory RT, Gayle RG, Parent III FN, Demasi R, et al. Blunt injury of the abdominal aorta: a review. J Trauma. 1997;42(4):748–55.

11. Choit RL, Tredwell SJ, Leblanc JG, Reilly CW, Mulpuri K. Abdominal aortic injuries associated with chance fractures in pediatric patients. J Pediatr Surg. 2006;41(6):1184–90.

12. Heck JM, Bittles MA. Traumatic abdominal aortic dissection in a 16-month-old child. Pediatr Radiol. 2009;39(7):750–3.

13. Siavelis HA, Mansour MA. Aortoiliac dissection after blunt abdominal trauma: case report. J Trauma. 1997;43(5):862–4.

14. Crabb GM, McQuillen KK. Subtle abdominal aortic injury after blunt chest trauma. J Emerg Med. 2006;31(1):29–31.

15. Michaels AJ, Gerndt SJ, Taheri PA, Wang SC, Wahl WL, Simeone DM, et al. Blunt force injury of the abdominal aorta. J Trauma. 1996;41(1):105–9.

16. Marty-Ane CH, Alric P, Prudhomme M, Chircop R, Serres-Cousine O, Mary H. Intravascular stenting of traumatic abdominal aortic dissection. J Vasc Surg. 1996;23(1):156–61.

17. Leiser A, Furrer M, Leutenegger A. Blunt abdominal trauma with lesion of the abdominal aorta – a case report. Swiss Surg. 1997;3(4):181–4.

18. Vernhet H, Marty-Ane CH, Lesnik A, Chircop R, Serres-Cousine O, Picard E, et al. Dissection of the abdominal aorta in blunt trauma: management by percutaneous stent placement. Cardiovasc Intervent Radiol. 1997;20(6):473–6.

19. Kory LA. Thrombosis of the abdominal aorta in a child after blunt trauma. AJR Am J Roentgenol. 2000;175(2):553–4.

20. Henaine R, Baste JC, Diard N, Sibe M, Sassoust G, Midy D. Blunt trauma to the infrarenal abdominal aorta with neurologic lesions. Case report and review of the literature. J Mal Vasc. 2001;26(2): 111–5.

21. Berthet JP, Marty-Ane CH, Veerapen R, Picard E, Mary H, Alric P. Dissection of the abdominal aorta in blunt trauma: endovascular or conventional surgical management? J Vasc Surg. 2003;38(5):997–1003.

22. Meghoo CA, Gonzalez EA, Tyroch AH, Wohltmann CD. Complete occlusion after blunt injury to the abdominal aorta. J Trauma. 2003;55(4):795–9.

23. Stahlfeld KR, Mitchell J, Sherman H. Endovascular repair of blunt abdominal aortic injury: case report. J Trauma. 2004;57(3):638–41.

24. Teruya TH, Bianchi C, Abou-Zamzam AM, Ballard JL. Endovascular treatment of a blunt traumatic abdominal aortic injury with a commercially available stent graft. Ann Vasc Surg. 2005;19(4):474–8.

25. Vuorisalo S, Railo M, Lappalainen K, Aho P, Lepantalo M. Low-energy blunt abdominal aortic trauma in an underweighted man. Eur J Vasc Endovasc Surg. 2005;29(6):595–6.

26. Aidinian G, Karnaze M, Russo EP, Mukherjee D. Endograft repair of traumatic aortic transection in a 10-year-old – a case report. Vasc Endovascular Surg. 2006;40(3):239–42.

27. Diaz JA, Campbell BT, Moursi MM, Boneti C, Kokoska ER, Jackson RJ, et al. Delayed manifestation of abdominal aortic stenosis in a child presenting 10 years after blunt abdominal trauma. J Vasc Surg. 2006;44(5):1104–6.

28. Ghekiere O, Laffargue G, Bolivar J, Taourel P. Dissection of the infrarenal abdominal aorta in blunt trauma. JBR-BTR. 2006;89(1):49.

29. Halkos ME, Nicholas J, Kong LS, Burke JR, Milner R. Endovascular management of blunt abdominal aortic injury. Vascular. 2006;14(4):223–6.

30. Marti M, Pinilla I, Baudraxler F, Simon MJ, Garzon G. A case of acute abdominal aortic dissection caused by blunt trauma. Emerg Radiol. 2006;12(4):182–5.

31. Gunn M, Campbell M, Hoffer EK. Traumatic abdominal aortic injury treated by endovascular stent placement. Emerg Radiol. 2007;13(6):329–31.

32. McCarthy MC, Price SW, Rundell WK, Lehner JT, Barney LM, Ekeh AP, et al. Pediatric blunt abdominal aortic injuries: case report and review of the literature. J Trauma. 2007;63(6):1383–7.

33. Burjonrappa S, Vinocur C, Smergel E, Chhabra A, Galiote J. Pediatric blunt abdominal aortic trauma. J Trauma. 2008;65(1):E10–2.

34. Huang JT, Heckman JT, Gunduz Y, Ohki T. Endovascular management of stenosis of the infrarenal aorta secondary to blunt abdominal aortic trauma in a multiply injured patient. J Trauma. 2009;66(6):E81–5.

35. Voellinger DC, Saddakni S, Melton SM, Wirthlin DJ, Jordan WD, Whitley D. Endovascular repair of a traumatic infrarenal aortic transection: a case report and review. Vasc Surg. 2001;35(5):385–9.

36. Rosengart MR, Zierler RE. Fractured aorta – a case report. Vasc Endovascular Surg. 2002;36(6):465–7.

37. Albino P, Garcia C, Meireles N. Post-traumatic pseudo aneurysm of the infrarenal aorta. A clinical report. Rev Port Cir Cardiotorac Vasc. 2004;11(2):97–100.

38. Raghavendran K, Singh G, Arnoldo B, Flynn WJ. Delayed development of infrarenal abdominal aortic pseudoaneurysm after blunt trauma: a case report and review of the literature. J Trauma. 2004;57(5): 1111–4.

39. Muniz AE, Haynes JH. Delayed abdominal aortic rupture in a child with a seat-belt sign and review of the literature. J Trauma. 2004;56(1):194–7.

40. Katsoulis E, Tzioupis C, Sparks I, Giannoudis PV. Compressive blunt trauma of the abdomen and pelvis associated with abdominal aortic rupture. Acta Orthop Belg. 2006;72(4):492–501.

41. Lalancette M, Scalabrini B, Martinet O. Seat-belt aorta: a rare injury associated with blunt abdominal trauma. Ann Vasc Surg. 2006;20(5):681–3.

42. Amini M. Pseudoaneurysm of the abdominal aorta following blunt trauma. J Coll Physicians Surg Pak. 2008;18(2):115–7.

43. Kawai N, Sato M, Tanihata H, Sahara S, Takasaka I, Minamiguchi H, et al. Repair of traumatic abdominal aortic pseudoaneurysm using N-butyl-2-cyano-acrylate embolization. Cardiovasc Intervent Radiol. 2010;33(2):406–9.

44. Rubin S, Pages ON, Poncet A, Baehrel B. Endovascular treatment of an acute subdiaphragmatic aortic rupture. Ann Thorac Surg. 2006;82(6):2276–8.

45. McEwan L, Woodruff P, Archibald C. Lap belt abdominal aortic trauma. Australas Radiol. 1999;43(3):369–71.

46. Moniz L, Neves J, Pereira AC. Traumatic pseudoaneurysm of the abdominal aorta. Case report. Rev Port Cir Cardiotorac Vasc. 2005;12(4):245–7.

47. Jongkind V, Linsen MA, Diks J, Vos AW, Klinkert P, Rauwerda JA, et al. Aortoiliac reconstruction for abdominal aortic rupture after blunt trauma. J Trauma. 2009;66(4):1248–50.

48. Naude GP, Back M, Perry MO, Bongard FS. Blunt disruption of the abdominal aorta: report of a case and review of the literature. J Vasc Surg. 1997;25(5):931–5.

49. Qureshi A, Roberts N, Nicholson A, Johnson B. Three-dimensional reconstruction by spiral computed tomography to locate aortic tear following blunt abdominal trauma. Eur J Vasc Endovasc Surg. 1997;14(4):316–7.

50. Harkin DW, Kirk G, Clements WD. Abdominal aortic rupture in a child after blunt trauma on a soccer field. Injury. 1999;30(4):303–4.

51. Lin PJ, Jeng LB, Chen RJ, Kao CL, Chu JL, Chang CH. Femoro-arterial bypass using Gott shunt in liver transplantation following severe hepatic trauma. Int Surg. 1993;78(4):295–7.

52. Nucifora G, Hysko F, Vasciaveo A. Blunt traumatic abdominal aortic rupture: CT imaging. Emerg Radiol. 2008;15(3):211–3.

53. Sugimoto T, Omura A, Kitade T, Takahashi H, Koyama T, Kurisu S. An abdominal aortic rupture due to seatbelt blunt injury: report of a case. Surg Today. 2007;37(1):86–8.

54. Fox JT, Huang YC, Barcia PJ, Beresky RE, Olsen D. Blunt abdominal aortic transection in a child: case report. J Trauma. 1996;41(6):1051–3.

55. Feliciano DV. Abdominal vascular injuries. Surg Clin North Am. 1988;68(4):741–55.

56. Reisman JD, Morgan AS. Analysis of 46 intra-abdominal aortic injuries from blunt trauma: case reports and literature review. J Trauma. 1990;30(10):1294–7.

57. Sumpio BE, Gusberg RJ. Aortic thrombosis with paraplegia: an unusual consequence of blunt abdominal trauma. J Vasc Surg. 1987;6(4):412–4.

58. Bergqvist D, Takolander R. Aortic occlusion following blunt trauma of the abdomen. J Trauma. 1981;21(4):319–22.

59. Brunsting LA, Ouriel K. Traumatic fracture of the abdominal aorta. Rupture of a calcified abdominal aorta with minimal trauma. J Vasc Surg. 1988;8(2):184–6.

60. Dajee H, Richardson IW, Iype MO. Seat belt aorta: acute dissection and thrombosis of the abdominal aorta. Surgery. 1979;85(3):263–7.

61. Malhotra AK, Fabian TC, Croce MA, Weiman DS, Gavant ML, Pate JW. Minimal aortic injury: a lesion associated with advancing diagnostic techniques. J Trauma. 2001;51(6):1042–8.

62. Azizzadeh A, Keyhani K, Miller III CC, Coogan SM, Safi HJ, Estrera AL. Blunt traumatic aortic injury: initial experience with endovascular repair. J Vasc Surg. 2009;49(6):1403–8.

63. Mellnick VM, McDowell C, Lubner M, Bhalla S, Menias CO. CT features of blunt abdominal aortic injury. Emerg Radiol. 2012;19(4):301–7.

64. de Mestral C, Dueck AD, Gomez D, Haas B, Nathens AB. Associated injuries, management, and outcomes of blunt abdominal aortic injury. J Vasc Surg. 2012;56(3):656–60.

65. Wall Jr MJ, Tsai PI, Gilani R, Mattox KL. Open and endovascular approaches to aortic trauma. Tex Heart Inst J. 2010;37(6):675–7.

66. Sakran JV, Mukherjee D. Four-year follow-up of endograft repair of traumatic aortic transection in a 10-year-old. Vasc Endovascular Surg. 2009;43(6):597–8.

67. Gilani R, Saucedo-Crespo H, Scott BG, Tsai PI, Wall Jr MJ, Mattox KL. Endovascular therapy for overcoming challenges presented with blunt abdominal aortic injury. Vasc Endovascular Surg. 2012;46(4):329–31.

68. Yeh MW, Horn JK, Schecter WP, Chuter TA, Lane JS. Endovascular repair of an actively hemorrhaging gunshot injury to the abdominal aorta. J Vasc Surg. 2005;42(5):1007–9.

69. Hussain Q, Maleux G, Heye S, Fourneau I. Endovascular repair of an actively hemorrhaging stab wound injury to the abdominal aorta. Cardiovasc Intervent Radiol. 2008;31(5):1023–5.

70. Stannard A, Eliason JL, Rasmussen TE. Resuscitative endovascular balloon occlusion of the aorta (REBOA) as an adjunct for hemorrhagic shock. J Trauma. 2011;71(6):1869–72.

71. Starnes BW, Quiroga E, Hutter C, Tran NT, Hatsukami T, Meissner M, et al. Management of ruptured abdominal aortic aneurysm in the endovascular era. J Vasc Surg. 2010;51(1):9–17.

72. White JM, Cannon JW, Stannard A, Markov NP, Spencer JR, Rasmussen TE. Endovascular balloon occlusion of the aorta is superior to resuscitative thoracotomy with aortic clamping in a porcine model of hemorrhagic shock. Surgery. 2011;150(3):400–9.

73. Morrison JJ, Percival TJ, Markov NP, Villamaria C, Scott DJ, Saches KA, et al. Aortic balloon occlusion is effective in controlling pelvic hemorrhage. J Surg Res. 2012;177(2):341–7.

74. Karmy-Jones R, Jurkovich GJ. Blunt chest trauma. Curr Probl Surg. 2004;41(3):211–380.

75. Jurkovich GJ, Esposito TJ, Maier RV. Resuscitative thoracotomy performed in the operating room. Am J Surg. 1992;163(5):463–8.

Abdominal Vein Injuries

17

Harleen K. Sandhu and Kristofer M. Charlton-Ouw

Contents

H.K. Sandhu, MD
Department of Cardiothoracic and Vascular Surgery,
School of Public Health, University of Texas Health
Science Center at Houston, Houston, TX, USA

K.M. Charlton-Ouw, MD (✉)
Department of Cardiothoracic and Vascular Surgery,
University of Texas Medical School at Houston,
Houston, TX, USA
e-mail: kristofer.charltonouw@uth.tmc.edu

17.1   Introduction

Traumatic injury to the abdominal vasculature is a surgical challenge with high morbidity and mortality rates. Despite the advances in prehospital resuscitative trauma management, no significant improvement has occurred in the associated mortality over the past 30 years [1, 2]. Intra-abdominal venous injuries (IAVIs), though relatively rare, constitute a more insidious and technically demanding category of abdominal vascular injury. The reported major IAVI in order of decreasing incidence includes the inferior vena cava (IVC), superior mesenteric vein, inferior mesenteric vein, portal vein, retrohepatic cava and hepatic veins, renal, splenic, and iliac veins [3]. Penetrating injuries account for nearly 90 % of traumatic IAVI [3, 4]. It is estimated that 10–15 % of the abdominal penetrating injuries involve a major vein and 1 in every 50 gunshot wounds involves the IVC [5, 6].

Whether blunt or penetrating, these injuries can be lethal because of bleeding and associated injuries. Even after initial control of hemorrhage, patients succumb to delayed complications and mortality due to multiorgan failure, venous insufficiency, shock, acidosis, coagulopathy, reperfusion injuries, and their sequelae. A large percentage of these patients arrive hemodynamically abnormal, and more than half are pronounced dead at arrival. The associated fatality rates are over 50 % during prehospital care and 20–60 % in those who survive the initial resuscitation and make it to the hospital [3, 5, 6].

A. Dua et al. (eds.), *Clinical Review of Vascular Trauma*,
DOI 10.1007/978-3-642-39100-2_17, © Springer-Verlag Berlin Heidelberg 2014

The "damage control" or the "bail out" philosophy introduced by Stone et al. involves initial laparotomy to achieve rapid hemostasis followed by ongoing resuscitation to correct the often present hypothermia, acidosis, coagulopathy, and abdominal compartment syndrome [7]. Assessment of retroperitoneal bleeding is difficult and is further compounded by the potential for iatrogenic injury while performing rapid dissection. Several studies show that outcomes relate to the anatomical location of injury, severity of shock at presentation, need for emergency room thoracotomy, number of associated vascular injuries, method of repair, and bowel ischemia [3, 8–10]. Decision for definitive venous repair should be based on the patients' physiological status. Repair options include ligation, shunting, patch venoplasty, bypass grafting (autogenous or prosthetic), or primary suture.

Familiarity with surgical anatomy allows the trauma surgeon to isolate bleeding vessels during an emergency. This chapter reviews the current knowledge on the presentation, management options, and surgical techniques of major IAVI with a focus on IVC, renal, and hepatic venous injuries. Injuries to the mesenteric, splenic, and iliac veins are dealt with elsewhere. We followed the anatomical zones of the retroperitoneum to systematically approach surgical considerations for exposure of the corresponding venous injury.

17.2 Abdominal Injury Zones

Initially proposed by Feliciano, categorization of the abdomen into functional zones enables a systematic approach (Fig. 17.1) [9, 11].

This zonal division of retroperitoneum aides in predicting the potentially injured structures and conceptualizing the management plan. Note that we here only discuss retroperitoneal zonal structures since that is where is the major vasculature is located.

Zone 1

This is a midline or central zone that is subcategorized into supramesocolic and inframesocolic regions. It extends from the diaphragm to the sacral promontory. The major vascular structures implicated in a central hematoma include the aorta and its major visceral braches, the portal vein, the subhepatic IVC and its major tributaries, the SMV, IMV, and renal veins.

Zone 2

This is the lateral zone. An injury in this region results in hematomas associated with renal vascular or renal injuries. It contains the adrenal glands, ureters, renal hilum, and parenchyma.

Zone 3

This is the pelvic zone. Hematomas in the pelvis suggest injury to the iliac vessels.

Zone 4

This is referred to as the retrohepatic zone and suggests injury to the retrohepatic IVC and hepatic veins. Case fatality with such injuries is often rapid and is commonly due to intraoperative exsanguination, especially with blunt venous trauma [11–13].

17.2.1 Anatomy

17.2.1.1 Inferior Vena Cava

The confluence of common iliac veins at the level of L5 marks the origin of IVC just posterior to the right common iliac artery (Fig. 17.2). It ascends along the right border of the vertebral bodies as it traverses through the diaphragmatic hiatus to drain into the right atrium. It receives numerous tributaries along its path along with a rich network of collaterals in the region of its bifurcation. The intra-abdominal IVC is commonly classified into four sections, namely, infrarenal, juxtarenal/perirenal, suprarenal/subhepatic, and the retrohepatic IVC.

Juxtarenal IVC injuries involve the region from the level of renal veins to the inferior border of the liver and are located just posterior to the duodenum and pancreas. The short suprarenal/subhepatic segment of IVC extends in-between the juxtarenal and retrohepatic sections. Achieving control of injury in this region is technically challenging owing to its anatomical relations with the portal vein lying anteromedially, renal vessels posteriorly, and its close proximity to the liver superiorly.

Fig. 17.1 Zones of the retroperitoneum. *Zone 1* is a midline or central zone that is subcategorized into supramesocolic and inframesocolic regions. It extends from the diaphragm to the sacral promontory. *Zone 2* is the lateral zone. An injury in this region results in hematomas associated with renal vascular or renal injuries. *Zone 3* is the pelvic zone. Hematomas in the pelvis suggest injury to the iliac vessels. *Zone 4* is referred to as the retrohepatic zone and suggests injury to the retrohepatic IVC and hepatic veins (not illustrated)

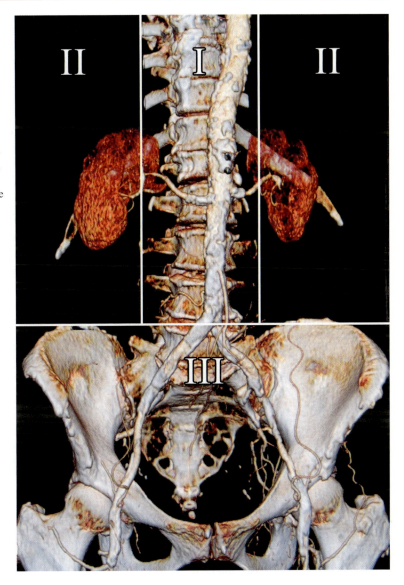

The retrohepatic IVC is defined as inferior to the phrenic veins, superior to the right adrenal vein, and running in a groove across the "bare area of the liver" – uncovered, without capsule [14]. The unique aspect of the retrohepatic IVC is its complete confinement in hepatic suspensory ligaments, posteriorly by diaphragm and anteriorly by liver; making it difficult to explore.

17.2.1.2 Hepatic Veins

Three major hepatic veins drain the liver parenchyma into the IVC. The left, right, and middle hepatic veins enter the IVC before it traverses the diaphragm below the atriocaval junction. There is usually less than 1 cm of IVC between the hepatic veins and the diaphragm. In many patients, this is a purely theoretical space and should not be considered for clamping. The accessory hepatic veins also join the retrohepatic IVC just inferior to this confluence, all together binding the cava to the liver surface. An avulsion injury can completely uproot the hepatic veins resulting in multiple lethal lacerations involving the cava and hepatic veins.

Fig. 17.2 The four zones of the inferior vena cava and major branches are illustrated

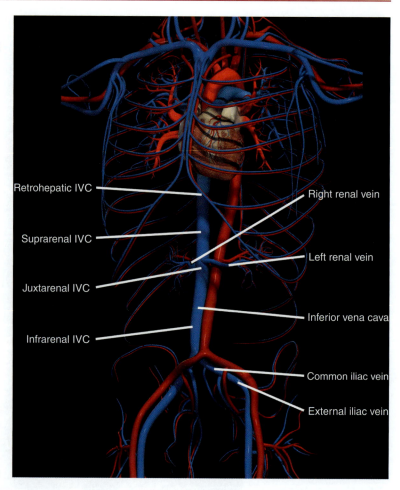

17.2.1.3 Renal Veins

One of the special aspects of the left renal vein is its contribution to the cardinal (collateral) network and that it is approximately three times longer than the right. It receives drainage from left gonadal, adrenal, and a lumbar vein before draining into the IVC, along with a connective channel to the azygous system [15, 16]. This collateral network enables left renal vein ligation without a nephrectomy. The right renal vein, on the other hand, lacks such collaterals.

17.3 Presentation and Patterns of Injury

17.3.1 Mechanisms of Injury

Injury to the IVC represents 30–40 % of all intra-abdominal vascular injuries and is associated with a 50 % mortality rate. It occurs in 0.5–5 % of penetrating and in 0.6–1 % of the blunt abdominal traumatic events [17, 18]. Penetrating injuries to the IVC, like gunshot or stab wounds, often involve other organ systems. In rare scenarios, complete transection of both IVC and aorta can result in an aortocaval fistula [19]. Blunt injuries resulting from shearing deceleration forces can tear off vascular structures from their pedicles, as seen with hepatic veins and retrohepatic cava (explained previously), and cause intraparenchymal laceration or compression or crush injuries as commonly seen with renal veins.

The mechanism of renal vein injury involves two possible patterns. One is due to the stretch exerted on the vessel during the decelerating forces of blunt trauma. This involves the left renal vein more commonly [16, 20]. The other form is secondary to compression against

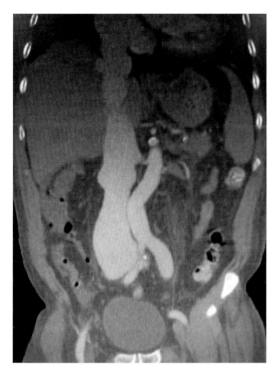

Fig. 17.3 Fistula between the common iliac artery and vein leading to significant distention of the inferior vena cava

vertebral bodies that can result in thrombosis and possible renal vein stenosis [16, 20].

17.3.2 Presentation and Diagnosis

A patient with an IAVI may present with normal vital signs or present with hypotension that may or may not be responsive to resuscitation. Because the venous system is low pressure, a majority of venous injuries will have a surrounding hematoma and present as a normotensive patient. This usually is the case with back or flank wounds. Most IVC injuries respond to intravenous fluid resuscitation even in cases of hemodynamic compromise [21]. Those with contained hematoma may be normotensive at arrival. Rarely, IVC injury may be associated with a simultaneous aortic injury presenting as aortocaval fistula that manifests as wide pulse pressure, hematuria, and an abdominal bruit (Fig. 17.3) [11, 22].

Most high-energy gunshot wounds, massive blunt hepatic parenchymal fractures, or avulsion injuries can present as massive unremitting hemorrhage. Such patients frequently exsanguinate before reaching the operating room. All patients presenting with shock and penetrating injuries should be surgical explored after initial resuscitation with resuscitation continuing in the operating room.

Current imaging protocols are not designed to specifically evaluate the venous system in trauma patients. Radiographic evaluation may include abdominal x-ray and contrast CT scan to define the extent of the contained hematoma [23, 24]. Multiplanar reformatted images tend to be more intuitive as they can be tailored to allow visualization of the specific anatomic structures in nonaxial planes. In addition to the direct signs of venous injury that include thrombosis, avulsion, tear/rupture, extravasation, or pseudoaneurysm, one should be mindful of the more indirect signs of venous injury such as a perivascular hematoma, fat stranding, and vessel wall irregularity. Although intravenous pyelography is a sensitive tool in diagnosis of renal vascular injuries in cases with flank wounds or suspected renal trauma, CT has largely replaced it since it has the added advantage of diagnosing concurrent injuries. A CT scan demonstrating an early filling of the hepatic veins with contrast material in a trauma patient raises the suspicion for an associated arteriovenous fistula and should be followed with arteriography [25].

17.4 Management

17.4.1 General Principles

17.4.1.1 Blunt Trauma

Except for zone 1, blunt traumas with stable, nonpulsatile, non-expanding hematomas should not be disrupted. Traditionally, all zone 1 blunt hematomas are explored since packing is difficult in this region. It is estimated that as many as 40 % patients exsanguinate after surgical disruption of hematomas [11, 26, 27]. Zone 4 hematomas are often not directly visualized on laparotomy, but packing of the anterior liver is prudent. Persistent bleeding or suspicion of arterial injury is grounds for exploration in any zone.

Patients presenting after blunt injury who have hematuria and a perirenal retroperitoneal hematoma on imaging are managed with a nonoperative approach. Nonoperative management is successful in 95 % of these blunt renal trauma patients [26]. There is widespread consensus on nonoperative management of these injuries as renal function becomes severely impaired after 3–6 h of ischemia and salvage rates are only 25–35 % [16].

17.4.1.2 Penetrating Trauma

Retroperitoneal hematomas secondary to penetrating injury are usually best managed by surgical exploration in zones 1 and 3.

Zone 2 penetrating injuries may be selectively managed by not disrupting a stable hematoma. In hemodynamically normal patients, it is prudent to pack stable zone 2 hematomas and treat concomitant injuries such as bowel lacerations. If a zone 2 hematoma is not explored, it is essential to exclude an ischemic kidney and injuries to the renal pelvis or ureters. Use of additional imaging postoperatively may help define these types of injuries and whether the kidney is adequately perfused.

Penetrating retroperitoneal zone 4 injuries involving the IVC or hepatic veins are identified by persistent bleeding with dark blood despite the Pringle maneuver and liver packing. Such injuries are often fatal, but patients surviving to laparotomy will require exploration for bleeding control.

17.4.2 Operative Approach

17.4.2.1 Surgical Exposures

Operative preparation should include an adequate supply of cross-matched blood, large-bore supradiaphragmatic venous access, rolled packs, sponges, suctions, intravascular balloon occlusion catheters, 4-0 vascular sutures, and warming blankets to avoid hypothermia. The patient is positioned in slight reverse Trendelenburg position to avoid venous air embolism [28, 29]. In emergent laparotomy, patients should be prepped from chin to knees, to enable exposure to chest,

groin, or for saphenous vein harvesting as autologous conduit.

Explore the abdomen via a long midline incision, extending from xiphoid process to pubic symphysis. The surgeon should expect distortion of normal anatomy due to significant displacement by a large retroperitoneal hematoma. All bleeding sites should be controlled with manual pressure, resection, or ligation of peripheral vessels, and all quadrants should be packed using laparotomy pads. The retroperitoneum is then evaluated for any IAVI or active bleeding.

Supramesocolic zone 1 hematomas require exploration by performing left medial visceral rotation that requires transection of the avascular line of Toldt in the left colon, incision of the lienosplenic ligament, and rotation of the colon, spleen, tail, and body of the pancreas as well as the stomach medially. This provides access to abdominal aorta and visceral vessels along with the left renal vascular pedicle. Alternatively, for juxta- and infrarenal IVC injuries, extended Kocher or Cattell-Braasch maneuver can be performed that involves transection along the avascular line of Toldt in the right colon and medial mobilization of the right colon, hepatic flexure, duodenum, and head of the pancreas. This exposes the superior mesenteric vessels and the infrahepatic/suprarenal IVC after incising the retroperitoneal tissue. The disadvantage of this maneuver is that there is a limited exposure to injuries at or above the level of supraceliac aorta and the hiatus. Venous hemorrhage can be controlled by finger or sponge-stick compression for proximal and distal control. Without imaging, the difficulty in zone 1 injuries is ascertaining whether left or right medial visceral rotation will give the best exposure. In general, right medial visceral rotation is best for IVC injuries, and left medial visceral rotation is best for aortic and other retroperitoneal zone 1 arterial injuries.

Exposure to the inframesocolic zone 1 hematomas involves cephalad displacement of the transverse colon and mesocolon, reflection of the small bowel to the right to locate the ligament of Treitz, and transecting it alongside the abdominal aorta until the left renal vein is located and the infrarenal aorta is exposed. The infrarenal IVC is exposed by transecting the avascular line of Toldt in the right colon along with a Kocher maneuver. Then the pancreas and duodenum are reflected to the left, and the retroperitoneal tissue covering the inferior vena cava is incised.

Exposure of the right/left lateral or zone 2 hematomas can be technically demanding. If the perirenal hematoma or active bleeding is located medially or if there is an expanding hematoma, vascular control at the level of the pedicle is advisable. It is performed by mobilization of the right colon and hepatic flexure, performing a Kocher maneuver thereby exposing the infrarenal inferior vena cava. The dissection is continued cephalad incising the tissues over the suprarenal infrahepatic inferior vena cava until the right renal vein is encountered. Similarly, for the left-sided exposure, the left colon and splenic flexure are mobilized, and the small bowel is reflected to the right. The ligament of Treitz is localized followed by cephalad mobilization of the transverse colon and mesocolon. The dissection is continued cephalad until the left renal vein is encountered over the abdominal aorta. Alternatively, the lateral aspects of Gerota's fascia can be incised along with lifting the kidney up and medially to locate the hemorrhage if a perirenal hematoma or bleeding is localized laterally.

Exposure to the zone 4 or retrohepatic cava and major hepatic veins requires a right thoracoabdominal incision or a median sternotomy and mobilization of the right triangular ligament along with the caval crossing point at the level of right adrenal vein [5]. For left-sided exposure, a full-length incision of the left triangular ligament is performed. Another approach is through bilateral subcostal incision with upper midline vertical extension, to the left of the xiphoid process, commonly used in liver transplantation, has been described in pediatric cases to gain exposure to juxtahepatic vasculature [30]. Evans et al. describe that this type of incision provides adequate exposure to repair associated splenic, pancreatic, renal, or intestinal injury. The tethering of the retrohepatic IVC to the liver surface by its numerous tributaries mandates extensive division of liver along the lobar planes to access this segment of IVC. Radical hepatic mobilization and division

further compounds the odds of fatality associated with retrohepatic cava and major hepatic venous trauma. Thus, this procedure is not recommended unless there is active bleeding that is not contained with perihepatic packing [5].

17.4.2.2 Control and Repair

Injuries to the infrahepatic, juxta-, and infrarenal IVC and renal veins can be repaired by lateral venorrhaphy using Allis or Babcock clamps for edge approximation during suture repair. Anterior caval injuries can be repaired primarily with transverse vascular sutures although posterior injuries require opening the anterior wall or extending the anterior injury. The repair of posterior infrahepatic/suprarenal IVC injuries often poses a challenge due to difficult exposure. Generally, these are repaired by extending the injury in the anterior wall and repairing the posterior wall from within. Saphenous vein patch angioplasty or interposition prosthetic grafts can be used for venous repair depending upon the extent of the defect. In some instances, a traumatic insult might result in a larger defect that, if repaired with lateral repair, might result in IVC stenosis. In such cases, PTFE or venous patch angioplasty is ideal. Venous ligation superior to the renal veins is not indicated due to higher incidence of renal failure. Through-and-through injuries are primarily repaired either by extending the laceration or by rotating the vessel. This often proves to be challenging and may involve ligation of numerous lumbar veins. In injuries involving massive destruction of infrarenal IVC, ligation as part of damage control is easily tolerated [4].

Injuries to the renal veins can be repaired with primary venorrhaphy or ligation. An unsuccessful right renal vein repair requires ligation but at the cost of a nephrectomy due to the lack of venous collaterals on the right (as previously discussed). Proximal ligation of the left renal vein is generally well tolerated, as the venous outflow is maintained via the venous collaterals.

Juxtahepatic venous injuries are associated with a high mortality rate. Some surgeons believe that such injuries should not be surgically explored given the high mortality associated with operative repair [5]. Others advocate that a single attempt at visualization for control and repair should be made and if it fails control should be limited to compression of the overlying liver. Some authors have advocated a vascular isolation of retrohepatic IVC and hepatic veins by clamping supra- and infrahepatic IVC, portal vein, and aorta in less severe injuries [31, 32]. However, the outcomes were not favorable in hypovolemic patients who reported an increased cardiac arrest rate. Schrock et al. originally proposed the use of an atriocaval shunt as an option to bypass these injuries during repair [33]. These shunts were designed to provide a bloodless field by directing the outflow of blood bypassing the retrohepatic cava along with the Pringle maneuver for inflow occlusion.

Though some authors advocate use of shunts as a last resort for salvage, the associated morbidity and mortality is extraordinarily high [5, 13, 34]. Their use was fraught with complications such as air embolism, perforation of vascular structures during manipulation, thrombosis, and pulmonary embolism. Anecdotal accounts have been reported in the literature on the success of venovenous bypass or cardiac bypass as a potential solution [35, 36]. This technique involves cannulation of femoral vein and axillary/internal jugular vein and placement on venous bypass during the course of operative repair. Others recommend tamponade and containment for hepatic venous injuries. In a prospective follow-up study, Fabian and colleagues reported attaining successful hemostasis with deep omental packing in blunt hepatic venous trauma patients with associated mortality of 20.5 % [37]. Such a mortality rate is significantly lower when compared with direct venous repair of comparable grade of injury [5]. Similar results were reported by Beal and colleagues in a cohort of severe juxtahepatic venous trauma, where perihepatic gauze packing was used as the tamponade strategy [38]. The associated mortality in such patients was 14 % with perihepatic packing as opposed to 70 % in those who underwent atriocaval shunting and direct venous repair [38]. Endovascular procedures like venous stenting and arterial embolization in cases with persistent juxtahepatic venous bleeding are theoretical options which are not possible given the rapidly of hemorrhage from these injuries.

17.4.2.3   Damage Control Approach

First promoted by Kocher and Billroth in the 1880s, evidence from modern literature suggests a reasonable survival rate with venous ligation if performed early in traumatic infrarenal caval transection patients [4, 39]. In a recent series of 100 patients with IVC injury, the ligation of infrarenal IVC performed as a damage control measure in 25 complex IVC injuries had an associated 59 % overall mortality, a longer hospital stay, and a more severe injury severity score (ISS) [40]. No long-term sequelae were seen in those who survived over the average follow-up period of 42 months. The authors concluded that infrarenal IVC ligation is an acceptable damage control measure. Other authors have shown similar results as well [41].

Use of straight vascular shunts that correspond to the size of the vessel lumen ranging from 8 to 16 French offers another option. After ligation or shunt placement, an abbreviated temporary closure with a vacuum closure device should be performed. After resuscitation to correct the acidosis, coagulopathy, and hypothermia, the patient is brought back to the operating room for definitive repair within 24–72 h. In cases of iliac or IVC ligation, prophylactic fasciotomies should be considered to avoid the development of compartment syndrome secondary to reperfusion injury, venous congestion, and ischemia [2, 40].

17.5   Endovascular Approach

Endovascular strategies offer an alternative approach as both temporary damage control measure as well as definitive repair of IAVI. Although long-term results are not available, small case reports and case series have reported successful repair of IVC and other venous trauma with endovascular techniques. Castelli et al. reported a successful account of IVC stent grafting without laparotomy or retroperitoneal dissection as an alternative to open surgery in cases of ruptured of the vena cava [42]. Others have reported use of fenestrated stent graft for traumatic juxtahepatic venous injuries [43]. Endovascular techniques such as stenting and balloon occlusion have documented success shown in scattered reports of patients presenting with IVC thrombosis, aneurysms, or pseudoaneurysms (contained hematoma) after blunt trauma. Although the long-term outcomes are variable, a surgeon should consider angioembolization and stenting as plausible treatment strategies when repair is felt to be required in a hemodynamically normal patient.

17.6 Outcomes and Consequences

A complication of massive resuscitation which is often associated with IAVI is development of abdominal compartment syndrome defined as an elevation of intra-abdominal pressure by 30 cm of H_2O. It presents as a tense abdomen along with organ dysfunction primarily renal and respiratory. The incidence of abdominal compartment syndrome is often reported in patients who underwent damage control procedures, had prolonged period of hypotension, required massive blood transfusions, had hypothermia, or underwent a tight abdominal closure. Treatment is avoiding initial abdominal closure or reopening a closed laparotomy until edema resolves and abdominal closure can occur safely.

A frequently reported morbidity associated with IVC injury is venous stasis distal to the site of ligation or repair and limb ischemia. Compression bandages and elevation are effective treatment options for the resulting edema due to venous insufficiency. Despite the lack of evidence in support of anticoagulant use, postoperative heparin or dextran infusion for 24–72 h is empirically given in patients with IVC narrowing following repair. Deep vein thrombosis and pulmonary embolism occur at sites of injury and repair.

Renal vascular injury is associated with a significant mortality of up to 54 % [4]. Irrespective of the outcomes of the reparative measures, the preoperative and intraoperative hypotension resulting from the injury incurs ischemic damage resulting in renal failure in the postoperative period. There is a small risk of delayed hypertension in such cases.

Conclusion

As many vascular surgeons know, venous injuries are often more troublesome than arterial injury. Retrohepatic IVC and hepatic vein injuries are best managed with packing to compress the liver posteriorly. Exposure should be performed for refractory bleeding but outcomes are poor. Outflow control of the IVC is best managed via right thoracoabdominal or medial sternotomy to access the intrapericardial supradiaphragmatic IVC. A Pringle maneuver with suprarenal IVC compression provides inflow control. Some blunt juxta- and infrarenal IVC injuries may be managed without retroperitoneal exploration unless there is active bleeding or suspicion of concomitant arterial injury, but most zone 1 retroperitoneal injuries should be explored. The left renal vein can be ligated if collaterals are intact. The right renal vein is short and usually requires repair or nephrectomy. Concomitant visceral and arterial injuries are common. Those with blunt trauma and a presentation of peritonitis, hemodynamic instability, or significant free abdominal fluid should be offered operative management. Survivors of both surgical and nonoperative management suffer venous thromboembolic events, proximal edema, and venous insufficiency.

References

1. Paul JS, Webb TP, Aprahamian C, Weigelt JA. Intraabdominal vascular injury: are we getting any better? J Trauma. 2010;69(6):1393–7.
2. Webb TP. Diagnosis and management of abdominal vascular injuries. Trauma. 2013;15:51–63.
3. Asensio JA, Chahwan S, Hanpeter D, Demetriades D, Forno W, Gambaro E, Murray J, Velmahos G, Marengo J, Shoemaker WC, Berne TV. Operative management and outcome of 302 abdominal vascular injuries. Am J Surg. 2000;180(6):528–33; discussion 533–4.

4. Asensio JA, Soto SN, Forno W, Roldan G, Petrone P, Gambaro E, Salim A, Rowe V, Demetriades D. Abdominal vascular injuries: the trauma surgeon's challenge. Surg Today. 2001;31(11):949–57.

5. Buckman RF, Pathak AS, Badellino MM, Bradley KM. Injuries of the inferior vena cava. Surg Clin North Am. 2001;81(6):1431–47.

6. Wiencek RG, Wilson RF. Abdominal venous injuries. J Trauma. 1986;26(9):771–8.

7. Stone HH, Strom PR, Mullins RJ. Management of the major coagulopathy with onset during laparotomy. Ann Surg. 1983;197(5):532–5.

8. Asensio JA, Forno W, Roldán G, Petrone P, Rojo E, Ceballos J, Wang C, Costaglioli B, Romero J, Tillou A, Carmody I, Shoemaker WC, Berne TV. Visceral vascular injuries. Surg Clin North Am. 2002;82(1): 1–20, xix.

9. Feliciano DV. Abdominal vessels. In: Ivatury R, Cayten C, editors. The textbook of penetrating trauma. Baltimore: Williams and Wilkins; 1996. p. 702–16.

10. Hansen CJ, Bernadas C, West MA, Ney AL, Muehlstedt S, Cohen M, Rodriguez JL. Abdominal vena caval injuries: outcomes remain dismal. Surgery. 2000;128(4):572–8.

11. Buckman Jr RF, Miraliakbari R, Badellino MM. Juxtahepatic venous injuries: a critical review of reported management strategies. J Trauma. 2000; 48(5):978–84.

12. Cogbill TH, Moore EE, Jurkovich GJ, Feliciano DV, Morris JA, Mucha P. Severe hepatic trauma: a multicenter experience with 1,335 liver injuries. J Trauma. 1988;28(10):1433–8.

13. Rovito PF. Atrial caval shunting in blunt hepatic vascular injury. Ann Surg. 1987;205(3):318–21.

14. Nakamura S, Tsuzuki T. Surgical anatomy of the hepatic veins and the inferior vena cava. Surg Gynecol Obstet. 1981;152(1):43–50.

15. Kabalin J, Tanagho E. Surgical anatomy of the genitourinary tract. In: Retik P, Walsh A, Stamey T, Vaughan E, editors. Campbell's urology. 6th ed. Philadelphia: WB Saunders; 1992. p. 39–45.

16. Tillou A, Romero J, Asensio JA, Best CD, Petrone P, Roldan G, Rojo E. Renal vascular injuries. Surg Clin North Am. 2001;81(6):1417–30.

17. Burch JM, Feliciano DV, Mattox KL, Edelman M. Injuries of the inferior vena cava. Am J Surg. 1988;156(6):548–52.

18. Mattox KL, Feliciano DV, Burch J, Beall Jr AC, Jordan Jr GL, De Bakey ME. Five thousand seven hundred sixty cardiovascular injuries in 4459 patients. Epidemiologic evolution 1958 to 1987. Ann Surg. 1989;209(6):698–705.

19. Mattox KL, Whisennand HH, Espada R, Beall Jr AC. Management of acute combined injuries to the aorta and inferior vena cava. Am J Surg. 1975; 130(6):720–4.

20. Bruce LM, Croce MA, Santaniello JM, Miller PR, Lyden SP, Fabian TC. Blunt renal artery injury: incidence, diagnosis, and management. Am Surg. 2001;67(6):550–4; discussion 555–6.

21. Feliciano DV. Approach to major abdominal vascular injury. J Vasc Surg. 1988;7(5):730–6.

22. Linker RW, Crawford Jr FA, Rittenbury MS, Barton M. Traumatic aortocaval fistula: case report. J Trauma. 1989;29(2):255–7.

23. Boyle Jr EM, Maier RV, Salazar JD, Kovacich JC, O'Keefe G, Mann FA, Wilson AJ, Copass MK, Jurkovich GJ. Diagnosis of injuries after stab wounds to the back and flank. J Trauma. 1997;42(2):260–5.

24. Biffl WL, Moore EE. Management guidelines for penetrating abdominal trauma. Curr Opin Crit Care. 2010;16(6):609–17. doi:10.1097/MCC.0b013e32833 f52d2.

25. Holly BP, Steenburg SD. Multidetector CT of blunt traumatic venous injuries in the chest, abdomen, and pelvis. Radiographics. 2011;31(5):1415–24. doi:10.1148/rg.315105221.

26. Feliciano DV. Management of traumatic retroperitoneal hematoma. Ann Surg. 1990;211(2):109–23.

27. Tieu B, Zhou M, Trunkey DD. Abdominal vascular injury. In: Flint L, Meredith JW, Schwab CW, Trunkey DD, Rue LW, Taheri PA, editors. Trauma: contemporary principles and therapy, vol. 43. 1st ed. Philadelphia: Lippincott Williams & Wilkins; 2008. p. 451–62.

28. Bricker DL, Morton JR, Okies JE, Beall Jr AC. Surgical management of injuries to the vena cava: changing patterns of injury and newer techniques of repair. J Trauma. 1971;11(9):725–35.

29. Bricker DL, Wukasch DC. Successful management of an injury to the suprarenal inferior vena cava. Surg Clin North Am. 1970;50(5):999–1002.

30. Evans S, Jackson RJ, Smith SD. Successful repair of major retrohepatic vascular injuries without the use of shunt or sternotomy. J Pediatr Surg. 1993; 28(3):317–20.

31. Waltuck TL, Crow RW, Humphrey LJ, Kauffman HM. Avulsion injuries of the vena cava following blunt abdominal trauma. Ann Surg. 1970;171(1): 67–72.

32. Yellin AE, Chaffee CB, Donovan AJ. Vascular isolation in treatment of juxtahepatic venous injuries. Arch Surg. 1971;102(6):566–73.

33. Schrock T, Blaisdell FW, Mathewson Jr C. Management of blunt trauma to the liver and hepatic veins. Arch Surg. 1968;96(5):698–704.

34. Beal SL, Ward RE. Successful atrial caval shunting in the management of retrohepatic venous injuries. Am J Surg. 1989;158(5):409–13.

35. Biffl WL, Moore EE, Franciose RJ. Venovenous bypass and hepatic vascular isolation as adjuncts in the repair of destructive wounds to the retrohepatic inferior vena cava. J Trauma. 1998;45(2): 400–3.

36. Kaoutzanis C, Evangelakis E, Kokkinos C, Kaoutzanis G. Successful repair of injured hepatic veins and inferior vena cava following blunt traumatic injury, by using cardiopulmonary bypass and hypothermic circulatory arrest. Interact Cardiovasc Thorac Surg. 2011;12(1):84–6.

37. Fabian TC, Croce MA, Stanford GG, Payne LW, Mangiante EC, Voeller GR, Kudsk KA. Factors affecting morbidity following hepatic trauma. A prospective analysis of 482 injuries. Ann Surg. 1991;213(6):540–7.

38. Beal SL. Fatal hepatic hemorrhage: an unresolved problem in the management of complex liver injuries. J Trauma. 1990;30(2):163–9.

39. Gazzaniga AB, Colodny AH. Long-term survival after acute ligation of the vena cava above the renal veins. Ann Surg. 1972;175(4):563–8.

40. Sullivan PS, Dente CJ, Patel S, Carmichael M, Srinivasan JK, Wyrzykowski AD, Nicholas JM, Salomone JP, Ingram WL, Vercruysse GA, Rozycki GS, Feliciano DV. Outcome of ligation of the inferior vena cava in the modern era. Am J Surg. 2010;199(4):500–6. doi:10.1016/j.amjsurg.2009.05.013. Epub 2010 Jan 15.

41. Mullins RJ, Lucas CE, Ledgerwood AM. The natural history following venous ligation for civilian injuries. J Trauma. 1980;20(9):737–43.

42. Castelli P, Caronno R, Piffaretti G, Tozzi M. Emergency endovascular repair for traumatic injury of the inferior vena cava. Eur J Cardiothorac Surg. 2005;28(6):906–8.

43. Watarida S, Nishi T, Furukawa A, Shiraishi S, Kitano H, Matsubayashi K, Imura M, Yamazaki M. Fenestrated stent-graft for traumatic juxtahepatic inferior vena cava injury. J Endovasc Ther. 2002;9(1):134–7.

Mesenteric Vascular Injuries

18

Leslie M. Kobayashi, Todd W. Costantini, and Raul Coimbra

Contents

18.1 Introduction

Abdominal vascular trauma is a rare entity accounting for 0.01–0.1 % of all traumas and 15–30 % of vascular trauma in civilian and 2–2.9 % in military series [1–3]. The lower incidence in military settings is likely due to the low probability of surviving evacuation to reach medical personnel. Even in modern military series injuries to named central vascular structures are nearly uniformly lethal [4].

Penetrating mechanisms are responsible for the vast majority of vascular injuries in the abdomen accounting for 70–95 % of patients in most series [1, 2, 5–12]. Gunshot and shotgun wounds are more common penetrating mechanisms than stab wounds [7]. Of blunt causes motor vehicle crashes are the most common, followed remotely by direct abdominal impact and falls [1, 7]. The most commonly injured abdominal vessels are the aorta, superior mesenteric (SMA) and iliac arteries and inferior vena cava (IVC), portal, and iliac veins [6, 9, 11, 12].

18.1.1 Visceral Aortic Branches

The aorta has three major visceral branches which include the celiac and superior and inferior mesenteric arteries (SMA/IMA). Celiac artery

L.M. Kobayashi, MD • T.W. Costantini, MD
R. Coimbra, MD, PhD (✉)
Division of Trauma, Surgical Critical Care and Burns, Department of Surgery, University of California San Diego Health Sciences, San Diego, CA, USA
e-mail: rcoimbra@ucsd.edu

A. Dua et al. (eds.), *Clinical Review of Vascular Trauma*,
DOI 10.1007/978-3-642-39100-2_18, © Springer-Verlag Berlin Heidelberg 2014

injuries are exceedingly rare, with an incidence of 0.01 % (Fig. 18.1). Associated injuries are common with these vascular injuries. The rarity and severity of celiac artery injury result in a high mortality in most series, ranging from 38 to 75 % [11, 13, 14]. Mortality correlates with advancing AAST-OIS grading, hypotension, need for resuscitative thoracotomy, and presence of associated injuries [11]. Historically, the presence of "black bowel" or visceral ischemia at the time of laparotomy was also associated with a poor prognosis, but this finding has been rare in modern series.

Injuries to the SMA are also exceedingly rare accounting for approximately 0.09 % of all traumas, the majority result from penetrating mechanisms, which account for 52–77 % of cases [5, 15]. There has been little change in SMA-associated mortality in the past four decades. In a series of six studies from 1972 to 1986, the overall survival was 57.7 % compared to four studies spanning 1990–2000 with a survival of 58.7 % [2]. Independent predictors of mortality include transfusion >10 units of PRBCs, acidosis, dysrhythmias, and multisystem organ failure. Additionally, mortality correlates with more advanced Fullen Classification and AAST-OIS grades of injury (Tables 18.1 and 18.2). Mortality is increased in patients with complex vascular reconstructions as compared to primary repair or ligation. Whether this is due to the complexity of the injury or the repair itself is not clear. Associated injuries which commonly include aortic, portal vein, liver, pancreatic, duodenal, renal, and splenic significantly increase mortality.

Injuries to the IMA/IMV are rare. Generally, isolated injuries are well tolerated if they are surgically addressed quickly. Mortality ranges from 0 to 100 % and is highly dependent on physiologic derangements at the time of admission and associated injuries [1].

18.1.2 Visceral Veins

Injuries to the portal (PV) and superior mesenteric veins (SMV) are rare, highly lethal injuries occurring in less than 1 % of all traumas [16, 17]. Most injuries occur as a result of penetrating

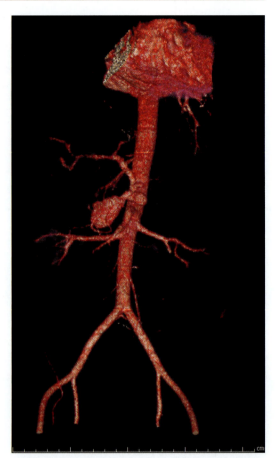

Fig. 18.1 Three-dimensional reconstruction of CT scan images obtained from a patient with a celiac artery pseudoaneurysm following blunt injury

trauma [16–20]. Because the PV and SMV are centrally located, nearly all patients have associated injuries, averaging 3 or more per patient [17, 19]. Mortality after PV injury ranges from 40 to 70 %, and mortality after SMV injury ranges from 0 to 83 % [2, 11, 16–20]. Mortality is increased by associated injuries, as well as hypotension on arrival and active hemorrhage at laparotomy [17, 19]. The vast majority of patients present with hypotension or peritonitis requiring emergent laparotomy, an additional minority will require resuscitative thoracotomy. The need to undergo either emergency department or operating room thoracotomy is associated with an increased risk of death. Advanced AAST-OIS grade and injuries spanning greater than 50 % or completely transecting the vessel wall are also associated with worse outcomes.

Table 18.1 Fullen anatomic classification of superior mesenteric artery injury [24]

Zone	Segment SMA	Grade	Ischemic category	Bowel affected	Mortality Asensio et al. [15] (%)	Mortality Asensio et al. [5, 7] (%)
I	Trunk proximal to first branch	1	Maximal	Jejunum, ileum, right colon	100	76.5
II	Trunk between inferior pancreaticoduodenal and middle colic	2	Moderate	Major segment, small bowel, right colon	43	44.1
III	Trunk distal to middle colic	3	Minimal	Minor segment or segments, small bowel or right colon	25	27.5
IV	Segmental branches (jejunal, ileal, colic)	4	None	None	25	23.1

SMA superior mesenteric artery

Table 18.2 AAST-OIST grading abdominal vascular injury [2]

Grade	Injury	Mortality Asensio et al. [15] (%)	Mortality Asensio et al. [7]
I	Non-named mesenteric arterial/venous branches, phrenic artery/vein, lumbar artery/vein, gonadal artery/vein, ovarian artery/vein, other non-named small artery/vein requiring ligation	0	16.4
II	Right, left, or common hepatic artery, splenic artery/vein, right or left gastric, GDA, IMA/IMV, primary named branches of SMA/SMV	20	25.5
III	SMV trunk, renal artery/vein, iliac artery/vein, hypogastric artery/vein, infrarenal IVC	0	40
IV	SMA trunk, celiac axis, suprarenal or infrahepatic IVC, infrarenal aorta	59	53.6
V	Portal vein, extraparenchymal hepatic vein, retrohepatic or suprahepatic IVC, suprarenal aorta	88	89.5

SMA superior mesenteric artery, *SMV* superior mesenteric vein, *IVC* inferior vena cava, *IMA* inferior mesenteric artery, *IMV* inferior mesenteric vein, *GDA* gastroduodenal artery

18.1.3 Inferior Vena Cava

IVC injuries occur after both blunt and penetrating trauma and are among the most common of intra-abdominal vascular injuries. Mortality can be high ranging from 36 to 70 % and increases with increasing associated injuries [6, 11, 12, 21, 22]. Mortality is also increased following blunt trauma, if there is release of the retroperitoneal tamponade with free hemorrhage into the abdominal cavity and in the presence of shock or acidosis [21, 23].

18.2 Anatomy and Physiology

The majority of abdominal vascular structures are located in the retroperitoneum which is divided into three zones. Zone I spans the midline of the abdomen and contains the aorta and its branches and the inferior vena cava (IVC). Zone II is located in the paracolic gutters bilaterally and contains the renal vessels and kidneys. Zone III begins at the sacral promontory and contains the iliac arteries and veins. This chapter will focus on the vessels contained within zone I as well as the portal and superior mesenteric veins (SMV) which along with the IVC provide the route for venous blood to return to the heart from the mesentery and lower extremities.

18.2.1 Visceral Aortic Branches

The mesenteric branches of the abdominal aorta include the celiac artery, SMA, and IMA. The celiac artery arises from the proximal abdominal aorta above the transverse mesocolon. The vessel ranges from 1 to 1.5 cm in length in most adults before dividing into the hepatic, splenic, and gastric branches. It is surrounded by a dense plexus of nervous and lymphatic tissue [1, 2]. The hepatic artery passes to the right posteriorly and enters the hepatoduodenal ligament just superior to the pylorus to the left of the common bile duct. The splenic artery, the largest of the celiac branches, courses inferiorly and to the left, posterior to the pancreas in the upper portion of the gland. The splenic artery gives off several dorsal pancreatic branches as well as the left gastroepiploic artery before entering the lienorenal ligament and dividing into the terminal splenic branches at the hilum of the spleen. The splenic artery also gives rise to the short gastric branches throughout its course. The left gastric artery ascends cephalad and laterally to the left to enter the lesser curvature of the stomach.

The SMA arises from the anterior aorta in close proximity to the celiac artery in the supramesocolic region of zone I. The first portion of the SMA passes first under the neck of the pancreas crossing the splenic vein, then over the uncinate process and third portion of the duodenum to enter the small bowel mesentery. SMA injuries can be classified according to the schema created by Fullen et al. in 1972, or by the AAST-OIS (Tables 18.1 and 18.2) [24]. The Fullen classification divides the SMA into the trunk, proximal branches (between the inferior pancreaticoduodenal and middle colic), middle branches (those distal to the middle colic), and terminal or segmental branches such as the jejuna and ileal arcades.

The IMA arises from the inframesocolic infrarenal abdominal aorta and travels in close proximity to the aorta as it courses caudad to emerge in the left lateral aspect of the colonic mesentery. Within the colonic mesentery, it gives off the left colic, sigmoidal, and superior rectal branches.

18.2.2 Visceral Veins

The portal venous system is created by the confluence of the SMV and splenic veins behind the neck of the pancreas at the level of the second lumbar vertebra. The IMV anatomy varies, but in general it will drain into either the splenic vein or less commonly into the SMV prior to their confluence. The portal vein forms at the superior aspect of the pancreas and enters the hepatoduodenal ligament where it travels posterior and lateral to the hepatic artery and common bile duct before entering the parenchyma of the liver in the hilum. The portal vein branches into left and right portal veins, the right then subsequently divides into superior and inferior branches.

18.2.3 Inferior Vena Cava

The IVC courses along the right paravertebral portion of the retroperitoneum, and injuries are classified by location, as infrarenal, suprarenal, or retrohepatic/suprahepatic. The suprahepatic and retrohepatic IVC extend from the diaphragmatic hiatus through the liver. The suprarenal IVC extends from just below the inferior liver edge to the level of the renal vein insertion sites. The infrarenal IVC is defined by the portion of the IVC below the renal veins inferiorly to the bifurcation into the common iliac veins. A previous retrospective review of IVC injuries stratified by location showed no significant difference in mortality between suprarenal and infrarenal IVC injuries if retrohepatic IVC injuries were excluded [12]. Due to massive hemorrhage and a difficult operative approach, injuries to the retrohepatic and suprahepatic IVC carry the highest mortality rates even in experienced trauma centers [8, 9, 12, 23, 25, 26].

18.3 Clinical Assessment and Initial Management

Presentation is dependent on whether the injury has resulted in tamponade or free rupture into the peritoneal cavity. If the hematoma has ruptured into the peritoneum, the patient may present in extremis as rapid exsanguination is possible. If the injury is contained in the retroperitoneum, the patient may present with normal hemodynamics in relatively stable condition. Other signs of abdominal vascular injury include a distended tender abdomen, lack of a femoral pulse, and gross hematuria.

Most patients will be in hemorrhagic shock, and immediate large-bore intravenous access, resuscitation, and rapid surgical control of bleeding are essential. Massive transfusion protocols should be instituted as soon as abdominal vascular injury is suspected, and resuscitation of the patient should be aggressive with 1:1 transfusion for adequate replacement of intravascular clotting factors [27]. Most patients with abdominal vascular injuries will undergo significant operative blood loss ranging from 5 to 10 L, and adjuncts such as cell saver or other blood reclamation techniques should be utilized [13, 14]. Every effort should be made to maintain normothermia as a core temperature of less than 34 °C has been found to be a significant predictor of mortality among these patients [12].

18.4 Diagnostic Testing

The majority of patients with major abdominal vascular injury are hypotensive upon presentation. Patients are commonly triaged according to the results of the Focused Assessment with Sonography for Trauma (FAST) scan. Patients with evidence of significant hemoperitoneum are taken for operative exploration while those with minimal or no peritoneal fluid should be resuscitated while other sources of hemorrhage are sought. In the rare cases where patients are hemodynamically normal, computed tomography (CT) has become the diagnostic tool of choice for detection of vascular injury [28, 29]. There is now growing support for the use of CT scanning in the triage of even hypotensive patients with abdominal and pelvic trauma. A large study of patients with both pelvic and abdominal trauma revealed an increasing use of preoperative/pre-angiographic CT for triage even among patients presenting in shock. This study revealed no increase in mortality nor significant delay to angiography or laparotomy as a result of CT scanning [30].

18.5 Operative and Interventional Management

18.5.1 Celiac Artery

Exposure of the celiac artery is best approached via left medial visceral rotation [1, 2, 7]. In order to obtain proximal control of the supraceliac aorta proximal to the celiac root, it may be necessary to divide the median arcuate ligament and crura of the diaphragm. This exposure allows visualization of the left lateral and anterior aspect of the upper abdominal aorta as well as the roots of the celiac and SMA origins. Alternatively, exposure of the celiac root can be performed through the gastrohepatic ligament. This requires division of the left triangular ligament and mobilization of the left lobe of the liver to the right and the esophagus to the left. Once the injury is exposed and proximal and distal control obtained, the surgical options include ligation or repair. The celiac artery can be ligated safely if the SMA is patent due to extensive collateral circulation. In a series by Asensio, among 13 patients, 11 underwent ligation and 1 underwent primary repair, of the patients who underwent ligation 4 survived. The single patient who underwent primary repair in this series also survived. Graham reported on 13 patients with celiac injury of which 4 patients underwent ligation with a survival rate of 50 % [14]. Asensio and his group found no survivors among their extensive literature search who underwent complex repair, reanastomosis, or reimplantation [13]. There are no reports of significant bowel ischemia following celiac ligation; however, ischemia and necrosis of the gallbladder after ligation is described, and cholecystectomy is advocated in all patients [2, 13]. Injury to branches of the celiac artery is also rare. The gastric and gastroduodenal branches can generally be ligated with little ill effects due to the extensive collateral flow from other celiac branches, as well as from SMA branches.

Hepatic artery ligation is generally well tolerated owing to the dual blood supply of the liver in conjunction with the portal vein and collateral flow from the gastroduodenal artery (GDA) if the ligation occurs distal to the GDA. When ligation occurs proximal to the GDA, decreased arterial blood flow to the liver may cause transient increase in liver transaminases, as opposed to elevations seen solely with parenchymal liver damage; this ischemic hepatitis is also associated with elevations in lactate dehydrogenase. Compromised arterial flow can also lead to biliary strictures as the arterial flow provides the primary blood supply to the ductal epithelium. Although rare, this can result in biliary strictures and cholangiectasis with resultant obstructive jaundice and occasionally cholangitis [31].

Splenic artery ligation just proximal to its terminal branch point is well tolerated if required for irreparable injury or uncontrollable bleeding. Although most often performed in conjunction with splenectomy as associated solid organ injury is common, the spleen if undamaged and not ischemic can be left in situ following ligation of the splenic artery. Most studies of splenic artery ligation for trauma have occurred in children where splenic salvage is common following both blunt and penetrating trauma. These studies demonstrate that in the majority of patients the spleen is viable following ligation and has normal immunological function [32, 33]. One study of splenic artery ligation without splenectomy in adult trauma patients had similar outcomes with no deaths and no need for reoperation following ligation [33].

18.5.2 SMA

Surgical approach to the SMA varies somewhat according to the location of injury. Injuries to Fullen zone I are best approached via a left medial visceral rotation [2]. Fullen zone II injuries are approached via visceral rotation, but transection of the neck of the pancreas may be necessary to visualize the injury and gain distal vascular control. Injuries in this location may also be approached by opening the root of the mesentery beneath the pancreas via the lesser sac [3]. Fullen zone III injuries are approached by dividing the ligament of Treitz to expose the suprarenal aorta and distal SMA trunk. They can also be exposed by performing an extended Kocher maneuver, mobilizing the duodenal C-loop until the SMA

is encountered as it comes out from beneath the neck of the pancreas. Fullen zone IV injuries are best approached directly through the mesentery. Once the injury is exposed, proximal and distal control should be obtained [1, 3, 6, 7].

In hemodynamically normal patients primary repair is utilized for injuries in all zones if possible, this can be accomplished in 22–40 % of cases [5, 15]. The edges of the injury are debrided to healthy tissue and re-approximated with monofilament nonabsorbable sutures. Large defects, however, are unlikely to come together primarily as branching of the SMA makes significant mobilization impossible. In these cases techniques such as vein patch, interposition graft, and reimplantation have all been described.

In hemodynamically abnormal patients rapid primary repair may be considered; however, if the defect is large or difficult to expose, it should be ligated or shunted. Historically, ligation of the SMA is reported to be well tolerated in the proximal trunk because of collateral flow through the celiac axis, while ligation of distal injuries was discouraged due to the risk of bowel ischemia [3]. However, in two large series by Asensio, the authors found ligation to be commonly used in distal injuries. Ligation of both proximal and distal injuries was tolerated, but mortality was higher when ligating proximal compared to distal injuries [5]. It should be kept in mind that bowel ischemia may result if multiple distal injuries are ligated.

Temporary intravascular shunts (TIVSs) are an alternative to ligation. Shunting of the SMA was first described by Reilly in 1995, when a Javid shunt was used to temporize a Fullen zone II injury. The shunt remained patent until definitive repair with an interposition graft on postoperative day two [34]. Since that time, TIVSs have rarely been reported in the treatment of SMA injuries [5, 15]. In a single institution's experience with shunts, Subramanian reported use in truncal injuries for only six patients, of these 33 % were SMA injuries. Compared to extremity injury, truncal TIVSs are associated with significantly higher transfusion requirements and higher rates of thrombosis [35].

Though only reported in 21–40 % of cases, strong consideration should be given to temporary abdominal closure (TAC) [5, 6, 11, 15]. SMA injuries in particular may benefit from TAC and second-look procedures due to the high risk of ischemic complications, abdominal compartment syndrome, and high rate of associated injuries [5].

In very rare cases patients with SMA injuries may present in stable condition and undergo imaging to diagnose their injuries prior to laparotomy. There have been four case reports of patients diagnosed with SMA injuries who subsequently underwent angioembolization. Embolization was successful in controlling hemorrhage in all four cases, with no reports documenting bleeding, ischemia, or perforation that required subsequent laparotomy [36–39]. Angiography is limited because it cannot diagnose or address associated injuries, but it may have a role as a surgical adjunct. Patients with stable hematomas or who respond to packing may benefit from angiography to delineate and embolize or stent these difficult to expose lesions.

18.5.3 IMA/IMV

The IMA/IMV can be exposed by elevating the transverse colon and incising the ligament of Treitz exposing the anterior aspect of the infrarenal abdominal aorta. The periaortic tissue should be ligated in order to prevent lymph leaks. The IMA can then be found arising from the left lateral aspect of the aorta approximately 3–4 cm above the aortic bifurcation. Generally IMA/IMV injuries are primarily repaired if amenable or ligated. Ligation is generally well tolerated because of the extensive collateral circulation [3]. However, the presence of back bleeding should be assessed, and while rare this injury can be complicated by rectal or colonic ischemia, particularly in patients with advanced atherosclerotic disease [2].

18.5.4 SMV/Portal Vein

Vascular control of PV and SMV injuries begins with performing a Pringle maneuver. An atraumatic vascular clamp should be placed on the porta hepatis. Once the hematoma and areolar tissue in the hepatoduodenal ligament are dissected, clear vascular clamps or vessel loops should be placed above and below the injury. The ability to gain proximal and distal control is limited by the short length of the porta hepatis. Extra length and access to more distal SMV injuries can be gained by dividing the neck of the pancreas if necessary. A wide Kocher or a Cattell-Braasch maneuver can be performed for exposure improved vascular control.

It is essential to obtain good exposure of the injury prior to any attempt at repair or ligation due to the close proximity of the bile duct and hepatic artery. PV injuries can be addressed by repair, reanastomosis, interposition graft, portosystemic shunt, or ligation. Ligation can be tolerated as long as the hepatic artery is patent, with mortality ranging from 20 to 90 % [17–20, 40]. If ligation is necessary it should be undertaken immediately after identification of a severe injury, as early ligation is associated with improved survival [40]. Ligation of the PV may result in splanchnic hypervolemia and systemic hypovolemia causing hemodynamic compromise; it is therefore important to carefully monitor preload and anticipate the need for aggressive intravascular volume replacement. SMV injuries can be treated with ligation or repair. In a large series by Asensio, repair was associated with a survival advantage; however, patients undergoing repair were significantly less injured and had fewer associated injuries than those undergoing ligation [19]. Another study by Fraga demonstrated similar outcomes among SMV injuries that were ligated and those that were treated with primary repair [17]. If ligation is performed it should be kept in mind that the syndrome of splanchnic hypervolemia/systemic hypovolemia is a significant risk although less common following SMV ligations than PV ligations [18].

Damage control laparotomy is particularly suited to PV and SMV ligation as a second-look operation to assess bowel viability is mandatory, and the risks of development of the abdominal compartment syndrome may be decreased with temporary abdominal closure techniques [16, 17]. Previous studies of these rare injuries have suggested the utility of TIVS in complex or long-segment injuries to diminish the risks of bowel ischemia; however, the literature lacks even one case report [16, 17].

18.5.5 IVC

The most common approach to the infrahepatic IVC is a right-sided medial visceral rotation (Cattell-Braasch maneuver). The white line of Toldt is divided lateral to the right colon, and the mesentery of the large and small bowel is dissected off of the retroperitoneum to its root. The duodenum is mobilized medially and superiorly, the right kidney is generally left in its normal anatomic location. This maneuver exposes the IVC from the inferior border of the liver to its bifurcation (Fig. 18.2). Infrarenal IVC injuries are considered the easiest to repair, carry the lowest mortality rate, and are usually controlled with compression directly above and below the injury digitally or with sponge sticks [41]. Tangential occlusion clamps (Satinsky clamp) can be used for vascular control with care to avoid tearing the IVC and enlarging the defect. The majority of injuries to the IVC are repaired with lateral venorrhaphy using 4-0 or 5-0 Prolene suture. The back wall should be inspected for through-and-through injuries. Posterior defects can be repaired by rotating the vessel or through the anterior defect [42]. In circumstances where the caval defect is large, either saphenous vein or prosthetic patches can be utilized to repair the defect. For those patients who are coagulopathic or in shock, ligation of the infrarenal IVC is possible (Fig. 18.3). Four-compartment lower extremity fasciotomies should be considered in cases of ligation as compartment syndrome is common. The bilateral lower extremities should be elevated in all cases in order to decrease accumulation of edema. A retrospective review of patients undergoing ligation of the IVC found that there were no surviving patients that experienced significant lower extremity edema or lower extremity dysfunction at a mean follow-up of 42 months after injury [43].

Infrahepatic, suprarenal injuries of the IVC are approached in a similar fashion as infrarenal

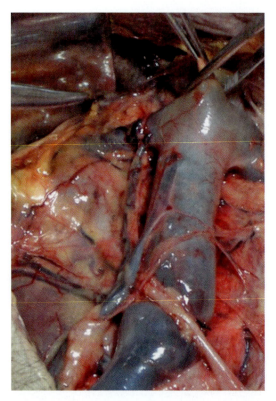

Fig. 18.2 Exposure of the infrarenal inferior vena cava (IVC) following right-sided medial visceral rotation. The ureter is seen crossing over the IVC at the bifurcation of the common iliac veins

injuries; however, exposure of the suprarenal IVC can be more difficult. In contrast to infrarenal IVC injuries, the suprarenal IVC should not be ligated in cases of severe injury as this would preclude renal outflow and result in renal failure.

Patient with evidence of hemorrhage near the liver, in whom a Pringle maneuver does not control bleeding, should be suspected of having a retrohepatic IVC injury. Surgical control can be achieved by complete liver mobilization and visualization of the retrohepatic IVC (Fig. 18.4). An atriocaval shunt can be used as a temporizing measure to bypass the area of injury while adequate mobilization and repair is undertaken [44]. Placement of an atriocaval shunt requires access to the chest via a right thoracotomy or median sternotomy. The shunt, usually a 36-French chest tube, is placed through the right atrial appendage and into the vena cava, where the shunt can bypass the area of injury, limit bleeding, and

Fig. 18.3 Ligation of the inferior vena cava (IVC) for an infrarenal IVC injury. IVC ligation can be considered for patients who are coagulopathic or in shock

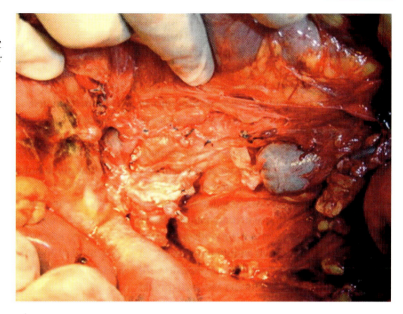

Fig. 18.4 Exposure of the retrohepatic inferior vena cava (IVC). Medial mobilization of the liver and partial hepatectomy have exposed the retrohepatic segment of the IVC. The right hepatic vein has been ligated. Clips have been placed on the short hepatic veins in order to control hemorrhage

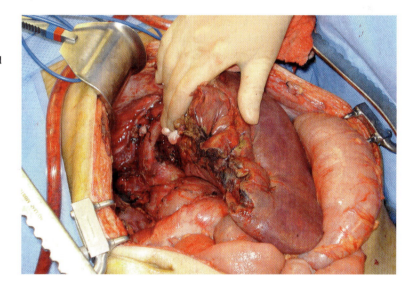

maintain venous return to the heart. Atriocaval shunts are rarely used and are associated with very high mortality [45]. Another damage control option is total hepatic isolation in which the suprahepatic IVC below the diaphragm or within the pericardium, the infrahepatic IVC, and the descending aorta is clamped while a Pringle is performed. This allows identification of the injury for repair or shunting in a theoretically bloodless field. It often results in arrest or severe shock as venous return to the heart is severely diminished, and outcomes are generally poor [8, 18, 21, 25].

18.6 Postoperative Management, Complications, and Outcomes

Mortality from abdominal vascular injuries remains high (20–60 %) and increases with increasing number of vessels injured and in the presence of associated nonvascular injuries (Tables 18.3 and 18.4). Mortality has not changed significantly over time despite advanced trauma systems and modern operative and ICU technologies. Mortality can be separated into early and late, with the majority of early deaths due to exsanguinations and late deaths due to multisystem organ failure [46].

Increased early mortality has been associated with shock (SBP ≤90 mmHg) on admission, acidosis, hypothermia ($T < 34°$), decreased Trauma Score, and need for either resuscitative thoracotomy or damage control procedures. Mortality is also increased by certain intraoperative and injury characteristics such as free intraperitoneal bleeding, need for transfusion greater than 10 units of packed red blood cells, suprarenal loca-

tion of injuries, advanced American Association for the Surgery of Trauma Organ Injury Scale (AAST-OIS) grade, and increased Injury Severity Score (ISS) [3, 11, 12, 21].

Conclusion

Abdominal vascular injuries are associated with high morbidity and mortality, with patients usually presenting in shock. Surgeons caring for trauma patients need to be knowledgeable in techniques to access the major, named vascular structures within the abdomen. Important basic principles of vascular surgery such as gaining proximal and distal control of the injured vessel, repairing vessels without significant narrowing of the vessel lumen, and when to consider patch angio-

Table 18.3 Mortality in abdominal vascular injury and isolated named vessel injuries [6, 11, 12, 21, 22]

Study	Overall mortality (%)	IVC (%)	Portal/SMV (%)	Celiac (%)	SMA (%)
Paul et al. [11]	28.5	44	Portal 69 SMV 60	75	33
Allison et al [47] *Pediatric	20	36–64	Portal 50	NR	0
Eachempati et al. [22]	38.7	67	NR	NR	NR
Tyburski et al. [12]	45	57	Portal: 69 SMV: 44	NR	51
Davis et al. [9]	Artery 54 Vein 36	53.4	SMV: 29	NR	44
Asensio et al. [6]	54	70.1	Portal 100 SMV 53	50	48
Coimbra et al. [8]	57	37	NR	NR	NR

IVC inferior vena cava, *SMA* superior mesenteric artery, *SMV* superior mesenteric vein, *NR* not reported
* study is of pediatric rather than adult patients

Table 18.4 Mortality stratified by number of vessels injured [6, 11, 12, 21]

Study	Mortality 1 vessel (%)	Mortality 2 vessels (%)	Mortality 3 vessels (%)	Mortality 4 vessels (%)	Mortality 5 vessels (%)
Paul et al. [11]	21.4	35.1	62.5	0	100
Tyburski et al. [12]	33	56	59	100	NR
Asensio et al. [6]	45	60	73	100	100
Asensio et al. [15] (SMA)	50	33–67	75	NR	NR

NR not reported

plasty versus interposition grafting are crucial in dealing with abdominal vascular injuries. Damage control techniques such as temporary intravascular shunting, knowledge of which vessels may be safely ligated, and temporary abdominal closure options are critically important in treating the severely injured, unstable patient.

References

1. Asensio JA, Forno W, Roldan G, et al. Visceral vascular injuries. Surg Clin North Am. 2002;82:1–20, xix.
2. Dente C, Feliciano D. Abdominal vascular injury. In: Feliciano DV, Mattox KL, Moore EE, editors. Trauma. New York: McGraw Hill; 2008. p. 737–57.
3. Hoyt DB, Coimbra R, Potenza BM, et al. Anatomic exposures for vascular injuries. Surg Clin North Am. 2001;81:1299–330, xii.
4. Stannard A, Brown K, Benson C, et al. Outcome after vascular trauma in a deployed military trauma system. Br J Surg. 2011;98:228–34.
5. Asensio JA, Britt LD, Borzotta A, et al. Multiinstitutional experience with the management of superior mesenteric artery injuries. J Am Coll Surg. 2001;193:354–65; discussion 365–56.
6. Asensio JA, Chahwan S, Hanpeter D, et al. Operative management and outcome of 302 abdominal vascular injuries. Am J Surg. 2000;180:528–33; discussion 533–4.
7. Asensio JA, Soto SN, Forno W, et al. Abdominal vascular injuries: the trauma surgeon's challenge. Surg Today. 2001;31:949–57.
8. Coimbra R, Yang J, Hoyt DB. Injuries of the abdominal aorta and inferior vena cava in association with thoracolumbar fractures: a lethal combination. J Trauma. 1996;41:533–5.
9. Davis TP, Feliciano DV, Rozycki GS, et al. Results with abdominal vascular trauma in the modern era. Am Surg. 2001;67:565–70; discussion 570–1.
10. Hoyt DB, Shackford SR, McGill T, et al. The impact of in-house surgeons and operating room resuscitation on outcome of traumatic injuries. Arch Surg. 1989;124:906–9; discussion 909–10.
11. Paul JS, Webb TP, Aprahamian C, et al. Intraabdominal vascular injury: are we getting any better? J Trauma. 2010;69:1393–7.
12. Tyburski JG, Wilson RF, Dente C, et al. Factors affecting mortality rates in patients with abdominal vascular injuries. J Trauma. 2001;50:1020–6.
13. Asensio JA, Petrone P, Kimbrell B, et al. Lessons learned in the management of thirteen celiac axis injuries. South Med J. 2005;98:462–6.
14. Graham JM, Mattox KL, Beall Jr AC, et al. Injuries to the visceral arteries. Surgery. 1978;84:835–9.
15. Asensio JA, Berne JD, Chahwan S, et al. Traumatic injury to the superior mesenteric artery. Am J Surg. 1999;178:235–9.
16. Pearl J, Chao A, Kennedy S, et al. Traumatic injuries to the portal vein: case study. J Trauma. 2004; 56:779–82.
17. Fraga GP, Bansal V, Fortlage D, et al. A 20-year experience with portal and superior mesenteric venous injuries: has anything changed? Eur J Vasc Endovasc Surg. 2009;37:87–91.
18. Coimbra R, Filho AR, Nesser RA, et al. Outcome from traumatic injury of the portal and superior mesenteric veins. Vasc Endovascular Surg. 2004;38:249–55.
19. Asensio JA, Petrone P, Garcia-Nunez L, et al. Superior mesenteric venous injuries: to ligate or to repair remains the question. J Trauma. 2007;62:668–75; discussion 675.
20. Jurkovich GJ, Hoyt DB, Moore FA, et al. Portal triad injuries. J Trauma. 1995;39:426–34.
21. Coimbra R, Hoyt D, Winchell R, et al. The ongoing challenge of retroperitoneal vascular injuries. Am J Surg. 1996;172:541–4; discussion 545.
22. Eachempati SR, Robb T, Ivatury RR, et al. Factors associated with mortality in patients with penetrating abdominal vascular trauma. J Surg Res. 2002;108:222–6.
23. Coimbra R, Prado PA, Araujo LH, et al. Factors related to mortality in inferior vena cava injuries. A 5 year experience. Int Surg. 1994;79:138–41.
24. Fullen WD, Hunt J, Altemeier WA. The clinical spectrum of penetrating injury to the superior mesenteric arterial circulation. J Trauma. 1972;12:656–64.
25. Hansen CJ, Bernadas C, West MA, et al. Abdominal vena caval injuries: outcomes remain dismal. Surgery. 2000;128:572–8.
26. Rosengart MR, Smith DR, Melton SM, et al. Prognostic factors in patients with inferior vena cava injuries. Am Surg. 1999;65:849–55; discussion 855–6.
27. Holcomb JB, Wade CE, Michalek JE, et al. Increased plasma and platelet to red blood cell ratios improves outcome in 466 massively transfused civilian trauma patients. Ann Surg. 2008;248:447–58.
28. Taourel P, Vernhet H, Suau A, et al. Vascular emergencies in liver trauma. Eur J Radiol. 2007;64:73–82.
29. Vu M, Anderson SW, Shah N, et al. CT of blunt abdominal and pelvic vascular injury. Emerg Radiol. 2010;17:21–9.
30. Fang JF, Shih LY, Wong YC, et al. Angioembolization and laparotomy for patients with concomitant pelvic arterial hemorrhage and blunt abdominal trauma. Langenbecks Arch Surg. 2011;396:243–50.
31. Martin de Carpi J, Tarrado X, Varea V. Sclerosing cholangitis secondary to hepatic artery ligation after abdominal trauma. Eur J Gastroenterol Hepatol. 2005; 17:987–90.
32. Conti S. Splenic artery ligation for trauma. An alternative to splenectomy. Am J Surg. 1980;140:444–6.
33. Keramidas D, Buyukunal C, Senyuz O, et al. Splenic artery ligation: a ten-year experience in the treatment of selected cases of splenic injuries in children. Jpn J Surg. 1991;21:172–7.

34. Reilly PM, Rotondo MF, Carpenter JP, et al. Temporary vascular continuity during damage control: intraluminal shunting for proximal superior mesenteric artery injury. J Trauma. 1995;39:757–60.

35. Subramanian A, Vercruysse G, Dente C, et al. A decade's experience with temporary intravascular shunts at a civilian level I trauma center. J Trauma. 2008;65:316–24; discussion 324–6.

36. Asayama Y, Matsumoto S, Isoda T, et al. A case of traumatic mesenteric bleeding controlled by only transcatheter arterial embolization. Cardiovasc Intervent Radiol. 2005;28:256–8.

37. Hagiwara A, Takasu A. Transcatheter arterial embolization is effective for mesenteric arterial hemorrhage in trauma. Emerg Radiol. 2009;16:403–6.

38. Demirel S, Winter C, Rapprich B, et al. Stab injury of the superior mesenteric artery with life threatening bleeding – endovascular treatment with an unusual technique. Vasa. 2010;39(3):268–70. doi:10.1024/0301-1526/a000041.

39. Kakizawa H, Toyota N, Hieda M, et al. Traumatic mesenteric bleeding managed solely with transcatheter embolization. Radiat Med. 2007;25:295–8.

40. Stone HH, Fabian TC, Turkleson ML. Wounds of the portal venous system. World J Surg. 1982;6:335–41.

41. Feliciano DV. Management of traumatic retroperitoneal hematoma. Ann Surg. 1990;211:109–23.

42. Carr JA, Kralovich KA, Patton JH, et al. Primary venorrhaphy for traumatic inferior vena cava injuries. Am Surg. 2001;67:207–13; discussion 213–4.

43. Sullivan PS, Dente CJ, Patel S, et al. Outcome of ligation of the inferior vena cava in the modern era. Am J Surg. 2010;199:500–6.

44. Schrock T, Blaisdell FW, Mathewson Jr C. Management of blunt trauma to the liver and hepatic veins. Arch Surg. 1968;96:698–704.

45. Burch JM, Feliciano DV, Mattox KL. The atriocaval shunt. Facts and fiction. Ann Surg. 1988;207:555–68.

46. Trunkey DD. Trauma. Accidental and intentional injuries account for more years of life lost in the U.S. than cancer and heart disease. Among the prescribed remedies are improved preventive efforts, speedier surgery and further research. Sci Am. 1983;249:28–35.

47. Allison ND, Anderson CM, Shah SK, et al. Outcomes of truncal vascular injuries in children. J Pediatric Surg. 2009:44:1958–1964

Part V

Pelvis

Karen J. Brasel and Kellie Brown

Iliac Artery Injuries

19

Nicolas H. Pope, William F. Johnston,
and Gilbert R. Upchurch Jr.

Contents

19.1 Introduction

Despite numerous advances and refinement in the care of trauma patients since the World War II, injuries to the iliac arteries remain highly lethal and difficult to treat [1–5]. The first modern, published attempts at repair of major vascular injuries came during World War II. DeBakey and Simeone reported 2,471 arterial injuries, including 43 to the iliac arteries, the vast majority of which were treated with simple ligation in order to prevent fatal hemorrhage. Over the course of the war, they attempted 81 arterial repairs consisting of 78 lateral suture repairs and only three end-to-end anastomoses with a 49 % amputation rate [6]. During the Vietnam conflict, advances in evacuation of injured personnel to forward surgical hospitals and increased availability of transfusion led to a better experience with these previously fatal injuries and a decrease in the amputation rate to 13 % [7].

The overall incidence of wartime iliac artery injury has been relatively unchanged from World War II to the Iraq-Afghanistan conflicts of the past decade, ranging from 1.7 to 3.8 % [6, 8–11]. The incidence of penetrating iliac artery injury in the civilian setting, however, has risen from the mid-1980s to the present day, most secondary to an overall increase of violence in urban settings [10]. The overall incidence of penetrating iliac artery injury as the result of gunshot wounds is near 10 % in the urban, civilian setting. Injury from stab wounds accounts for 2 % of iliac artery injuries [1, 10, 12, 13].

N.H. Pope, MD • W.F. Johnston, MD
Department of Surgery, University of Virginia,
Charlottesville, VA, USA

G.R. Upchurch Jr., MD (✉)
Division of Vascular and Endovascular Surgery,
Department of Surgery, Molecular Physiology
and Biological Physics, University of Virginia,
Charlottesville, VA, USA
e-mail: gru6n@virginia.edu

A. Dua et al. (eds.), *Clinical Review of Vascular Trauma*,
DOI 10.1007/978-3-642-39100-2_19, © Springer-Verlag Berlin Heidelberg 2014

Blunt injury represents approximately 5 % of all injuries to the iliac arteries [2]. Injury resulting from blunt trauma occurs more commonly in the internal iliac system, although blunt injuries to the common iliac arteries have been reported [14–16]. These injuries are thought to be the result of arterial stretching across bony structures within the displaced pelvis [17, 18]. Intimal disruption and resultant thrombosis are more common than transection [19, 20]. Patients with large atherosclerotic plaque burden are thought to be more likely to suffer these types of injuries [15, 16, 21, 22].

Associated venous injury is common in both mechanisms, complicating between 32 and 45 % of all iliac artery injuries [4, 23–25]. Concomitant injury to nearby visceral organs is common in penetrating trauma. The most frequent synchronously injured organs are the small bowel, colon, and urinary bladder [4, 23, 26, 27]. As will be discussed later, injury to these structures often complicates the repair and makes the decision to use prosthetic grafts more difficult, but not impossible.

19.2 Anatomy and Physiology

19.2.1 Anatomy

The abdominal aorta bifurcates into the right and left common iliac arteries at the level of the fourth lumbar vertebrae. From there, each artery courses laterally and downwards to the level of the sacroiliac joint, where each again bifurcates into the internal (hypogastric) and external iliac artery.

Owing to the position of the abdominal aorta to the left of midline, the right common iliac artery is slightly longer than the left and crosses the final lumbar vertebrae at a more oblique angle. Important structures that are at risk of concomitant injury are the inferior vena cava and right common iliac vein laterally and posteriorly, the cecum and terminal ilium anteriorly, and the ureter which courses lateral to medial, traversing the common iliac artery near the iliac bifurcation. Posteriorly, it is abutted by the fifth lumbar

vertebral body and the psoas major muscle more laterally. In rare instances, the right common iliac artery is absent, and the right internal and external iliac arteries arise directly from the abdominal aorta [4, 10, 24, 28].

The left common iliac artery is shorter and courses laterally at a more acute angle than the right common iliac artery. The left common iliac artery runs anterior to the right common iliac vein proximally and lateral and anterior to the left common iliac vein more distally. Other structures which are at risk for concomitant injury include the sigmoid colon anteriorly and the left ureter, which lies anterior to the iliac bifurcation. Posteriorly and laterally, it is supported by the body of the final lumbar vertebrae and the psoas major. Although more commonly shorter in length, it more commonly bifurcates into the internal and external iliac arteries lower down in the pelvis than its right counterpart [4, 10, 24, 28].

The internal iliac artery follows the line of the sacroiliac joint into the internal ring of the pelvis where it gives off the iliolumbar and lateral sacral arteries before dividing into an anterior and posterior trunk. Arteries of the anterior trunk, including the obturator, uterine, and internal pudendal arteries, arise just medial to the acetabula to supply visceral structures within the pelvis. Collateralization is typically excellent, through the inferior mesenteric artery via the superior hemorrhoidal arteries and by means of the uterine, ovarian, and vesical arteries of the contralateral side, such that ligation of a single, or even bilateral, internal iliac arteries for uncontrolled hemorrhage is generally well tolerated [4, 10, 28–32]. Injuries that result in damage to the lumbar vertebrae, sacroiliac joints, or acetabula should raise suspicion for arterial injury of the internal iliac system [4, 10, 24, 28].

The external iliac artery exits the abdomen and supplies arterial flow to the leg as the common femoral artery. Prior to crossing under the inguinal ligament, the external iliac artery gives rise to two potential sources for collateralization: the inferior epigastric and the deep circumflex iliac arteries. The inferior epigastric runs superiorly along the posterior surface of the rectus abdominis muscle and joining the superior epigastric artery. The deep circumflex iliac arteries provide further collateral circulation with the last lumbar artery. While these areas of collateralization may prove of great importance to patients with chronic aortoilio-occlusive disease, they are generally too small to significantly supply arterial flow to the lower extremity in the setting of an acute vascular injury [4, 28, 33].

19.2.2 Physiology

Many patients having suffered iliac arterial injury present to trauma centers in profound hemorrhagic shock [2, 4, 10, 23, 24, 26, 27, 31, 32, 34]. These patients represent a challenge not only due to the anatomic location of their injuries but also secondary to the profound metabolic derangements resulting from massive blood loss. The aptly named "triangle of death," acidosis, hypothermia, and coagulopathy, have frustrated countless trauma surgeons and led to the development of "damage control" techniques to minimize operative time in such moribund patients [35–38].

As expected, presenting physiologic parameters predict outcomes. Cushman et al. reviewed the records of 53 patients with iliac vessel injury taken for emergent laparotomy. A significant difference was found between preoperative and postoperative temperature and base deficit among survivors as compared with non-survivors [26]. Other factors that were found to adversely influence survival include the number of major vascular injuries, concomitant iliac venous injury, and injury to visceral structures [26].

Haan et al. were able to quantify these observations and correlated overall survival for patients with iliac vessel injury to their associated Injury Severity Score (ISS). Those with a higher ISS had more complications and an overall decreased survival. Asensio et al. demonstrated, not surprisingly, that as American Association for the Surgery of Trauma Organ Injury Scale (AAST-OIS) increased, survival sharply decreased from 65 % for grade III to 21 % for grade V injuries [2, 34].

19.3 Clinical Assessment

A high suspicion for iliac artery injury is necessary in order to make a timely and potentially lifesaving diagnosis. Most (61–84 %) patients with iliac artery injury present to trauma centers in hemorrhagic shock [23, 27]. Patients with penetrating injuries of the abdomen or pelvis, particularly to the lower abdomen or pelvis, with persistent hypotension despite resuscitation should be suspected of having an abdominal vascular injury. The triad of abdominal distention, hypotension, and absent unilateral lower extremity pulses is virtually pathognomonic for iliac artery injury [10]. The presence of peripheral pulses does not, however, rule out iliac arterial injury, as up to 25 % of patients with iliac artery injury may have a palpable distal pulse on the side of injury [39, 40].

19.4 Diagnostic Testing

When a high index for suspicion of iliac artery injury is present, operative intervention should not be delayed in order to obtain further diagnostic studies. In patients sustaining blunt trauma, anterior-posterior (AP) views of the pelvis obtained in the trauma bay may reveal pelvic fractures that should raise concern for iliac vessel injury [17]. Particular fracture patterns are associated with a higher likelihood of iliac vessel injury. Patients with both anterior rami and sacroiliac joint injury have been reported to be at high risk for iliac vascular injury [4, 17, 18, 41, 42].

Focused Assessment with Sonography for Trauma (FAST) examination may suggest iliac artery injury with positive pelvic windows. The absence of blood in the pelvis does not, however, rule out the possibility of iliac arterial injury, as retroperitoneal bleeding is poorly visualized with the FAST exam.

Angiography has become an important tool in the management of blunt iliac artery injury. Because of the difficult anatomic location and the high frequency of concomitant injury, endovascular techniques have become the treatment of choice for bleeding pelvic vessels that are the result of blunt trauma. While digital subtraction angiography (DSA) had been the preferred diagnostic tool to detect pelvic arterial injuries resulting from blunt trauma, improvements in computed tomography angiography (CTA) in detecting both arterial and venous injury have led to a shift towards CTA for the initial diagnostic test in this patient population [43, 44].

Advantages of CTA include the ability to obtain full-body imaging to assess for other injuries, an ability to distinguish between arterial and venous injuries, and the ability to frequently differentiate between ongoing bleeding and a stable pelvic hematoma. Modern CTA is able to detect arterial dissection, pseudoaneurysm, and arteriovenous fistula [45]. The most obvious disadvantage of CTA is the lack of interventional capability.

19.5   Initial Management

Initial management is focused on balanced resuscitation and early diagnosis in the emergency department. Although definitive treatments of blunt and penetrating injuries differ, the initial establishment of adequate intravenous access and resuscitation does not.

Suspicion of iliac artery injury should lead to early activation of hospital protocols to make available adequate quantities of blood and blood products. If a massive transfusion is required, resuscitation according to massive transfusion protocols, with emphasis on preventing dilutional coagulopathy, has been shown to improve survival [46–48]. The placement of lower extremity venous lines for resuscitation should be avoided. Presence of concomitant iliac vein injury is common and may complicate attempted resuscitation efforts through ipsilateral femoral venous catheters [4]. In the absence of head injury, hypotensive resuscitation should be considered, avoiding attempts to normalize blood pressure until definitive control of bleeding is achieved. In patients requiring operative intervention, resuscitation should begin before, but not delay, transport to the operating room.

Methods to avoid the development of hypothermia should be instituted. Use of intravenous fluid warmers and forced warm air heating devices should be instituted early and continued throughout treatment. Avoidance of hypothermia and associated coagulopathy and acidosis has become part of the "damage control" practice in the severely injured and begins before any incision is made.

19.6   Operative Management

19.6.1 Endovascular Therapies

Patients with blunt iliac arterial injuries can frequently be best managed with endovascular techniques. The majority of patients found to have ongoing pelvic arterial bleeding on CTA require subsequent DSA-guided embolization [45]. Although this requires additional intra-arterial contrast media, there is evidence to suggest that by defining the area of injury, CTA prior to DSA may reduce the total contrast requirement [49, 50]. Arterial bleeding resulting from pelvic fractures in blunt trauma typically arises from the internal iliac distribution. Embolic therapy for these injuries has become the preferred method of treatment, as surgical ligation can prove difficult given the high degree of collateralization (Fig. 19.1). In addition, surgical ligation sacrifices some of the tamponade effect provided by the intact abdominal wall [45, 51]. When selective embolization of arterial bleeding fails, temporary angiographic embolization of bilateral internal iliac arteries has been reported 97 % effective at controlling refractory bleeding without ischemic complications [52].

Large arterial wall defects may be amenable to endovascular stent-grafting with covered stent-grafts in order to exclude the injured segment. Arterial access may be established through the ipsilateral or contralateral femoral system, as well as through an axillary approach. Delivery of stent-grafts typically requires relatively large arterial sheaths and may be made more difficult by calcification of the potential access sites. In addition, adequate landing zones are required

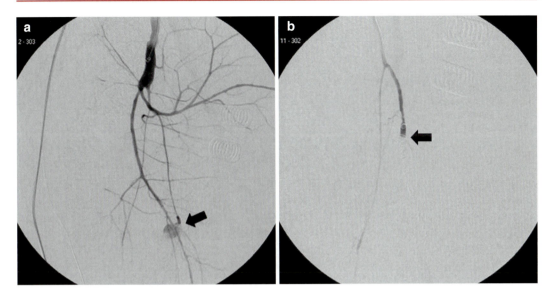

Fig. 19.1 (**a**) Active extravasation (*arrow*) of contrast seen arising from a branch of the left internal iliac artery in a patient with multiple pelvic fractures after blunt trauma. (**b**) Successful coil embolization (*arrow*) of the bleeding vessel. Initial diagnosis of active bleeding was made with CTA

proximally and distally to the area of injury in order to ensure correct stent placement and to avoid stent-graft migration.

Failure of endovascular attempts to control ongoing arterial hemorrhage requires surgical exploration. Temporary aortic occlusion balloons placed in the angiography suite may be used under such circumstances to slow the rate of hemorrhage while operative resources are mobilized [10].

The role for angiography in penetrating iliac arterial injury is limited. The majority of these patients present in hemorrhagic shock and with multiple other associated injuries which require immediate operative intervention [2, 10, 12, 13, 23, 24, 26, 27, 34, 53]. While great advances in endovascular therapy have taken place over the past 20 years, most trauma centers still lack hybrid interventional-operative suites to attempt combined open and endovascular treatment [10].

Although fortunately a rare complication, iatrogenic injury to the iliac arteries most commonly occurs either as the result of laparoscopic trocar insertion or pedicle screw placement during lumbar spine surgery. Successful placement of a covered, self-expanding, or balloon-expandable endovascular stent-graft to exclude the site of injury has been reported [14, 54]. Unlike patients who suffer iliac artery injuries in the field, these injuries occur in the operating suite and resuscitation can begin immediately, and the incidence of concomitant injury and physiologic derangement is low. Emergent transport to the angiography suite for endovascular treatment may be preferred over open management of these injuries in this particular patient population.

19.6.2 Operative Treatments

Patients with penetrating injury require immediate operative management. These patients, along with patients who have a blunt mechanism and indication for operation, should be brought to the operating room with adequate stores of blood and blood products immediately available. Normothermic measures should be continued throughout the operative period. The patient is placed in the supine position and is prepped and draped in the standard trauma fashion—from chin to knees and to the OR table on the sides. Both axillae should be within the field if

Fig. 19.2 Left-to-right medial visceral rotation (Mattox maneuver). Mobilization of the left colon along the line of Toldt provides excellent access to the abdominal aorta (Adapted from Lee and Bongard [4], with permission)

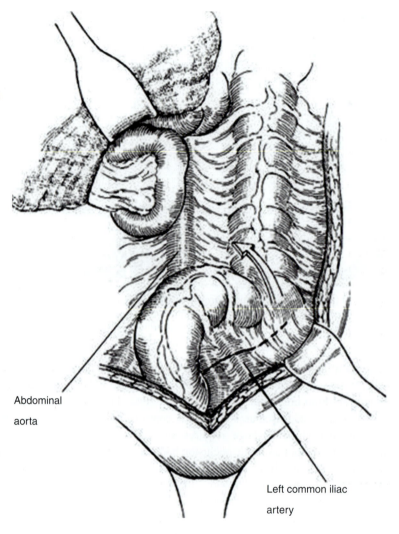

Abdominal

aorta

Left common iliac

artery

the need for axillofemoral bypass arises. A groin towel is placed with care not to obscure access to the femoral arterial system on either side of the patient. Preoperative antibiotics should be administered prior to incision.

Exposure begins through a midline laparotomy incision extending from the xyphoid to the symphysis pubis. Once the peritoneal cavity has been entered, packing of solid organ injuries should proceed along standard trauma principles. Presence of a zone III retroperitoneal hematoma in the setting of penetrating trauma is not uncommon in patients with iliac arterial injury and requires exploration. If the iliac artery bleeds freely into the abdomen, direct manual compression to the artery lesion or proximal artery can

stop bleeding until proximal and distal control can be achieved.

Exposure of the iliac system is best achieved through a left-to-right medial visceral rotation (Mattox maneuver) [55]. The peritoneal attachments of the left colon are mobilized along the avascular line of Toldt, and the left colon is rotated medially to expose the aorta and iliac vessels (Fig. 19.2). Alternatively, if injury to the right iliac artery is suspected, right-to left medial visceral rotation provides easy access to the right common and external iliac arteries. Care must be taken to avoid injury to the ureters during dissection.

The discovery of massive hemorrhage on entering the abdomen requires immediate action to attempt to gain proximal and distal control of the bleeding vessels. Temporary manual compression of the distal aorta against the vertebral bodies and of the common femoral arteries just beyond the inguinal ligament may slow the rate of hemorrhage while formal proximal and distal control can be established [4, 24]. This is best achieved through pelvic vascular isolation either with vascular clamps or vessel loops.

Proximal control is obtained by carefully placing vascular clamps across the distal aorta and inferior vena cava proximal to their bifurcations. Distal control is obtained by placing a single clamp across the distal external iliac artery and vein bilaterally [4, 56, 57]. This maneuver allows for further identification of areas of both arterial and venous injury. As injuries are identified, the clamps are moved more near to the area of injury thus reestablishing flow to uninjured vessels.

Injury to the distal external iliac artery may require an inguinal incision to gain adequate distal control. This incision should be made longitudinally and can be extended distally to transect the inguinal ligament if necessary. Alternative proximal control can be obtained by transecting the hepatoduodenal ligament and cross-clamping the supraceliac aorta. This not only compromises mesenteric and renal blood flow but also allows for greater collateral flow to the injured artery and should only be used as a temporizing measure while more proximal control can be obtained closer to the site of injury.

Once the area of injury has been identified and isolated, devitalized tissue should be debrided to allow for a full assessment of the extent of injury and allow for proper choice of the type of repair that should be attempted. Simple disruptions involving less than 50 % of the circumference of the arterial wall may be closed primarily in a transverse fashion with interrupted polypropylene suture. Attempting primary repair of more extensive lesions may result in stenosis at the site of anastomosis.

Such lesions may be treated with excision of the injured segment and end-to-end anastomosis. This should only be attempted if mobilization of the proximal and distal artery can provide for a tension-free repair. Distances greater than 1 cm are generally not amenable to end-to-end anastomosis [4]. Autologous saphenous vein grafts are rarely large enough caliber for use in the iliac arteries [10]. Alternatively, autologous femoral vein may be used for interposition grafting of the iliac arteries [58, 59]. The femoral vein is typically of adequate diameter for interposition grafting of the iliac arteries. Unlike the saphenous vein, its length may be of concern should a particularly long segment of artery require excision. Either the ipsilateral or the contralateral superficial femoral vein is chosen if concomitant injury is absent. Also, consider the likelihood of adequate venous outflow from the chosen donor leg if distal injuries are present. The proximal and distal superficial femoral vein is clamped and side branches are ligated. The homograft is then excised leaving adequate cuffs near both clamps for definitive closure of the venous stumps. Valves are stripped or the direction of the conduit is reversed before reanastomosis. The interposition graft is placed using polypropylene sutures with care to avoid excess tension, torque, or redundancy.

If a tension-free repair cannot be accomplished with the available length of femoral autograft, the use of polytetrafluoroethylene (PTFE) grafts provides an excellent option for reconstruction. These are typically readily available in most hospitals in various sizes. As compared with grafts for more distal arteries, the use of PTFE grafts in the iliac system has better primary and secondary patency rates [60]. An appropriately sized PTFE graft is anastomosed proximally and distally with 4-0 or 5-0 polypropylene suture. The clamps are flashed both proximally and distally to minimize thromboembolism prior to completing the anastomosis. Reconstruction of more complex injuries occurring near areas of bifurcation can be accomplished either with arterial transposition or extra-anatomic bypass.

Arterial transposition involves removing the common iliac artery near the aorta, excising the injured segment, and reimplanting the arterial stump to the contralateral common iliac artery. This technique allows for tension-free repair of injuries occurring near the aortic bifurcation. To

Fig. 19.3 Two-layer closure of iliac arterial stump. Polypropylene suture is used to close the artery in a horizontal mattress stitch. A second running layer is imbricated over the distal arterial stump (Adapted from Lee and Bongard [4], with permission)

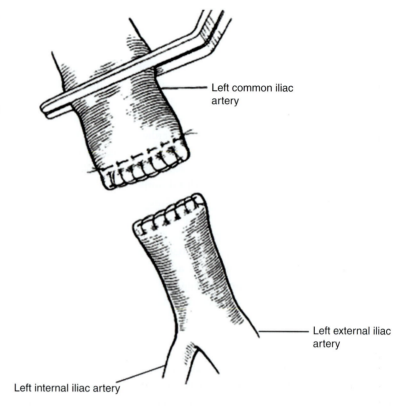

Left common iliac artery

Left external iliac artery

Left internal iliac artery

accomplish this, the aortic cross-clamp is carefully placed immediately proximal to the aortic bifurcation. Vascular clamps are then placed across both common iliac arteries distal to the area of injury and with enough space on the contralateral side to allow for easy reanastomosis. The injured vessel is divided near the aorta and the proximal iliac artery stump is closed with 3-0 or 4-0 polypropylene suture in two layers (Fig. 19.3). The injured portions of the explanted artery are debrided, and an arteriotomy is made in the contralateral common iliac artery. The anastomosis is carried out with 4-0 or 5-0 polypropylene suture [4].

Injuries to the external iliac artery near the iliac bifurcation can be repaired using the uninjured ipsilateral hypogastric artery as an interposition graft. Proximal control is obtained with a vascular clamp placed carefully across the proximal common iliac artery. Care must be taken during this dissection to identify and protect the ureter as it crosses into the pelvis at the iliac bifurcation. Control of outflow may require a

separate inguinal incision and division of the inguinal ligament should mobilization transabdominally fail to provide adequate length to perform a tension-free repair. The ipsilateral hypogastric artery is then mobilized and divided at the level of the middle hemorrhoidal artery [4]. The injured segment of the external iliac artery is then excised and both proximal and distal stumps are oversewn in two layers with polypropylene suture. The hypogastric artery is then reimplanted to the external iliac artery distal to the area of injury (Fig. 19.4).

The advantage of such arterial transposition techniques is that they avoid the need for prosthetic material when operating in a contaminated field. The most obvious drawback to such techniques is that they require longer operative times and are more technically complex than either simple repair or prosthetic interposition grafting.

Concomitant injury to visceral or urologic structures is common [4, 12, 23, 26, 27]. The use of prosthetic material for vascular repair in the setting of abdominal contamination remains

Fig. 19.4 Ipsilateral hypogastric arterial transposition is used to perfuse the lower extremity in patients with injuries to the proximal external iliac artery (Adapted from Lee and Bongard [4], with permission)

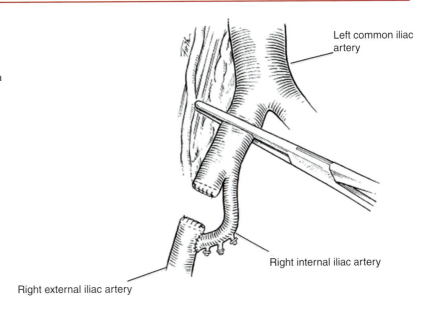

Left common iliac artery

Right internal iliac artery

Right external iliac artery

controversial. In the largest series to date, Burch reported the use of prosthetic arterial interposition grafts in five patients with associated colorectal injuries. Of these patients, there were no graft infections and all grafts remained patent without thrombosis [10, 23]. In the setting of visceral injury, thorough irrigation of the peritoneal cavity should precede any definitive vascular repair. The avoidance of prosthetic material in the setting of gross fecal contamination is reasonable as long as this decision does not significantly lengthen the operative time or exceed the technical expertise of the surgeon.

Extra-anatomic revascularization with either femoral-femoral or axillofemoral bypass represents an additional option in the setting of gross contamination. These techniques have been long used in the non-trauma population in the setting of contamination; however, they are generally time-consuming and have lower long-term patency rates than local repairs [23]. In the majority of patients with iliac artery injuries, extra-anatomic bypass should not be attempted at the initial operation and should be reserved for only those with significant fecal contamination that makes the use of local prosthetic grafts suboptimal.

Attempts at definitive repair of iliac artery injuries at initial operation must be made

judiciously. Asensio and colleagues have demonstrated a reliable set of variables, including Injury Severity Score (ISS) ≥ 25, systolic blood pressure <70 mmHg, pH <7.10, or temperature <34 °C, the presence of any which predict poor outcomes so a damage control approach is recommended [37]. Given the significant physiologic derangement often seen at initial presentation, the use of damage control techniques, including temporary intravascular shunts (TIVS), should be utilized if patients demonstrate significant acidosis or hypothermia [2, 23, 26, 61].

The TIVS provides fast and reliable perfusion to the lower extremity in situations where ligation would have previously been considered for uncontrolled hemorrhage in the unstable patient. The use of these synthetic shunts both controls hemorrhage and prevents critical limb ischemia. Whereas unilateral internal iliac artery ligation is generally well tolerated, ligation of the external iliac artery as a lifesaving maneuver results in limb loss in 50 % of patients, and there is an associated 90 % overall mortality [6, 23, 62]. TIVS can range in complexity from small chest tubes or red-rubber catheters to heparin-bonded Argyle shunts designed for such a purpose. Selection of a device for TIVS should be based upon their rapid availability and arterial caliber. Shunts are placed after first obtaining proximal and distal control of the injured segment. Thrombectomy is performed with appropriately sized Fogarty balloons and the shunt is placed in the proximal artery. The shunt is then flushed with blood and placed in the distal artery. Both ends are secured using heavy silk ties [62]. Arterial clamps are then removed and blood flow to the distal extremity assessed by confirming distal Doppler signals. Definitive repair is generally attempted 24–48 h after initial operation once the patient has been adequately warmed and resuscitated. Fasciotomies should be performed in the distal leg anytime prolonged ischemia to the extremity is suspected. The specific order in which these multidisciplinary repairs should proceed is discussed elsewhere in this textbook.

19.7 Postoperative Management

Patients with iliac arterial injuries or who have undergone iliac artery repair should be monitored initially in an intensive care setting. Peripheral pulses on the side of injury should be carefully monitored and documented. Suspicion of a developing compartment syndrome should prompt a return to surgery for fasciotomy. Particular attention should be paid to the fluid status of these patients as most have suffered massive blood loss with varying degrees of resuscitation during treatment. Use of central venous catheters to monitor central venous pressure and guide ongoing fluid replacement is commonly indicated.

Routine systemic anticoagulation for patients who have undergone large-vessel (aorta, iliac) reconstruction is not indicated. For those patients who have undergone more distal bypasses, the use of systemic anticoagulants should be weighed against the risk of bleeding depending on what other injuries the patient has suffered.

For patients without hollow viscous or urologic injury, standard perioperative antibiotic therapy alone is warranted. Broad-spectrum antibiotic therapy is recommended for those with intestinal spillage or an open abdomen. For patients with gastrointestinal contamination and synthetic material used for reconstruction, prophylactic antibiotic therapy should be continued longer.

19.8 Complications and Pitfalls

The vast majority of mortality associated with iliac artery injuries results from complications of hemorrhagic shock within the first 24 h of injury [2, 23, 25, 26, 61, 63]. Failure to control hemorrhage or to adequately resuscitate these frequently moribund patients leads to poor outcomes.

Vascular complications related to the repair of iliac artery injuries are dependent upon the type of repair. In the largest series to date, Burch et al. reported an overall arterial complication rate of 10.5 % among patients surviving greater than 24 h. In this series, a single patient undergoing end-to-end anastomosis experienced arterial thrombosis postoperatively. Four patients (25 %) treated with PTFE interposition grafts experienced graft thrombosis; however, all grafts were successfully opened at a second operation. Four patients (67 %) treated with ligation of the common or external iliac artery with extra-anatomic bypass suffered arterial complications, including graft thrombosis (33 %), compartment syndrome (50 %), and ultimate amputation (50 %) [23]. It should be noted that this later group of patients had suffered significantly greater blood loss and were much more likely to remain hypotensive following repair than in other treatment groups.

Other vascular complications following repair include aneurysmal dilatation or pseudoaneurysm formation, arterial stenosis (leading to claudication), arteriovenous fistula formation, and graft infection. Avoidance of the former can be accomplished by carefully and appropriately sizing patches as not to cause either stenosis or the potential for dilatation [1, 10, 11, 53, 64]. Pseudoaneurysms can typically be treated endovascularly by exclusion with covered stents, even in the event of rupture [65].

Graft infection, particularly under circumstances where grafts were placed in a contaminated field, presents a challenging problem. Burch has described the use of PTFE for interposition grafting in five patients with associated colorectal injuries, all of whom were treated with copious irrigation prior to graft placement and prophylactic antibiotic therapy. Of these five patients, there were four survivors and infections were prevented [23]. Antimicrobial therapy for graft infections is tailored to the specific organism. The duration of treatment is determined by the presence of septicemia or abscess, both of which require a minimum of 6 weeks of therapy [66]. For chronic graft infections, treatment options include explanting the infected device with extra-anatomic bypass or in situ exchange with antibiotic-bonded vascular grafts. Rifampin-bonded aortic grafts have shown some promise; however, their success has varied depending upon the infectious organism [67].

19.9 Outcomes

Despite great advances in both the transportation of the injured and advanced trauma care, the overall mortality from iliac artery injuries remains between 24 and 40 % [4, 23–27, 34, 53, 61]. Ongoing hemorrhage represents the most common cause of death in the first 24 h of injury [2, 23, 25, 26, 61, 63]. For patients who present in extremis and require a damage control approach to initial operation, TIVS has largely replaced external iliac ligation, nearly eliminating the high rate of limb loss associated with this maneuver [6, 23, 62].

Conclusion

Injury to the iliac arteries remains a devastating injury with significant morbidity and mortality that continues to challenge trauma surgeons. Patients typically present in significant metabolic disarray as a result of massive hemorrhage. Damage control techniques, including TIVS, should be employed for patients who are coagulopathic, hypothermic, or acidotic. Definitive arterial repair can be accomplished by various techniques, selection of which should depend upon the extent and location of injury. Penetrating injury typically requires open repair, whereas most blunt injuries are today amenable to endovascular therapies. Early communication between the trauma surgeon, vascular surgeon, and interventional radiologist is necessary. Fasciotomies should be strongly considered in patients with injury to the common or external iliac arteries or in patients with crush injury in order to avoid development of compartment syndrome.

References

1. Asensio JA, Chahwan S, Hanpeter D, Demetriades D, Forno W, Gambaro E, Murray J, Velmahos G, Marengo J, Shoemaker WC, Berne TV. Operative management and outcome of 302 abdominal vascular injuries. Am J Surg. 2000;180:528–33; discussion 533–4.
2. Asensio JA, Petrone P, Roldan G, Kuncir E, Rowe VL, Chan L, Shoemaker W, Berne TV. Analysis of 185 iliac vessel injuries: risk factors and predictors of outcome. Arch Surg. 2003;138:1187–93; discussion 1193–4.
3. Feliciano DV. Abdominal vascular injuries. Surg Clin North Am. 1988;68:741–55.
4. Lee JT, Bongard FS. Iliac vessel injuries. Surg Clin North Am. 2002;82:21–48.
5. Mullins RJ, Huckfeldt R, Trunkey DD. Abdominal vascular injuries. Surg Clin North Am. 1996;76:813–32.
6. De BM, Simeone FA. Battle injuries of the arteries in World War II; an analysis of 2,471 cases. Ann Surg. 1946;123:534–79.
7. Rich NM, Hughes CW. Vietnam vascular registry: a preliminary report. Surgery. 1969;65:218–26.
8. Clouse WD, Rasmussen TE, Peck MA, Eliason JL, Cox MW, Bowser AN, Jenkins DH, Smith DL, Rich NM. In-theater management of vascular injury: 2 years of the balad vascular registry. J Am Coll Surg. 2007;204:625–32.
9. Hughes CW. Arterial repair during the Korean war. Ann Surg. 1958;147:555–61.
10. Ksycki M, Ruiz G, Perez-Alonso AJ, Sciarretta JD, Gonzalo R, Iglesias E, Gigena A, Vu T, Asensio JA. Iliac vessel injuries: difficult injuries and difficult management problems. Eur J Trauma Emerg Surg. 2012;38:347–57.
11. White JM, Stannard A, Burkhardt GE, Eastridge BJ, Blackbourne LH, Rasmussen TE. The epidemiology of vascular injury in the wars in Iraq and Afghanistan. Ann Surg. 2011;253:1184–9.
12. Bongard F, Dubrow T, Klein S. Vascular injuries in the urban battleground: experience at a metropolitan trauma center. Ann Vasc Surg. 1990;4:415–8.
13. Mattox KL, Feliciano DV, Burch J, Beall Jr AC, Jordan Jr GL, De Bakey ME. Five thousand seven hundred sixty cardiovascular injuries in 4459 patients. Epidemiologic evolution 1958 to 1987. Ann Surg. 1989;209:698–705.
14. Dell'Erba A, Di Vella G, Giardino N. Seatbelt injury to the common iliac artery: case report. J Forensic Sci. 1998;43:215–7.

15. Lyden SP, Srivastava SD, Waldman DL, Green RM. Common iliac artery dissection after blunt trauma: case report of endovascular repair and literature review. J Trauma. 2001;50:339–42.

16. Tsai FC, Wang CC, Fang JF, Lin PJ, Kao CL, Hsieh HC, Chu JJ, Chen RJ, Chang CH. Isolated common iliac artery occlusion secondary to atherosclerotic plaque rupture from blunt abdominal trauma: case report and review of the literature. J Trauma. 1997;42:133–6.

17. Carrillo EH, Wohltmann CD, Spain DA, Schmieg Jr RE, Miller FB, Richardson JD. Common and external iliac artery injuries associated with pelvic fractures. J Orthop Trauma. 1999;13:351–5.

18. Thomford NR, Curtiss PH, Marable SA. Injuries of the iliac and femoral arteries associated with blunt skeletal trauma. J Trauma. 1969;9:126–34.

19. Brathwaite CE, Rodriguez A. Injuries of the abdominal aorta from blunt trauma. Am Surg. 1992;58:350–2.

20. Lock JS, Huffman AD, Johnson RC. Blunt trauma to the abdominal aorta. J Trauma. 1987;27:674–7.

21. Gupta N, Auer A, Troop B. Seat belt-related injury to the common iliac artery: case report and review of the literature. J Trauma. 1998;45:419–21.

22. Roth SM, Wheeler JR, Gregory RT, Gayle RG, Parent 3rd FN, Demasi R, Riblet J, Weireter LJ, Britt LD. Blunt injury of the abdominal aorta: a review. J Trauma. 1997;42:748–55.

23. Burch JM, Richardson RJ, Martin RR, Mattox KL. Penetrating iliac vascular injuries: recent experience with 233 consecutive patients. J Trauma. 1990;30:1450–9.

24. Mattox KL, Rea J, Ennix CL, Beall Jr AC, DeBakey ME. Penetrating injuries to the iliac arteries. Am J Surg. 1978;136:663–7.

25. Ryan W, Snyder 3rd W, Bell T, Hunt J. Penetrating injuries of the iliac vessels. Early recognition and management. Am J Surg. 1982;144:642–5.

26. Cushman JG, Feliciano DV, Renz BM, Ingram WL, Ansley JD, Clark WS, Rozycki GS. Iliac vessel injury: operative physiology related to outcome. J Trauma. 1997;42:1033–40.

27. Degiannis E, Velmahos GC, Levy RD, Wouters S, Badicel TV, Saadia R. Penetrating injuries of the iliac arteries: a South African experience. Surgery. 1996;119:146–50.

28. Gray H, Standring S, Ellis H, Berkovitz BKB. Gray's anatomy: the anatomical basis of clinical practice. Edinburgh: Elsevier Churchill Livingstone; 2005.

29. Joshi VM, Otiv SR, Majumder R, Nikam YA, Shrivastava M. Internal iliac artery ligation for arresting postpartum haemorrhage. BJOG. 2007;114:356–61.

30. Papathanasiou K, Tolikas A, Dovas D, Fragkedakis N, Koutsos J, Giannoylis C, Tzafettas J. Ligation of internal iliac artery for severe obstetric and pelvic haemorrhage: 10 year experience with 11 cases in a university hospital. J Obstet Gynaecol. 2008;28:183–4.

31. Patterson FP, Morton KS. The cause of death in fractures of the pelvis: with a note on treatment by ligation of the hypogastric (internal iliac) artery. J Trauma. 1973;13:849–56.

32. Ravitch MM. Hypogastric artery ligation in acute pelvic trauma. Surgery. 1964;56:601–2.

33. Rich NM, Mattox KL, Hirshberg A. Vascular trauma. 2nd ed. Philadelphia: Elsevier; 2004.

34. Haan J, Rodriguez A, Chiu W, Boswell S, Scott J, Scalea T. Operative management and outcome of iliac vessel injury: a ten-year experience. Am Surg. 2003;69:581–6.

35. Danks RR. Triangle of death. How hypothermia acidosis & coagulopathy can adversely impact trauma patients. JEMS. 2002;27:61–6, 68–70.

36. Moore EE, Thomas G. Orr memorial lecture. Staged laparotomy for the hypothermia, acidosis, and coagulopathy syndrome. Am J Surg. 1996;172:405–10.

37. Asensio JA, McDuffie L, Petrone P, Roldan G, Forno W, Gambaro E, Salim A, Demetriades D, Murray J, Velmahos G, Shoemaker W, Berne TV, Ramicone E, Chan L. Reliable variables in the exsanguinated patient which indicate damage control and predict outcome. Am J Surg. 2001;182:743–51.

38. Burch JM, Ortiz VB, Richardson RJ, Martin RR, Mattox KL, Jordan Jr GL. Abbreviated laparotomy and planned reoperation for critically injured patients. Ann Surg. 1992;215:476–83; discussion 483–4.

39. Gelenber RH, Menson J, Fromek A. The peripheral pulse following arterial injury. J Trauma. 1980;20:948–50.

40. Kennedy F, Cornwell EE, Lockett C, Demetriades D. Blunt injury to the left common iliac artery. Am Surg. 1995;61:360–2.

41. Cryer HM, Miller FB, Evers BM, Rouben LR, Seligson DL. Pelvic fracture classification: correlation with hemorrhage. J Trauma. 1988;28:973–80.

42. Smejkal R, Izant T, Born C, Delong W, Schwab W, Ross SE. Pelvic crush injuries with occlusion of the iliac artery. J Trauma. 1988;28:1479–82.

43. Ben-Menachem Y, Handel S, Ray R. Embolization procedures in trauma: a matter of urgency. Semin Interv Radiol. 1985;2:107–17.

44. Kertesz JL, Anderson SW, Murakami AM, Pieroni S, Rhea JT, Soto JA. Detection of vascular injuries in patients with blunt pelvic trauma by using 64-channel multidetector CT. Radiographics. 2009;29:151–64.

45. Niola R, Pinto A, Sparano A, Ignarra R, Romano L, Maglione F. Arterial bleeding in pelvic trauma: priorities in angiographic embolization. Curr Probl Diagn Radiol. 2012;41:93–101.

46. Gonzalez EA, Moore FA, Holcomb JB, Miller CC, Kozar RA, Todd SR, Cocanour CS, Balldin BC, McKinley BA. Fresh frozen plasma should be given earlier to patients requiring massive transfusion. J Trauma. 2007;62:112–9.

47. Malone DL, Hess JR, Fingerhut A. Massive transfusion practices around the globe and a suggestion for a

common massive transfusion protocol. J Trauma. 2006;60:S91–6.

48. Mohan D, Milbrandt EB, Alarcon LH. Black hawk down: the evolution of resuscitation strategies in massive traumatic hemorrhage. Crit Care. 2008; 12:305.

49. Mirvis SE. Imaging of acute thoracic injury: the advent of MDCT screening. Semin Ultrasound CT MR. 2005;26:305–31.

50. Mirvis SE. Thoracic vascular injury. Radiol Clin North Am. 2006;44:181–97, vii.

51. van Urk H, Perlberger RR, Muller H. Selective arterial embolization for control of traumatic pelvic hemorrhage. Surgery. 1978;83:133–7.

52. Velmahos GC, Chahwan S, Hanks SE, Murray JA, Berne TV, Asensio J, Demetriades D. Angiographic embolization of bilateral internal iliac arteries to control life-threatening hemorrhage after blunt trauma to the pelvis. Am Surg. 2000;66:858–62.

53. Davis TP, Feliciano DV, Rozycki GS, Bush JB, Ingram WL, Salomone JP, Ansley JD. Results with abdominal vascular trauma in the modern era. Am Surg. 2001;67:565–70; discussion 570–1.

54. Nyman U, Uher P, Lindh M, Lindblad B, Brunkwall J, Ivancev K. Stent-graft treatment of iatrogenic iliac artery perforations: report of three cases. Eur J Vasc Endovasc Surg. 1999;17:259–63.

55. Fry WR, Fry RE, Fry WJ. Operative exposure of the abdominal arteries for trauma. Arch Surg. 1991;126: 289–91.

56. Carrillo EH, Bergamini TM, Miller FB, Richardson JD. Abdominal vascular injuries. J Trauma. 1997;43: 164–71.

57. Feliciano DV, Bitondo CG, Mattox KL, Burch JM, Jordan Jr GL, Beall Jr AC, De Bakey ME. Civilian

trauma in the 1980s. A 1-year experience with 456 vascular and cardiac injuries. Ann Surg. 1984;199: 717–24.

58. Aljafri A, Kingsnorth A. Advanced surgical practice. Cambridge University Press, New York, NY; 2002, pp 601–2.

59. Sternbergh 3rd WC, Money SR. Iliac artery stent infection treated with superficial femoral vein. J Vasc Surg. 2005;41:348.

60. Feliciano DV, Mattox KL, Graham JM, Bitondo CG. Five-year experience with PTFE grafts in vascular wounds. J Trauma. 1985;25:71–82.

61. Carrillo EH, Spain DA, Wilson MA, Miller FB, Richardson JD. Alternatives in the management of penetrating injuries to the iliac vessels. J Trauma. 1998;44:1024–9; discussion 1029–30.

62. Ball CG, Feliciano DV. Damage control techniques for common and external iliac artery injuries: have temporary intravascular shunts replaced the need for ligation? J Trauma. 2010;68:1117–20.

63. Asensio J. Exsanguination. Trauma Q. 1990;6:1–25.

64. Paul JS, Webb TP, Aprahamian C, Weigelt JA. Intraabdominal vascular injury: are we getting any better? J Trauma. 2010;69:1393–7.

65. Yeh MW, Horn JK, Schecter WP, Chuter TA, Lane JS. Endovascular repair of an actively hemorrhaging gunshot injury to the abdominal aorta. J Vasc Surg. 2005;42:1007–9.

66. Darouiche RO. Treatment of infections associated with surgical implants. N Engl J Med. 2004;350:1422–9.

67. Hayes PD, Nasim A, London NJ, Sayers RD, Barrie WW, Bell PR, Naylor AR. In situ replacement of infected aortic grafts with rifampicin-bonded prostheses: the Leicester experience (1992 to 1998). J Vasc Surg. 1999;30:92–8.

Iliac Vein Injuries

20

William F. Johnston, Nicolas H. Pope,
and Gilbert R. Upchurch Jr.

Contents

W.F. Johnston, MD • N.H. Pope, MD
Department of Surgery, University of Virginia,
Charlottesville, VA, USA

G.R. Upchurch Jr., MD (✉)
Division of Vascular and Endovascular Surgery,
Department of Surgery, Molecular Physiology
and Biological Physics, University of Virginia,
Charlottesville, VA, USA
e-mail: gru6n@virginia.edu

20.1   Introduction

Iliac vein injuries are some of the most lethal injuries in trauma surgery and are among the most challenging injuries managed by trauma surgeons. Given their anatomic position deep in the pelvis, injuries to the iliac veins are rare, but are difficult to isolate and repair when they occur. Furthermore, iliac vessel injuries are frequently complicated by uncontrolled hemorrhage and multiple associated injuries. Therefore, surgeons must be able to diagnose iliac vein injuries quickly and have an understanding of iliac vessel anatomy and physiology.

20.2   Background/Epidemiology

During World War I, World War II, and the Vietnam War, the incidence of iliac vessel injury ranged from 0.4 to 2.6 % [1]. In the civilian arena, iliac vein injuries are frequently seen in major urban trauma centers with an incidence of 5.0 % of trauma patients with major cardiac or vascular injuries [2]. The incidence of iliac vein injuries is increasing, and damage to iliac veins has been discovered in up to 20 % of abdominal vascular trauma [3]. Injury to the iliac vein is seen mostly with penetrating trauma from gunshot wounds, followed by penetrating trauma from stab wounds [4]. Although less frequent, damage to the iliac veins can occur with blunt trauma. Between 10 and 25 % of iliac vein injuries occur secondary to blunt injury [5, 6]. While penetrating injury is

A. Dua et al. (eds.), *Clinical Review of Vascular Trauma*,
DOI 10.1007/978-3-642-39100-2_20, © Springer-Verlag Berlin Heidelberg 2014

most frequently seen in young male patients, blunt injury is more commonly seen in older patients with an even distribution between men and women [1, 6, 7]. Iliac vein injuries are at least as common as iliac artery injuries and may occur either as an isolated injury or in combination with iliac artery injury [8, 9]. With penetrating trauma, iliac venous injury most commonly involves the common iliac vein (41 %) followed by the external iliac vein (27 %) and the internal iliac vein (16 %) [7].

20.3   Anatomy/Physiology

The iliac veins provide a critical role in venous drainage from the lower extremities and pelvis. The iliac vessels are located in the pelvic retroperitoneum and are therefore relatively protected, explaining why injuries to the iliac vessels are infrequent but often lethal. The surgeon must have a functional understanding of the anatomic relationship of the iliac arterial and venous systems to perform a repair. The right and left common iliac veins converge to form the inferior vena cava at the level of the fifth lumbar vertebrae below the level of the aortic bifurcation and directly posterior to the right common iliac artery. The common iliac vein forms from the confluence of the internal and external iliac veins. The left common iliac vein passes posterior to the right common iliac artery, and the right common iliac vein travels inferiorly to the right iliac artery to reside medially to the right external iliac artery (Fig. 20.1). The external iliac vein travels with the external iliac artery and is a continuation of the common femoral vein as it passes under the inguinal ligament to drain the lower extremity. The internal iliac vein (also called the hypogastric vein) forms from a coalescence of pelvic veins, including the gluteal vein, internal pudendal vein, and obturator veins joining pelvic venous plexuses and sacral veins to drain blood from the pelvis and surrounding tissue. The right iliac vessels are located near the terminal ileum and cecum, while the left iliac vessels are near the sigmoid colon. The ureters cross anteriorly over the external iliac artery and vein just distal to the iliac bifurcation and must be identified and

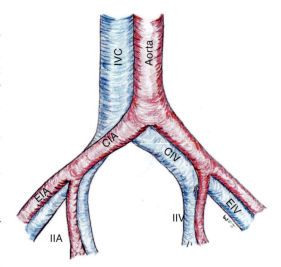

Fig. 20.1 Normal anatomy of the iliac arteries and veins. *IVC* inferior vena cava, *CIV* common iliac vein, *EIV* external iliac vein, *IIV* internal iliac vein, *CIA* common iliac artery, *EIA* external iliac artery, *IIA* internal iliac artery

Table 20.1 Associated injuries with iliac vein injury

Small bowel	46.4–77.6 %
Colon	24.0–57.1 %
Bladder	6.1–10.2 %
Ureter	3.9–10.1 %
Liver	1.7–12.0 %
Kidney	1.1–4.1 %
Pelvic fracture	1.1–6.7 %

From Burch et al., Wilson et al., Oliver et al., and Haan et al. [5–7, 10]

protected during exploration. Collateral flow to the iliac vein includes transpelvic collaterals (anastomosis of the hemorrhoidal veins to the superior hemorrhoidal veins of the inferior mesenteric vein, opposite sides of the gonadal veins, and sacral veins) and paravertebral collaterals.

Given the anatomically protected location of the iliac vessels, injuries with enough force to cause iliac vessel injuries are frequently complicated by associated damage to surrounding organs [1]. Many patients will have more than one vascular injury and may have combined arterial and venous injuries. In patients with penetrating trauma to the iliac vein, 34–57 % will have a concomitant injury to the iliac artery [4–6, 10]. Associated nonvascular injuries occur in almost all patients and most frequently include the small bowel, colon, bladder, and ureter (Table 20.1).

20.4 Clinical Assessment

On initial evaluation, patients are often hypotensive and tachycardic secondary to blood loss following either penetrating or blunt trauma. Full exposure is required to identify penetrating injuries. With blunt trauma, the diagnosis is especially challenging but is often associated with pelvic fractures. The most critical component to patient survival is rapid recognition of hemorrhagic shock and rapid transport to a trauma center with notification of the trauma surgery team.

20.5 Diagnostic Testing

Laboratory testing frequently demonstrates mild acidosis and anemia [5]. If the diagnosis of iliac vessel injury is delayed, the patient will become progressively more acidotic, anemic, and coagulopathic. Iliac vein injuries can present with retroperitoneal hematoma, free intraperitoneal hemorrhage, or both. The Focused Assessment with Sonography for Trauma (FAST) exam is commonly employed in most major trauma centers to detect major intra-abdominal free fluid with over 90 % sensitivity and specificity reported in initial studies [11]. However, controversy exists as more recent studies have suggested that the FAST exam has a much lower sensitivity for detecting intra-abdominal bleeding, highlighting the importance for continued clinical evaluation of the patient even if the FAST is negative [12]. In regard to the iliac vessels, the FAST exam is not sensitive for retroperitoneal hemorrhage or pelvic evaluation in the setting of a pelvic fracture [13, 14]. The retroperitoneum is best evaluated with CT scanning in hemodynamically stable patients and laparotomy in hemodynamically unstable patients. If an iliac vessel injury is initially suspected, a FAST may be performed as it has minimal morbidity, is quickly performed, and may detect free intra-abdominal hemorrhage. However, if the FAST is equivocal or does not correspond with the patient's hemodynamic status, consideration should be given to diagnostic peritoneal lavage (DPL), the less invasive technique of diagnostic peritoneal aspiration, or early laparotomy to detect intra-abdominal bleeding [12].

20.6 Initial Treatment

In the emergency department, hemorrhagic shock must be promptly diagnosed with notification of the trauma surgical team. Large-bore intravenous access should be obtained along with arterial blood pressure monitoring to guide resuscitation measures. Hypotensive resuscitation should be employed in the absence of head injury, avoiding a normal blood pressure until hemostasis is achieved [15, 16]. As the pelvis can accommodate significant hemorrhage from vessels unable to be easily compressed, avoidance of clot disruption is essential. Early use of blood, plasma, and platelets is required in patients in whom there is a high likelihood of massive transfusion.

20.7 Blunt Trauma

Although injury to iliac veins from blunt pelvic trauma is uncommon, blunt iliac vein injuries occur and are highly lethal. Vascular injuries with blunt trauma are frequently seen in the setting of pelvic fractures as the iliac vessels stretch over the bony pelvis. Wilson et al. reported only one incident of blunt trauma in their series of 49 patients with iliac vein injuries [10]. However, a higher incidence of iliac vein injury has recently been reported in patients following blunt trauma with pelvic fractures [17]. Iliac vein injuries are most commonly found in patients with pelvic fractures who do not improve after pelvic compression or arteriography with transarterial embolization. Pelvic compression with fracture reduction by an external fixator or a wrapping with a bedsheet can tamponade minor venous bleeding and decrease pelvic volume (Table 20.2) [18]. Angiography with transarterial embolization is a highly effective and safe method of controlling arterial bleeding from pelvic fractures that are difficult to manage with surgery [19]. However, neither pelvic fixation nor transarterial embolization can effectively manage injuries to the iliac veins due to their size and location. To complicate the issue, injury to the iliac veins has also been reported in the absence of a pelvic fracture [20]. Therefore, a high index of clinical suspicion must be maintained for iliac vein injury in

Table 20.2 Out-of-hospital vascular clamps in control of junctional bleeding of the groin

Name	Combat ready clamp	Abdominal aortic tourniquet	Junctional emergency treatment tool	SAM junctional tourniquet
Nickname	CRoC	AAT	JETT	SJT
Maker	Combat Medical Systems	Compression Works	North American Rescue Products	SAM Medical Products
City, state	Fayetteville, NC	Hoover, AL	Greer, SC	Wilsonville, OR
510(k) date	8/11/10	10/18/11	1/3/13	3/18/13
FDA number	K102025	K112384	K123194	K123694
NSN	6515-01-589-9135	6515-01-616-4999	6515-01-616-5841	Pending
Cost ($ USD, est. USG)	450	475	220	279
Weight (gm)	799	485	651	499
Cube (L)	0.8	1.4	1.6	1.5
Indication	Battlefield, difficult inguinal bleeds	Battlefield, difficult inguinal bleeds	Difficult inguinal bleeds	Difficult inguinal bleeds, pelvic fracture immobilization

USG federal government, *NSN* National Stock Number, *FDA* Food and Drug Administration, *USD* United States dollar, *est.* estimated

patients with blunt trauma who do not respond appropriately to resuscitation. A multidisciplinary approach involving all members of the trauma team should be involved in determining the proper order of care, procedure selection, using the optimally positioned incisions, and coordinating overall care.

The algorithm for pelvic fractures associated with hemorrhagic shock is pelvic compression with a bedsheet or a commercially available device, with early transfusion of red blood cells, plasma, and platelets. If the patient does not respond appropriately, angiography is performed to evaluate the iliac and pelvic arteries. If the patient continues to decompensate despite arterial embolization, the patient is rapidly taken to the operating room for exploratory laparotomy.

The role of diagnostic venography following angiography but prior to laparotomy has been evaluated [17]. In a review of 11 patients with pelvic fractures that failed pelvic compression and angiographic embolization, significant venous extravasation from the iliac veins was identified in 9 patients (82 %). These patients were then treated with laparotomy ($n=1$, no survivors), retroperitoneal gauze packing ($n=3$, 1 survivor), or endovascular stent placement ($n=3$, 3 survivors). The remaining two patients died prior to treatment. The authors concluded that venography is a useful tool to diagnose iliac vein

injury and identify the site of hemorrhage. In patients who remain hemodynamically unstable following blunt pelvic injury despite pelvic compression and arterial embolization, venography should be considered in an effort to diagnose and treat major iliac vein trauma.

20.8   Iatrogenic Injury

In addition to trauma, iliac vein injury is a known complication of anterior exposure for spine surgery with an incidence of approximately 4 % [21]. Anterior exposure of L4–L5 or L5–S1 vertebral levels requires mobilization of the iliac vessels to access the underlying spine. The left common iliac vein is the most dorsally located and the most likely to be injured during anterior spinal exposure [22]. Injuries are more likely to occur in patients with soft tissue inflammation (such as osteomyelitis, osteophyte formation, and previous anterior spine surgery) that causes the overlying blood vessels to be relatively fixed in position and more challenging to dissect. The majority of injuries to the iliac vein are avulsed branches of the left common iliac vein or common iliac vein lacerations [23]. Large injuries are amenable to suture repair, while smaller injuries may be treated by suture repair or topical hemostatic agents.

20.9   Operative Management

An unstable trauma patient with an iliac vein injury is best treated by rapid recognition and operative repair. In the operating room, the patient should be prepared from thighs to chin. As associated vascular injuries are common, the patient's legs should be prepared for potential saphenous vein harvest. A standard trauma midline laparotomy is performed with temporary packing of all four quadrants for hemostasis. Mesenteric sources of bleeding are controlled with suture ligation. A large retroperitoneal hematoma extending to the pelvic brim will usually be the first sign of iliac vessel injury. Exposure of the iliac vessels requires dividing the avascular line of Toldt of both the right and left colon to reflect both sides of the colon medially with a combination of blunt and sharp dissection [24]. Proximal and distal control of the vessel is paramount but is frequently challenging to obtain due to the large associated retroperitoneal hematomas. Burch et al. describe a method of total pelvic vascular isolation that can be employed when no clear source of hemorrhage can be identified: the aorta, right and left external iliac arteries and veins, and the inferior vena cava are sequentially occluded with clamps to limit pelvic circulation [7]. When the hematoma extends deep into the pelvis or there is suspected injury to the distal external iliac vessels, distal control is best established through a separate groin incision overlying the femoral vessels [25]. The inguinal ligament can be divided and later repaired, if necessary.

Following pelvic vascular isolation, bleeding may continue from the internal iliac vessels, requiring direct tamponade. As the dissection progresses, the clamps are advanced progressively closer to the injury until the injury is isolated with no back bleeding. Occasionally, the right common iliac artery or either internal iliac artery must be divided for adequate exposure of the iliac vein (Fig. 20.2). Division of the arterial system is needed when there is any injury to the confluence of the common iliac veins behind the right common iliac artery or to the junction of the internal and external iliac veins behind the internal iliac arteries. Division of the iliac arteries is uncomfortable for the surgeon to perform but can decrease the overall morbidity to the patient by improving exposure, speeding hemorrhage control, and allowing faster vein repair. Following venous repair, the artery can be reanastomosed.

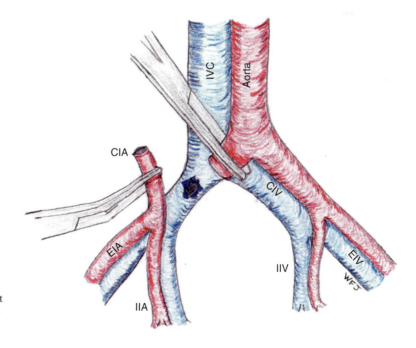

Fig. 20.2 Division of the right common iliac artery reveals an injury to the right common iliac vein facilitating repair

Since the internal iliac vein can be ligated without significant consequence, it may be sacrificed to facilitate repair of the main iliac vessels. Once control of the source of hemorrhage is obtained and the patient is hemodynamically stable, temporary repair of enteric defects and removal of gross spillage should be accomplished prior to final vascular repair. The bowel may then be packed out of the field with intent to return for definitive repair at a later time.

If an iliac vein injury is suspected, the veins can be compressed by a sponge stick or finger compression until the overlying arterial system is fully mobilized. Attempts to clamp the iliac vein prior to adequate dissection can result in an injury to the posterior wall of the iliac vein and an even more challenging repair [26]. Given the potential for venous injury with passage of the clamp posterior to the vein, alternative methods have been described, including the passage of endovascular balloons from either groin to occlude the origin of the common iliac vein and distally in the external iliac vein [27]. Endovascular balloon occlusion does not require an angiographic table and can be performed under direct visualization and palpation. The endovascular occlusion technique allows improved visualization of the injury because there are fewer instruments in the operative field. After the injury is isolated and vascular control is achieved, the vein should be locally irrigated with heparinized saline to remove thrombus.

Iliac vein injuries can be treated with repair or ligation. Repair with lateral venorrhaphy, patch venoplasty, or direct end-to-end anastomosis is preferred over ligation. Venous repair allows continued venous drainage and decreased incidence of postoperative lower extremity edema [7, 25]. Lateral venorrhaphy can be performed with 4-0 to 6-0 monofilament suture with attention given to narrow the vein as little as possible. Since the walls of the vein are delicate, minimal force must be applied. If the injury is not amenable primary venorrhaphy, patch venoplasty can be considered with harvested saphenous vein [25]. Patch venoplasty with saphenous vein graft is an autogenous graft that will not narrow the iliac vein,

but this procedure does require additional time to harvest and prepare the saphenous vein. Rarely, end-to-end iliac vein anastomoses can be performed, but tension on the anastomosis must be avoided. If the injury is more complex and not amenable to simple suture repair or a tension-free anastomosis, an interposition graft may be used. Autogenous graft material is preferred to synthetic material due to better patency rates. Autogenous options include saphenous vein, basilic vein, internal jugular vein, or femoral vein [28]. If the diameter of the vein is insufficient, panel grafts and spiral grafts may be constructed from saphenous vein wrapped around a chest tube of desired diameter [29]. Preparation of panel and spiral grafts is time-consuming and may not be suitable during emergent repair. Synthetic interposition grafts with PTFE have been reported but have poor patency rates and are associated with chronic lower extremity edema [30, 31]. Synthetic grafts have been safely used in cases with associated intestinal injuries without subsequent graft infection [4]. Therefore, if autogenous graft material is not available, a synthetic interposition graft should be utilized.

If vascular repair cannot be promptly performed, temporary vascular shunts may be used to provide temporary continuation of venous blood flow until the vein can be definitively repaired. From the military trauma experience in Iraq, vascular shunts have been successfully used as a temporizing measure until the patient could undergo repair at a central hospital [32]. Impressively, Rasmussen et al. reported that all temporary venous shunts remained patent without thrombosis until patients could undergo definitive repair [32].

An alternative method of repair is ligation of the injured iliac vein. Many groups advocate ligation of the injured iliac veins over venorrhaphy because ligation is the most rapid method of repair and is associated with minimal long-term postoperative complications [1, 5, 10, 24]. Ligation should be considered in patients with severe hemodynamic instability secondary to hemorrhage, extensive local injury, or massive contamination. Ligation is performed with nonabsorbable suture.

Following vascular repair or ligation, the peritoneum should be closed over the repair when feasible for a layer of protection. The abdomen should be irrigated copiously with warmed saline with antibiotic irrigation and temporarily closed, while the patient is taken to the intensive care unit for further resuscitation with correction of acidosis and coagulopathy. Time should not be taken to definitively repair associated injuries to the bowel or urologic system. Definitive repair of associated injuries can be performed in 24–48 h during the second-look operation.

20.10 Postoperative Management

Postoperatively, patients with injuries to the common or external iliac veins should have their legs elevated with elastic compression to alleviate edema until they are ambulatory. For isolated venous injuries, fasciotomies are not needed. Intraoperative blood loss is extensive, averaging over 5–6 L per patient [1, 7]. Therefore, attention must be paid to maintain core body temperature and avoid hypothermia.

20.11 Complications

A complicated postoperative course should be expected following iliac vessel repair due to the severity of the injury leading to iliac vein damage. The most common complications include coagulopathy, arrhythmias, hypothermia, and acidosis due to hemorrhage and massive blood transfusion. Specifically related iliac vessel complications following repair include infection (17 %), multiple system organ failure (11 %), deep venous thrombosis (7 %), and arteriovenous fistula (3 %) [1]. Amputations are not common with venous injury but may be required if there is a combined arteriovenous injury. Lower extremity edema is relatively common in the immediate postoperative period and is more common in

patients treated with venous ligation than with lateral suture repair. Fortunately, the majority of patients treated with ligation have resolution of their edema within 1–3 months. The incidence of chronic venous insufficiency following ligation varies, with some groups reporting intractable edema or venous insufficiency with leg ulceration in 8–21 % of patients treated with ligation and other groups reporting no significant edema following ligation [5, 7, 10]. Resolution of edema is possible due to the extensive collateral network of veins. With such an extensive collateral system, ligation of the inferior vena cava can even be tolerated with a low incidence of long-term swelling [33]. Lateral suture repair of the iliac vein has a lower incidence of edema than ligation with an incidence of approximately 3 %. Those patients with edema following lateral suture repair should expect resolution within 1 month of discharge.

The occurrence of a deep venous thrombosis (DVT) following iliac vein repair is 3.0 % without therapeutic anticoagulation [7]. Due to the risk of continued hemorrhage from associated injuries, prophylactic anticoagulation is often held until the patient can be stabilized. There is a concern for thrombosis to form at the site of repair following lateral venorrhaphy, and pulmonary emboli have rarely been reported [7]. Venous ligation is also associated with a risk of venous thrombosis from decreased blood flow, which may result in pulmonary embolization [4, 34]. Overall, there does not appear to be a difference in terms of the risk of pulmonary emboli between ligation and lateral suture repair. Regarding isolated repair of the internal iliac vein, DVT and postoperative swelling are infrequent regardless of the method of repair.

20.12 Endovascular Treatment

Endovascular attempts at repair of iliac venous injuries are not widely reported because most patients with iliac vessel injury arrive in shock and are taken directly to the operating room [35].

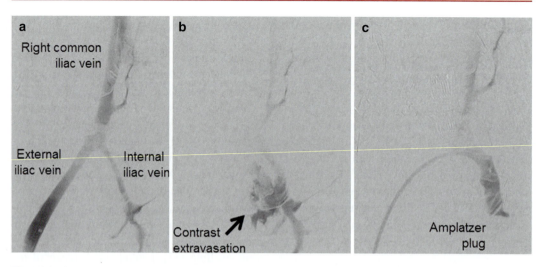

Fig. 20.3 Contrast angiography demonstrating right internal iliac vein injury with delayed extravasation of contrast (**a**, **b**) treated with Amplatzer plug (**c**)

Patients in shock are best treated in the operating room rather than on the angiography table. However, laparotomy with retroperitoneal exposure for iliac vein injury is technically challenging, and the retroperitoneal incision can release the tamponade and may increase venous bleeding that will obscure the surgical field. Therefore, the concept of the hybrid operating room with combined capability for angiographic and open procedures is useful in managing trauma patients with significant vascular injury. In a hybrid operating room, endovascular techniques, such as stenting, can supplement open techniques to seal the vein from the vessel lumen while maintaining the effect of the tamponade.

Venography for evaluation of the iliac veins following pelvic fracture was first described in 1970 to assist with diagnosis [36]. Since that time, the field of endovascular surgery has progressed dramatically and is now able to offer multiple therapeutic options. Pelvic venography can be performed through the injection of 40–50 cc of contrast via transfemoral access with a 9-Fr catheter sheath with a balloon occlusion catheter in the inferior vena cava. The balloon is inflated just above the confluence of the common iliac veins and contrast is infused through a side port [17]. With this method, all iliac veins, including the internal iliac veins, may be evaluated. If extravasation is seen, the injury may be treated with endovascular embolization or stent placement. Embolization may be performed to treat injuries to the internal iliac vein with no significant sequelae due to the extensive network of pelvic collateral veins (Fig. 20.3). Covered stents have also been used to treat spontaneous iliac vein rupture and iliac vein injury secondary to blunt trauma [37]. Once contrast extravasation is seen on diagnostic venography, a hydrophilic soft-tip wire (such as a glide wire) can be carefully advanced into the inferior vena cava with covered stents placed to extend from the common iliac vein to the external iliac vein. When covered stents are unavailable, uncovered stents can successfully treat iliac vein injuries (Fig. 20.4) [17, 18]. Uncovered stents improve venous flow and pressure secondary to relieving the narrowing of the vein due to the external compressing hematoma [38]. Despite being uncovered, the stents achieve hemostasis because the venous system is a low-pressure system. For sizing, stents are oversized by 10–20 %, as most patients are hypovolemic and hypotensive at stent placement. Following stent placement, patients are placed on oral aspirin for life.

Urogenital and Retroperitoneal Injuries

21

David R. King and John O. Hwabejire

Contents

D.R. King, MD (✉) • J.O. Hwabejire, MD
Division of Trauma, Emergency Surgery
and Surgical Critical Care, Department of Surgery,
Massachusetts General Hospital,
165 Cambridge Street, Boston, MA, USA
e-mail: dking3@partners.org, david.king16@us.army.mil

21.1 Introduction

The kidneys, ureters, and bladder (KUB), together with the urethra, constitute an anatomically and physiologically contiguous urinary system. However, such organ injuries have very distinct epidemiology, clinical presentation, management, and outcomes following trauma. For practical purposes therefore, the clinical considerations regarding trauma to the vasculature of these organs and other retroperitoneal structures are examined separately.

A. Dua et al. (eds.), *Clinical Review of Vascular Trauma*,
DOI 10.1007/978-3-642-39100-2_21, © Springer-Verlag Berlin Heidelberg 2014

21.2 Kidney

21.2.1 Background/Incidence/ Epidemiology

Injuries to the renal vasculature (renovascular injuries) are relatively uncommon, but when they do occur, they require expeditious diagnosis and management because of the relatively high morbidity and mortality that result. The mortality rate is between 19 and 44 %, although associated injuries are common and severe hemorrhagic shock from these other injuries may be the cause of death [1, 2]. Most renovascular injuries are due to penetrating rather than blunt trauma [3–5].

While renal injuries are said to occur in about 1.2 % of trauma cases in the USA, the overall incidence of renovascular injuries in the adult trauma population is put at 2.5–5 % of all renal injuries [3–5]. The specific incidence of renovascular injuries reported in the literature depends on the mechanism of injury, the blood vessel involved (renal artery or vein), the grade of renal injury, and the age group under consideration (adult vs. pediatric).

Bruce et al. retrospectively examined 36, 938 blunt trauma admissions over a 15-year period and estimated the incidence of blunt renal artery injury (BRAI) to be about 0.08 % [6]. In that study, the mean age of subjects was 32 years, most were female (64 %), motor vehicle crash was the cause of injury in 80 % of cases, and associated injuries, mainly to the spleen (50 %) and liver (43 %), were frequent. Knudson et al. in a multicenter study involving six level I trauma centers evaluated 89 patients with renovascular injuries and grades IV or V American Association for the Surgery of Trauma (AAST) renal injuries (Table 21.1) and estimated their mean age to be 30 years, with 51 % of these injuries resulting from penetrating trauma [7, 8]. Most (54 %) of these patients presented to the emergency department in shock. Associated injuries were present in almost 90 % of the patients, with 77 % of those with grade IV renal injuries and 72 % with grade V injuries having concomitant abdominal injuries. In the pediatric population, the incidence of renovascular injuries and grades IV or V renal injuries ranges from 9 to 31 % [8–15].

Table 21.1 AAST kidney injury scale

Kidney injury scale		
Grade[a]	Type of injury	Description of injury
I	Contusion	Microscopic or gross hematuria, urologic studies normal
	Hematoma	Subcapsular, nonexpanding without parenchymal laceration
II	Hematoma	Nonexpanding perirenal hematoma confirmed to renal Retroperitoneum
	Laceration	<1.0 cm parenchymal depth of renal cortex without urinary Extravasation
III	Laceration	<1.0 cm parenchymal depth of renal cortex without collecting system rupture or urinary extravagation
	Laceration	Parenchymal laceration extending through renal cortex, medulla and collecting system
IV	Vascular	Main renal artery or vein injury with contained hemorrhage
V	Laceration	Completely shattered kidney
	Vascular	Avulsion of renal hilum which devascularizes kidney

[a]Advance one grade for bilateral injuries up to grade III
From Moore et al. [83]; with permission

21.2.2 Anatomy/Physiology

The kidneys are a pair of bean-shaped retroperitoneal organs located in the paravertebral gutters, between the transverse processes of T12 and L3 vertebrae, having an average weight of 150 g in the male and 135 g in the female. The dimensions of the healthy kidney vary considerably, an average estimate being: length of 10 cm, width of 7 cm, and thickness of 3 cm [16, 17].

The right and left renal arteries, which provide blood supply to the right and left kidneys, respectively, are primary branches of the abdominal aorta. Each renal artery sequentially branches into the segmental arteries, interlobar arteries, arcuate arteries, and interlobular arteries. The interlobular arteries are end arteries that give rise to the afferent arterioles. The renal glomeruli are formed from the latter and play a dominant role in renal ultrafiltration. The glomeruli drain into the efferent arterioles which eventually give rise to peritubular capillaries. Filtered blood from these capillary networks flows into the interlobular veins, arcuate veins, interlobar veins, and finally the renal veins. The renal veins drain into the inferior vena cava.

The physiological functions of the kidneys include removal of excess salt, water, and metabolic wastes, blood pressure regulation through the renin-angiotensin-aldosterone system, regulation of blood pH, control of red blood cell synthesis through the production and release of erythropoietin, and regulation of calcium homeostasis through the production of 1, 25-dihydroxycholecalciferol [18]. These functions are severely compromised in acute or chronic renal failure.

21.2.3 Clinical Assessment

Diagnosis of renovascular injuries on the basis of clinical assessment alone is difficult. While hematuria – gross or microscopic – is the commonest clinical presentation, it is absent in about 18–36 % of patients [3, 4, 19]. Depending on the severity of injury and blood loss, affected patients may also present with symptoms and signs of hemorrhagic shock. However, signs of hemorrhagic shock are not specific for any injury type. Since associated injuries are common and attention is often diverted to these, the diagnosis of renovascular injuries is commonly delayed, and a high index of suspicion is necessary [2].

21.2.4 Diagnostic Testing

In patients with renovascular injury, diagnostic studies are frequently not done preoperatively, as these patients often have other renal and nonrenal injuries that require immediate surgery [3]. When the clinical conditions of the patient allow, i.e., if the patient is hemodynamically stable, several imaging options are available. Every attempt should be made to image both kidneys, as the degree of functionality of both kidneys may affect the definitive treatment options chosen.

21.2.4.1 Computerized Tomography (CT) Scan

Abdominal contrast-enhanced CT scan, particularly the helical type, has a relatively high accuracy when used for the diagnosis of renovascular injuries [6]. Its advantages include its rapidity, noninvasiveness, and ability to diagnose associated injuries [3]. Renal artery occlusion manifests on CT as "lack of enhancement or excretion often in the presence of normal renal contour, rim enhancement, central hematoma, and abrupt cutoff of an enhancing renal artery" [3]. The findings in renal venous injuries are similar (central hematomas, renal enhancement, and intact renal contours) but typically show anterior displacement of the renal hilum and parenchyma [3].

21.2.4.2 Angiography

Although angiography is invasive and time consuming compared to CT, it may be more specific for defining the exact location and degree of vascular injuries [20]. It is indicated when, in the absence of a CT scan, intravenous urography (IVU) shows no visualization of the kidneys, the common causes of nonvisualization being total avulsion of the renal vessels, renal artery thrombosis, and severe contusion causing major vascular spasm [20]. It is also indicated if pedicle injury is suspected and the findings on CT are equivocal [20].

21.2.4.3 Intravenous Urography

Prior to the advent of CT, IVU was commonly the initial imaging modality for renal trauma, its major finding being nonfunction of the affected kidney [3, 20]. However, nonfunction is not peculiar to renovascular injuries – in one study, out of 53 % with unilateral renal nonvisualization, only 40 % had injury to the renal pedicle [3, 21]. Therefore, whenever CT is available, it should be the preferred diagnostic technique.

21.2.4.4 Renal Scintigraphy

Renal scintigraphy can be used to evaluate the renal vasculature when CT is unavailable or if the patient is allergic to iodinated contrast material [20]. It provides a quantitative assessment of renal blood flow and renal function, although this is rarely used in the acute trauma discovery phase of care [7].

21.2.4.5 Urinalysis

In the patient with renovascular trauma, urinalysis may show gross or microscopic hematuria. Although hematuria is neither sensitive nor specific for renovascular trauma, findings of gross hematuria or findings of microscopic hematuria in the presence of shock mandate interrogation of the genitourinary system to exclude injury [20].

21.2.4.6 Serum Creatinine

For a trauma patient evaluated within 1 h of injury, the serum creatinine concentration obtained is a reflection of prior renal function, and an elevated level indicates pre-injury renal pathology [20]. Whatever the case, it is important to establish a baseline value, as serial measurement of creatinine will be required for patients with renovascular trauma.

21.2.5 Initial Management (ER)

As mentioned earlier, patients with renovascular trauma often have associated injuries. Therefore, as is this case with any other trauma patients, initial management in the emergency room should follow the basic principles of Advanced Trauma Life Support (ATLS), combined with sophisticated thinking and prioritization of injury management. During the primary survey, the airway must be kept patent and the cervical spine stabilized (if cervical spine injury is suspected), breathing and ventilation must be assured, the patient must be examined for signs of hemorrhagic shock and appropriately treated, and ongoing bleeding must be controlled. In renal trauma, control of hemorrhage may require immediate

surgical exploration. Having an operating room with imaging capabilities, especially CT scan, is particularly useful in these circumstances as they can aid rapid diagnosis. In the unlikely event that CT scan is not readily available, an IVU should be considered if the patient has gross hematuria [20]. However, the limitations of the IVU mentioned earlier should be borne in mind when this option is chosen.

21.2.6 Definitive Management

The Eastern Association for the Surgery of Trauma (EAST) reviewed the published literature on management of renovascular injuries and concluded that there was insufficient data to make any recommendations regarding management of renovascular trauma [22]. The treatment options described below are based on the available studies on the literature. Clinical outcomes and the factors that affect them are described in a subsequent section. Options for definitive management of renovascular trauma depend on the type of injury and the time of presentation, and include the following (Tables 21.2 and 21.3) [7]:
1. Observation
2. Renal angiography with arterial embolization
3. Vascular repair: primary vascular (arterial or venous) repair or revascularization with arterial bypass
4. Partial nephrectomy/parenchymal repair
5. Immediate (total) nephrectomy

21.2.6.1 Observation

In certain scenarios, observation can play a role in the management of renovascular injuries [23]. These scenarios include venous thrombosis with two kidneys present, segmental arterial injury, arterial thrombosis with two kidneys present, arterial intimal injury with two kidneys present (Fig. 21.1), or a delayed presentation with a nonfunctional kidney. Nephrectomy may be required in these cases, though it is rarely indicated acutely [23]. It may be necessary if the patient develops either subsequent infectious or hypertensive complications.

Table 21.2 Operative management of retroperitoneal hematomas after blunt abdominal trauma

Location	Approach
Midline supramesocolic	Open hematoma[a]
Midline inframesocolic	Open hematoma[a]
Lateral Perirenal	Do not open if preoperative IVP; ultrasound or CT reveals reasonably intact kidney
Paraduodenal	Open hematoma[a] to rule out duodenal (bile staining, crepitus) perforation
Pericolonic	Open hematoma to rule out colonic injury, if not associated with pelvic hematoma
Pelvic	Do not open if pelvic fracture is present, rate of expansion is slow, arterial pulsations intact in groins, and urethrogram and cystogram are normal
Portal and retrohepatic portal	Open hematoma to rule out injury to common bile duct or portal vein[a]
Retrohepatic	Controversial. Do not open in stable patient if not obvious active hemorrhage after hepatic injury treated

Modified from Feliciano [85]
[a]After obtaining proximal and, if possible, distal vascular control

Table 21.3 Operative management of retroperitoneal hematomas after penetrating abdominal trauma

Location	Approach
Midline supramesocolic	Open hematoma[a]
Midline inframesocolic	Open hematoma[a]
Lateral Perirenal	Open hematoma[a], unless preoperative CT allows for careful staging of renal parenchymal injury
Paraduodenal	Open hematoma[a]
Pericolonic	Controversial. No major structures located here, but steady bleeding from lumbar vessels or muscular branches has been a cause of reoperation
Pelvic	Open hematoma[a]
Portal and retrohepatic portal	Open hematoma[a]
Retrohepatic	Controversial. Do not open in stable patient if no obvious active hemorrhage after hepatic injury treated

Modified from Feliciano [85]
[a]After obtaining proximal and, if possible, distal vascular control

21.2.6.2 Renal Angiography with Arterial Embolization

There are a few case series that have described the use of angiography with arterial embolization for treatment of renovascular injuries. This option is used when the primary problem is arterial bleeding in a hemodynamically normal patient. In one study, all five patients with renovascular injuries underwent superselective arterial embolization, bleeding was controlled without recurrence, and serum creatinine concentration returned to pre-injury values within 10 days [24]. Similar results were obtained in another series with six patients [25]. The small sample sizes in these and other studies make outcome of this treatment option uncertain, and further studies are needed to define the exact group of renovascular trauma patients that would benefit from this technique.

21.2.6.3 Vascular Repair

Vascular repair is one of the "renal preservation strategies" and is especially indicated if a patient has a solitary kidney or in cases of bilateral renal injuries [7, 26–31]. Repair can be done primarily or by use of a bypass graft. Outcomes following repair are described below subsequently. The majority of authors suggest that success of arterial reconstruction depends on the duration and degree of ischemia and presence or absence of accessory renal arteries providing collateral flow, with irreversible damage occurring when the warm renal ischemia time exceeds 2 h [2, 32]. A lack of relationship between outcome and time to definitive surgery is also reported, because the time of warm ischemia that is tolerated is so short [7]. This is the primary consideration when deciding whether to undertake an interventional or observational approach to renal injury.

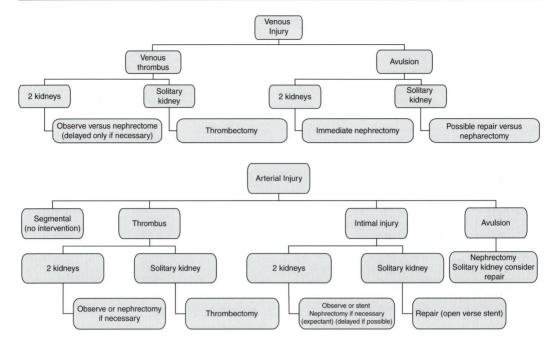

Fig. 21.1 Algorithm for the conservative management of renovascular injuries. *Top.* Venous injuries. *Bottom.* Arterial injuries (Santucci and Fisher [23]. With permission of The Journal of Trauma Injury, Infection, and Critical Care)

21.2.6.4 Partial Nephrectomy/Parenchymal Repair

Partial nephrectomy/parenchymal repair has both been used in the management of renovascular injuries [7]. The segmental vascular supply of the kidney makes this feasible, as one segment can be removed without compromising the functions of the other segments.

21.2.6.5 Immediate (Total) Nephrectomy

Immediate nephrectomy can be used as the primary treatment modality in severe renovascular injury of the grade IV/V variety. It is also indicated when there is failure of vascular repair with either infectious or hypertensive complications resulting from the nonfunctional kidney.

The operative approach to the vasculature of the right kidney usually requires a Cattell-Braasch maneuver (right medial visceral rotation) for exposure of the kidney, renal vessels, and associated right-sided retroperitoneal vascular structures. For the left kidney and vascular structures, a Mattox maneuver (left-sided medial visceral rotation) is usually undertaken. These

approaches are used for addressing renal vascular injuries or when a partial nephrectomy is to be done. The primary technical consideration for total nephrectomy is whether vascular control is obtained prior to entering Gerota's fascia and mobilizing the kidney. From a practical standpoint, this is usually dictated by the patient's hemodynamic status. In patients with rapidly expanding hematomas, it is usually most expeditious to enter Gerota's fascia, quickly mobilize the kidney, and control the bleeding with manual pressure or clamps once the kidney and renal vasculature are mobilized. If the patient's hemodynamic status allows, the approach above to the renal vessels preserves the option of a partial nephrectomy.

21.2.7 Postoperative Management (Including Rehabilitation/Follow-Up)

21.2.7.1 Follow-Up Imaging Studies

These may include abdominal CT scan, angiography, or renal scintigraphy [7]. Renal scintigraphy provides a quantitative assessment of renal function, especially when attempts have been made to salvage the kidneys [7, 33]. The patient with renal dysfunction becomes symptomatic when renal function drops below 25 %. When renal function drops below 10–15 %, dialysis is required to sustain life [34].

21.2.7.2 Serial Measurement of Blood Pressure

Blood pressure monitoring helps to detect the onset of renovascular hypertension. If this occurs, it may be controlled with medication but ultimately often requires nephrectomy.

21.2.7.3 Serum Chemistry

Serial measurement of serum creatinine and electrolytes is important to monitor renal function. However, if the patient has one normal kidney, the serum creatinine may not change even with no function of the contralateral kidney, so this must not be used as the sole measure to follow renal function.

21.2.8 Complications and Pitfalls

21.2.8.1 Renovascular Hypertension

The incidence of posttraumatic renovascular hypertension in the literature ranges from 3.2 to 50 %, with the true incidence reported to be close to about 5 % [7, 37–42]. Several explanations have been proposed to describe the mechanism of hypertension following renovascular trauma, including renal artery stenosis or occlusion resulting from thrombosis, compression, or an intimal flap, as well as the development of a restrictive fibrous capsule around the traumatized kidney that compresses the renal parenchyma and limits normal blood flow [35, 37, 43]. Both of these result in activation of the renin-angiotensin-aldosterone system, with subsequent salt and water retention and widespread vasoconstriction of arterioles. Intractable renovascular hypertension is amenable to nephrectomy, and surgery may be the optimal treatment option [7, 19, 44–47].

21.2.8.2 Diminished Renal Function

Renal dysfunction may be reversible or may progress to acute or chronic renal failure. Serial measurement of serum creatinine is extremely insensitive to changes in renal function of the injured kidney in the presence of a normal contralateral kidney.

21.2.9 Outcomes

Post-injury renal function with poor outcome was defined by Knudson et al. as any of the following [7]:

- Renal failure (defined as requiring dialysis or serum creatinine ≥ 2 mg/dL)
- Renal scan showing less than 25 % function of the injured kidney
- Post-injury hypertension requiring medication
- Delayed nephrectomy, i.e., nephrectomy performed greater than 24 h after injury but during the index hospitalization

Similar clinical outcome measures have also being used by other investigators [34].

Factors affecting outcome include:

Mechanism of Injury: Knudson et al. showed that patients with blunt renovascular injuries were about 2.29 times more likely to have a poor outcome compared to those with penetrating injuries [7].

Type of Vascular Repair: In the same study, for patients with grade IV injuries, outcomes were significantly worse in patients who had arterial repairs compared to those with venous repairs [7]. Other studies have supported this finding [48].

Grade of Renal Injury: For those with grade IV injuries, outcomes were significantly better in those who had a partial nephrectomy or parenchymal repair, compared to those who had a total nephrectomy [7]. For those with grade V injuries, outcomes were significantly better in those who had immediate nephrectomy, compared to those who underwent arterial repair and those who had no renal surgery. In fact, in patients with grade V injuries, attempts at arterial repair or bypass were 15 times more likely to result in a poor outcome, compared with immediate nephrectomy.

Age: Some investigators have reported that immediate nephrectomy (85.7 % good outcomes) and arterial repairs (66.7 % good outcomes) produce the best results in the pediatric population with grades IV and V renal injuries [7]. In this study, 40 % of children treated expectantly, i.e., nonoperatively, had a poor outcome. However, recent evidence suggests that in children with unilateral renovascular injury treated with either nephrectomy or renal preservation, the outcomes were comparable, providing a strong argument for renal preservation [34].

21.3   Ureter

21.3.1   Background/Incidence/ Epidemiology

Like renovascular injuries, injuries to the ureters are relatively rare. Injuries to the blood vessels that supply the ureters do not occur in isolation from ureteral injuries themselves. Therefore, a snapshot of ureteral trauma is provided, with specific highlights of vascular considerations as applicable. This chapter focuses on ureteral injury due to external trauma rather than iatrogenic injuries.

The incidence of ureteral injuries from external trauma is estimated to range from less than 1 % to about 2.6 % of all genitourinary injuries, with blunt trauma accounting for about 61.5 % of cases and penetrating trauma accounting for the remaining 38.5 % [49, 50]. Siram et al. reported mortality rates of 6 % for penetrating trauma and 9 % for blunt trauma, although these differences were not statistically significant [49]. In that study, penetrating trauma patients had a higher incidence of vascular injuries (38 %). In patients with penetrating trauma, the most commonly injured vessels were the iliac vein (18 %), iliac artery (10 %), and the inferior vena cava (7 %), whereas, in the blunt trauma subset, the iliac artery (6 %), renal artery (4 %), and renal vein (3 %) were the most

commonly injured. Therefore, in the evaluation of any patient with ureteral trauma, a careful search for associated blood vessel injury should be carried out. Alternatively, and more commonly, the surgeon is operating for major vascular injury of the iliac or renal vessels, and after control of the vascular injuries, the surgeon is obliged to evaluate the ureter adjacent to the vascular injury.

21.3.2   Anatomy/Physiology

The ureters are a pair of tubular structures composed largely of smooth muscles that convey urine from the kidneys to the bladder where it is stored prior to micturition. In the adult, the ureter is about 25 cm in length and has a diameter of about 3 mm [51]. The ureter is retroperitoneal, with the upper half located in the abdomen, where it exits the kidney from the renal pedicle, and the lower half located in the pelvis, where it enters the bladder at an oblique angle. The ureter receives multiple blood supplies. The abdominal part is supplied by branches from the renal artery, the abdominal aorta, and the gonadal artery, whereas the pelvic part is supplied by the common iliac artery, internal iliac artery, inferior vesical artery (in the male), or uterine artery (in the female) [51]. The veins draining the ureter generally correspond to the arteries. The peristaltic actions of the ureteral smooth muscles help to actively convey urine from the kidney to the bladder. Reflux in the opposite direction is normally prevented by the oblique angling of the ureter as it enters the bladder.

21.3.3   Clinical Assessment

The diagnosis of ureteral injury is easy to miss as there are no specific symptoms or signs associated with it. Hematuria, the classic symptom of urinary tract injury, is present in only 50 % of patients with ureteral injury [20, 52]. Therefore, the diagnosis should be suspected in every patient with penetrating abdominal injury, especially those due to gunshot wounds and blunt trauma with sudden deceleration trauma in which the kidney and renal pelvis can be torn away from the ureter [20, 53]. As the later mechanism can also result in renovascular injuries, these should be actively sought [8].

21.3.4 Diagnostic Testing

Imaging techniques that can help to establish the diagnosis of ureteral injury include intravenous urography, retrograde pyelography, and ureteral catheterization [53]. CT scan, when used in the evaluation of the patient with abdominal trauma can also aid in the diagnosis and when combined with contrast, is the investigation of choice [20, 54]. The diagnosis can also be made in the absence of imaging when the patient's clinical condition warrants immediate laparotomy [20]. Urinalysis is not particularly useful, as hematuria may be absent in up to half of affected patients. As in all cases of urinary system trauma, serum creatinine levels should be obtained.

21.3.5 Initial Management (ER)

As discussed under the initial management of renovascular injuries, the emphasis when a patient with ureteral injury is first evaluated in the emergency room is to follow ATLS principles and ensure a patent airway with C-spine stabilization (if indicated), ensure that breathing and ventilation are adequate, and ensure that hemorrhage control is achieved. Only after these should a more definitive repair of ureteral injury be carried out.

21.3.6 Operative Management

Operative management of ureteral injury depends on the grade of injury. Grades I and II lesions can be managed with ureteral stenting or by placement of a nephrostomy tube to divert urine [20, 55]. For injury of higher grades, repair is indicated and the type of repair is determined by the site of injury, as shown below [20, 53]:

- *Upper third*
  - Ureteroureterostomy
  - Transureteroureterostomy
  - Ureterocalycostomy
- *Middle third*
  - Ureteroureterostomy
  - Transureteroureterostomy
  - Boari flap and reimplantation
- *Lower third*
  - Direct reimplantation
  - Psoas hitch
  - Blandy cystoplasty
- *Complete ureteral loss*
  - Ileal interposition (delayed)
  - Autotransplantation (delayed)

The damage control maneuver is always to intubate the proximal ureter with a red rubber catheter (or similar) and externalize it to the skin as a "tube ureterostomy." Definitive repair can be undertaken once physiologic derangement has been corrected.

21.3.7 Postoperative Management (Including Rehab/Follow-Up)

Postoperatively, intravenous urography or retrograde pyelography can be used to assess for urinary leak. Ultrasonography may be used to monitor the patient for the development of hydronephrosis, while renal scintigraphy can be used to quantitatively assess renal function [54]. Serum creatinine levels are also used to monitor patients for early signs of renal failure. The frequency and duration of follow-up depends on the severity of injury and the specific operative procedure, but may be up to 1 year [54].

21.3.8 Complications and Pitfalls

The complication rate after repair of traumatic ureteral injury is estimated at 25 % [49, 56, 57]. Possible complications of ureteral trauma and subsequent repair include urinary leak (presenting as urinoma, abscess, or peritonitis), ureteral stricture, hydronephrosis, and renal dysfunction

[20, 54, 58]. Adequate follow-up and appropriate management are crucially important.

21.3.9 Outcomes

In patients who are under surgery to repair the ureter after trauma, outcomes depend on the specific procedure, time to definitive diagnosis, and the presence of associated injuries [59]. Time to diagnosis affects the extent of renal dysfunction, underscoring the need to maintain a high index of suspicion.

21.4 Bladder

21.4.1 Background/Incidence/ Epidemiology

Injuries to the bladder account for about 2 % of all genitourinary injuries that require surgical repair [60]. Blunt trauma is a more common cause of bladder injury than penetrating trauma (67–86 % vs. 14–33 %) [20, 60–62]. It is estimated that 70–90 % of all patients with bladder injuries have associated pelvic fractures [20, 61, 63, 64]. This association is important because pelvic fracture is a major cause of additional bleeding. Therefore, any patient with evidence of bladder injury must be expeditiously evaluated for signs of hemorrhagic shock. Traumatic bladder rupture due to blunt mechanism may be classified as either extraperitoneal with leakage of urine limited to the perivesical space, or intraperitoneal, in which there is disruption of the peritoneal surface with urinary extravasation [20].

21.4.2 Anatomy/Physiology

The bladder is a pear-shaped retroperitoneal organ that is located within the bony pelvis. When distended, it projects into the abdomen, making it more susceptible to trauma. It is bounded anteriorly by the pubic symphysis, superiorly by coils of small intestine and the sigmoid colon, laterally by the levator ani and obturator internus muscles, and posteriorly (in the male) by the rectum, vasa deferentia, and seminal vesicles or (in the female) by the supravaginal part of the cervix [65]. The bladder connects inferiorly with the urethra through the bladder neck, which is its narrowest part. Both the internal and external urethral sphincters regulate the flow of urine from the bladder.

The blood supply of the bladder is through the superior and inferior vesical arteries, which are branches of the internal iliac artery, while it is drained by a plexus of veins (the vesical plexus) that empties into the internal iliac vein [65]. The bladder stores urine until the micturition reflex is activated. Usually, this occurs when it is distended to its maximum capacity of about 500–600 mL.

21.4.3 Clinical Assessment

Gross hematuria and abdominal tenderness are the commonest manifestation of bladder trauma, occurring in about 82 and 62 %, respectively, of affected patients [20, 61]. Patients may also present with difficulty or inability to void [66]. Physical examination findings include abdominal distension and signs of peritoneal irritation (guiding, rigidity, tenderness, rebound tenderness) [66]. A high-riding prostate indicates disruption of the bladder and proximal urethra [66]. There may also be evidence of a pelvic fracture.

21.4.4 Diagnostic Testing

Cystography is the gold standard for the diagnosis of bladder injury, with an accuracy of 85–90 % [20, 66]. An initial plain film is taken, followed by another film after the about 300–400 mL of contrast has been injected into the bladder via the ureter. A post-drainage film is taken thereafter. Some authors recommend taking a film after about 100 mL of contrast has been injected [66]. Extravasation of the contrast indicates bladder rupture.

Intravenous urography (*IVU*) has a low accuracy of about 15–25 % and a high false-negative rate of about 64–84 % and is not recommended [20, 67–70].

CT cystography can be reliably used in the diagnosis of bladder injury, as it has a sensitivity of 85 % and a specificity of 100 % [20, 71]. The added advantages of CT include its speed and less radiation exposure [72]. Since most patients suspected for bladder injury will undergo CT, CT cystography eliminates the additional cost of a conventional cystography [20].

21.4.5 Initial Management (ER)

Cass et al. examined 417 patients with bladder injuries and showed that 94 % of them had associated injuries [73]. Pelvic fracture was present in 83 % of these patients, fractured ribs in 17 %, severe head injury in 6 %, and fractured spine in 6 %. As with all trauma evaluations, implementing the ATLS principles while identifying and treating life-threatening injuries should take precedence over specific diagnosis and treatment of bladder injury. Pelvic fractures can be associated with significant hemorrhage, which must be expeditiously identified and controlled.

21.4.6 Operative Management

Treatment of bladder rupture depends on the type: intraperitoneal or extraperitoneal. Intraperitoneal bladder rupture requires emergency surgical exploration and repair [20, 74]. The Eastern Association for the Study of Trauma (EAST) recommends managing the majority of extraperitoneal bladder ruptures with catheter drainage alone, with the exception of bone fragments projecting into the bladder, open pelvic fractures, and bladder injuries associated with rectal perforations [22]. In these scenarios, surgical management is indicated. Presence of bone fragments can be determined by intraoperative cystoscopy, if laparotomy is not undertaken for another reason. If the exploration is being undertaken for another reason, the bladder is generally explored through a large vertical cystotomy, and the bladder is inspected from the inside and repair undertaken. Urinary drainage is generally required for several weeks by Foley catheter.

21.4.7 Postoperative Management (Including Rehabilitation/Follow-Up)

Postoperatively, intravenous antibiotics should be administered as the potential for infection is high [74]. A pelvic drain, if placed intraoperatively, should be removed within 48–72 h, at which time drainage would have reduced significantly. Cystography (CT or conventional) should be done 10–14 days after surgery to assess for leakage.

21.4.8 Complications and Pitfalls

Potential complications of bladder trauma include urinary incontinence, pelvic infection, fistula formation, and urinary extravasation [74, 75]. There are additional complications that may occur during or after surgical repair of a ruptured bladder. These include severe hemorrhage from violation of a pelvic hematoma and small capacity bladder from aggressive debridement of the bladder [74].

21.4.9 Outcomes

Mortality after bladder trauma is more often related to the effect of associated injuries rather than the bladder rupture itself. As mentioned earlier, severe hemorrhagic shock from a pelvic bleed, severe head injuries, and rib fracture with soft tissue injury are some of the concomitant events that accompany bladder trauma, any one of which can be a cause of death.

21.5 Other Retroperitoneal Structures

21.5.1 Background/Incidence/Epidemiology

There are numerous anatomical organs that can be described by the term "retroperitoneal structures." Specific incidence and management of these differ. For the purpose of this review, this section focuses on retroperitoneal hematomas, as they can result from trauma to the vasculature of any of these structures.

Based on etiology, the incidence of retroperitoneal hematoma is estimated at 67–80 % due to blunt trauma and 20–33 % due to penetrating trauma [76–79]. Allen et al. reported an incidence of 44 % in 171 patients admitted after blunt trauma [80]. The overall incidence following penetrating trauma is uncertain. Retroperitoneal hematomas have high mortality rates of about 18–33 % [78].

21.5.2 Anatomy

The retroperitoneum or retroperitoneal space is the part of the abdominal cavity that is posterior to the peritoneal cavity from the diaphragm to the pelvic inlet [81]. Its anterior boundary is the peritoneal fascia, while its posterior boundary is the transversalis fascia. Classically, the retroperitoneum is divided into the posterior pararenal space, the perirenal space, and the anterior pararenal space [81]. For practical purposes, the retroperitoneum is divided into three zones: zone 1 is the central part, located in the middle of the abdominal cavity, and zone 2 comprises of the right and left flanks, while zone 3 comprises of the entire pelvis. Retroperitoneal structures are organs whose anterior surfaces are covered by peritoneum. These include the kidneys; ureters; bladders; adrenal glands; abdominal aorta; inferior vena cava; the head, neck, and body of the pancreas; and parts of the esophagus, duodenum, colon, and rectum [81–83].

21.5.3 Clinical Assessment

The clinical presentation of retroperitoneal hematoma depends on the specific organ that is injured and may include pain in the anterior abdomen, flank, back, or pelvic area [76]. Signs of hemorrhagic shock (including hypotension, tachycardia with weak and thready pulse, hypothermia, tachypnea) may be present in patients with pelvic fracture or injuries to the abdominal aorta, inferior vena cava, or other large vessels [76].

Ecchymosis of the flanks (Grey Turner's sign) or ecchymosis of the inguinal ligaments (Fox's sign) are late manifestations [76].

21.5.4 Diagnostic Testing

CT scanning, particularly the multi-detector CT, is the investigation of choice for the diagnosis of retroperitoneal injuries and hematomas [81], especially if the patient is hemodynamically stable. A focused assessment with sonography for trauma (FAST) exam is useful in patients who are hemodynamically unstable, although the FAST will only be positive if the retroperitoneal hematoma has ruptured freely into the intraperitoneal space. If there is a suspicion of renal injury, a one-stop IVU to assess the functionality of the kidneys should be done.

21.5.5 Initial Management (ER)

As described in earlier sections, initial management of patients with suspected retroperitoneal hematomas should follow the ATLS principles. Particular attention should be paid to the identification and control of hemorrhage as the potential for hemorrhagic shock in these patients is very high. Appropriate fluid and blood product resuscitation should be rapidly instituted in the setting of profound hypotension while initiating some hemorrhage control maneuver. A patient with blunt abdominal trauma, hypotension, and a positive FAST or penetrating abdominal trauma with hypotension should be rapidly transported to the operating room for immediate exploratory laparotomy [84].

21.5.6 Definitive Management

The specific operative management depends on the etiology – blunt or penetrating – size and location of the hematoma, and underlying structure that is injured. These are well summarized by Feliciano [76]. Although traditional teaching recommends operative management for all central hematomas, the expanded use of CT scans for evaluation of abdominal trauma has allowed nonoperative management of small central hematomas in patients who are hemodynamically normal without other indications for operation. Interventional approaches are also possible as an alternative to operative management, although there is little data to guide decision-making.

21.5.7 Postoperative Management (Including Rehab/Follow-Up)

The postoperative management depends on the intraoperative findings. A patient with a retroperitoneal hematoma often has associated organ injuries. If there is bowel injury, antibiotics should be administered perioperatively. If there is renal injury, renal scintigraphy may be used to assess renal function postoperatively. The patient should also be proactively examined for signs of postoperatively hemorrhage.

21.5.8 Complications and Pitfalls

Expansion of the hematoma is the commonest complication.

21.5.9 Outcomes

As mentioned earlier, the mortality rate for retroperitoneal hematoma is relatively high. Death may result from rupture of the hematoma and subsequent hemorrhagic shock, or from associated injuries. Early diagnosis is key to reducing mortality.

Conclusion

Renovascular, ureteral, and bladder injuries are rare, and there is insufficient evidence in the literature to draw up robust guidelines regarding management. However, the goal of therapy should be to save the patient's life through expeditious control of hemorrhage and, as much as possible, to preserve renal function.

Retroperitoneal hematomas are relatively common after abdominal and pelvic trauma. Early diagnosis, appropriate resuscitation, and treatment are key in improving survival. Operative approach for massive retroperitoneal bleeding generally requires a wide exposure and direct inspection of the entire compartment.

References

1. Elliott SP, Olweny EO, McAninch JW. Renal arterial injuries: a single center analysis of management strategies and outcomes. J Urol. 2007;178(6):2451–5.
2. Santucci RA, Wessells H, Bartsch G, Descotes J, Heyns CF, McAninch JW, et al. Evaluation and management of renal injuries: consensus statement of the renal trauma subcommittee. BJU Int. 2004;93:937.
3. Carroll PR, McAninch JW, Klosterman P, Greenblatt M. Renovascular trauma: risk assessment, surgical management, and outcome. J Trauma. 1990;30:547–54.
4. Cass AS, Bubrick M, Luxenberg M, Gleich P, Smith C. Renal pedicle injury in patients with multiple injuries. J Trauma. 1985;25:892.
5. Wessells H, Suh D, Porter JR, Rivara F, MacKenzie EJ, Jurkovich GJ, et al. Renal injury and operative management in the United States: results of a population-based study. J Trauma. 2003;54:423.
6. Bruce LM, Croce MA, Santaniello JM, Miller PR, Lyden SP, Fabian TC. Blunt renal artery injury: incidence, diagnosis, and management. Am Surg. 2001;67(6):550–4.
7. Knudson MM, Harrison PB, Hoyt DB, Shatz DV, Zietlow SP, Bergstein JM, Mario LA, McAninch JW. Outcome after major renovascular injuries: a Western trauma association multicenter report. J Trauma. 2000;49(6):1116–22.
8. http://www.aast.org/Library/TraumaTools/InjuryScoringScales.aspx#ureter.
9. Thompson-Fawcett M, Kolbe A. Paediatric renal trauma: caution with conservative management of major injuries. Aust N Z J Surg. 1996;66:435–40.
10. Wessel LM, Scholz S, Jester I, et al. Management of kidney injuries in children with blunt abdominal trauma. J Pediatr Surg. 2000;35:1326–30.
11. Madour WA, Lai MK, Linke CA, Frank IN. Blunt renal trauma in the pediatric patient. J Pediatr Surg. 1981;16:669–76.
12. Kuzmarov IW, Morehouse DD, Gibson S. Blunt renal trauma in the pediatric population: a retrospective study. J Urol. 1981;126:648–9.
13. Ahmed S, Morris LL. Renal parenchymal injuries secondary to blunt abdominal trauma I childhood: a 10-year review. Br J Urol. 1982;54:470–7.
14. Emanuel B, Weiss H, Gollin P. Renal trauma in children. J Trauma. 1977;17:275–8.

15. Bass DH, Semple PL, Cywes S. Investigation and management of blunt renal injuries in children: a review of 11 years' experience. J Pediatr Surg. 1991; 26:196–200.
16. Hoenig DM. Kidney anatomy. 2013. http://emedicine.medscape.com/article/1948775-overview.
17. Wein AJ, Kavoussi LR, Novick AC, Partin AW, Peters CA. Campbell-Walsh urology, vol. I. 9th ed. Philadelphia: Saunders; 2007. p. 24.
18. http://download.videohelp.com/vitualis/med/kidneys_and_ureters.htm.
19. Bertini JE, Felchner SM, Miller P, et al. The natural history of traumatic branch renal artery injury. J Urol. 1986;135:228–30.
20. Lynch D, Martinez-Piñeiro L, Plas E, Serafetinidis E, Turkeri L, Hohenfellner M. Guidelines on urological trauma. European Association of Urology. 2003.
21. Cass AS, Luxenberg M. Unilateral nonvisualization on excretory urography after external trauma. J Urol. 1984;132:225–7.
22. Holevar M, Ebert J, Luchette F, Nagy K, Sheridan R, Spirnak P, Yowler C. Practice management guidelines for the management of genitourinary trauma. The EAST Practice Management Guidelines Work Group. 2003.
23. Santucci RA, Fisher MB. The literature increasingly supports expectant (conservative) management of renal trauma — a systematic review. J Trauma. 2005;59(2):493–503.
24. Poulakis V, Ferakis N, Becht E, Deliveliotis C, Duex M. Treatment of renal-vascular injury by transcatheter embolization: immediate and long-term effects on renal function. J Endourol. 2006;20(6):405–9.
25. Chatziioannou A, Brountzos E, Primetis E, Malagari K, Sofocleous C, Mourikis D, Kelekis D. Effects of superselective embolization for renal vascular injuries on renal parenchyma and function. Eur J Vasc Endovasc Surg. 2004;28(2):201–6.
26. Tillou A, Romero J, Asensio JA, Best CD, Petrone P, Roldan G, Rojo E. Renal vascular injuries. Surg Clin North Am. 2001;81(6):1417–30.
27. Klink BK, Sutherin S, Heyse P, McCarthy MC. Traumatic bilateral renal artery thrombosis diagnosed by computed tomography with successful revascularization: case report. J Trauma. 1992;32:259–62.
28. Greenholz SK, Moore EE, Peterson NE, Moore GE. Traumatic bilateral renal artery occlusion: successful outcome without surgical intervention. J Trauma. 1986;26:941–4.
29. Scalfani SJA. The diagnosis of bilateral renal artery injury by computed tomography. J Trauma. 1986; 26:295–6.
30. Peterson NE. Review article: traumatic bilateral renal infarction. J Trauma. 1989;29:158–67.
31. Unger JI, Bare C, Haight J. Traumatic bilateral renal artery thrombosis. J Trauma. 1977;17:64–8.
32. Culp DA. Renal arterial block. Surg Gynecol Obstet. 1969;129:114–5.
33. Wessells H, Deirmenjian J, McAninch JW. Preservation of renal function after reconstruction for trauma: quantitative assessment with radionuclide scintigraphy. J Urol. 1997;157:1583–6.
34. http://kidney.niddk.nih.gov/kudiseases/pubs/yourkidneys/.
35. Barsness KA, Bensard DD, Partrick D, Hendrickson R, Koyle M, Calkins CM, Karrer F. Renovascular injury: an argument for renal preservation. J Trauma. 2004;57(2):310–5.
36. Peterson NE. Complications of renal trauma. Urol Clin North Am. 1989;16:221–35.
37. Monstrey SJ, Beerthuizen GI, van der Werken C, et al. Renal trauma and hypertension. J Trauma. 1989; 29:65–70.
38. Stables DP, Fouche RF, DeVilliers JP, et al. Traumatic renal artery occlusion: 21 cases. J Urol. 1976; 115:229–33.
39. Haas CA, Dinchman KH, Nasrallah PF, Spirnak JP. Traumatic renal artery occlusion: a 15-year review. J Trauma. 1998;45:557–61.
40. Montgomery RC, Richardson JD, Harty JI. Posttraumatic renovascular hypertension after occult renal injury. J Trauma. 1998;45:106–10.
41. Watts RA, Hoffbrand BI. Hypertension following renal trauma. J Hum Hypertens. 1987;1:65–71.
42. Caine JG, Fields S, Rakotomalata H, et al. Renal trauma with posttraumatic hypertension in a neonate. J Pediatr Surg. 1992;27:520–2.
43. von Knorring J, Fyhrquist F, Ahonen J. Varying course of hypertension following renal trauma. J Urol. 1981;126:798–801.
44. Weaver FA, Kuehne JP, Papanicolaou G. A recent institutional experience with renovascular hypertension. Am Surg. 1996;62:241–5.
45. Slavis SA, Hodge EE, Novick AC, Maatman T. Surgical treatment for isolated dissection of the renal artery. J Urol. 1990;144:233–7.
46. Weimann S, Flora G, Dittrich P, et al. Traumatic renal artery occlusion: is late reconstruction advisable? J Urol. 1987;137:727–9.
47. Hansen KJ, Deitch JS, Oskin TC, et al. Renal artery repair: consequence of operative failures. Ann Surg. 1998;227:678–90.
48. Ivatury RR, Zubowski R, Stahl WM. Penetrating renovascular trauma. J Trauma. 1989;29:1620–3.
49. Elliott SP, McAninch JW. Ureteral injuries from external violence: the 25-year experience at San Francisco General Hospital. J Urol. 2003;170(4 Pt 1):1213–6.
50. Siram SM, Gerald SZ, Greene WR, Hughes K, Oyetunji TA, Chrouser K, Cornwell 3rd EE, Chang DC. Ureteral trauma: patterns and mechanisms of injury of an uncommon condition. Am J Surg. 2010;199(4):566–70.
51. http://medchrome.com/basic-science/anatomy/clinical-anatomy-ureter/.
52. Medina D, Lavery R, Ross SE, Livingston DH. Ureteral trauma: preoperative studies neither predict injury nor prevent missed injuries. J Am Coll Surg. 1998;186(6):641–4.

53. Lynch TH, Martínez-Piñeiro L, Plas E, Serafetinides E, Türkeri L, Santucci RA, Hohenfellner M, European Association of Urology. EAU guidelines on urological trauma. Eur Urol. 2005;47(1):1–15.

54. Santucci RA. Ureteral trauma workup. 2013. http://emedicine.medscape.com/article/440933-overview.

55. Armenakas NA. Ureteral trauma: surgical repair. Urol Clin North Am. 1998;6:71–84.

56. Bright 3rd TC, Peters PC. Ureteral injuries due to external violence: 10 years' experience with 59 cases. J Trauma. 1977;17(8):616–20.

57. Brandes SB, Chelsky MJ, Buckman RF, et al. Ureteral injuries from penetrating trauma. J Trauma. 1994;36(6):766–9.

58. Elliott SP, McAninch JW. Ureteral injuries: external and iatrogenic. Urol Clin North Am. 2006;33:55–66.

59. Ghali AM, El Malik EM, Ibrahim AI, Ismail G, Rashid M. Ureteric injuries: diagnosis, management, and outcome. J Trauma. 1999;46(1):150–8.

60. Corriere Jr JN, Sandler CM. Management of the ruptured bladder: seven years of experience with 111 cases. J Trauma. 1986;26(9):830–3.

61. Carroll PR, McAninch JW. Major bladder trauma: mechanisms of injury and a unified method of diagnosis. J Urol. 1984;132(2):254–7.

62. McConnell JD, Wilkerson MD, Peters PC. Rupture of the bladder. Urol Clin North Am. 1982;9(2):293–6.

63. Flancbaum L, Morgan AS, Fleisher M, Cox EF. Blunt bladder trauma: manifestation of severe injury. Urology. 1988;31(3):220–2.

64. Castle WN, Richardson Jr JR, Walton BJ. Unsuspected intraperitoneal rupture of bladder presenting with abdominal free air. Urology. 1986;28(6):521–3.

65. Ellis H. Clinical anatomy: a revision and applied anatomy for clinical students. Malden: Blackwell Publishing; 2006.

66. Rackley R. Bladder trauma. 2013. http://emedicine.medscape.com/article/441124-overview#a0112.

67. Festini G, Gregorutti S, Reina G, Bellis GB. Isolated intraperitoneal bladder rupture in patients with alcohol intoxication and minor abdominal trauma. Ann Emerg Med. 1991;20(12):1371–2.

68. Werkman HA, Jansen C, Klein JP, Ten Duis HJ. Urinary tract injuries in multiply-injured patients: a rational guideline for the initial assessment. Injury. 1991;22(6):471–4.

69. Carroll PR, McAninch JW. Major bladder trauma: the accuracy of cystography. J Urol. 1983;130(5):887–8.

70. MacMahon R, Hosking D, Ramsey EW. Management of blunt injury to the lower urinary tract. Can J Surg. 1983;26(5):415–8.

71. Deck AJ, Shaves S, Talner L, Porter JR. Computerized tomography cystography for the diagnosis of traumatic bladder rupture. J Urol. 2000;164(1):43–6.

72. Vaccaro JP, Brody JM. CT cystography in the evaluation of major bladder trauma. Radiographics. 2000;20(5):1373–81.

73. Cass AS. The multiple injured patient with bladder trauma. J Trauma. 1984;24(8):731–4.

74. Rackley R. Bladder trauma treatment and management. 2013. http://emedicine.medscape.com/article/441124-treatment#a1128.

75. http://www.merckmanuals.com/professional/injuries_poisoning/genitourinary_tract_trauma/bladder_trauma.html.

76. Feliciano DV. Management of traumatic retroperitoneal hematoma. Management of traumatic retroperitoneal hematoma. Ann Surg. 1990;211(2):109–23.

77. Grieco JG, Perry Jr JF. Retroperitoneal hematoma following trauma: its clinical significance. J Trauma. 1980;20:733–6.

78. Selivanov V, Chi HS, Alverdy JC, et al. Mortality in retroperitoneal hematoma. J Trauma. 1984;24:1022–7.

79. Henao F, Aldrete JS. Retroperitoneal hematomas of traumatic origin. Surg Gynecol Obstet. 1985;161:106–16.

80. Allen RE, Eastman BA, Halter BL, Conolly WB. Retroperitoneal hemorrhage secondary to blunt trauma. Am J Surg. 1969;118:558–61.

81. Daly KP, Ho CP, Persson DL, Gay SB. Traumatic retroperitoneal injuries: review of multidetector CT findings. Radiographics. 2008;28(6):1571–90.

82. Chung WK. Gross anatomy (board review). Hagerstown: Lippincott Williams & Wilkins; 2005. p. 256.

83. Moore KL, Dalley AF, Agur AMR. Clinically oriented anatomy. Hagerstown: Lippincott Williams & Wilkins; 2005. p. 1209.

84. Ernest EM, Feliciano DV, Mattox KL, editors. Trauma. 5th ed. New York: The McGraw-Hill Companies, Inc.; 2004. p. 758.

85. Feliciano DV. Abdominal trauma. In: Schwartz SI, Ellis H, editors. Mangot's abdominal operations. East Norwalk: Appleton & Lange; 1989.

Part VI

Lower Extremity

Anahita Dua, Martin A. Schreiber,
John F. Kragh Jr., and Melina R. Kibbe

Femoral and Above-Knee Popliteal Injuries

22

Charles J. Fox

Contents

C.J. Fox, MD, FACS
Department of Surgery,
Denver Health Medical Center,
University of Colorado School of Medicine,
777 Bannock Street, M.C. 0206,
Denver, CO 80204, USA
e-mail: charles.fox@dhha.org

22.1   Introduction

A changing resuscitative paradigm, newer approaches to deep soft tissue wounds, and the expanding application of endovascular therapies now represent the latest developments in the modern surgical management for femoral and popliteal arterial injury [1–5]. With nearly 50,000 US troops wounded in the wars of Iraq and Afghanistan as of 2012, an evidenced-based approach to treating lower extremity arterial injury has been the subject of numerous reports, and a summary of recent teachings is the focus of this chapter [6].

22.2   Epidemiology

In the Vietnam War, vascular injuries accounted for 2–3 % of battle-related injuries [7]. Published reports over a decade of war demonstrate that the rate of vascular injury has been steadily increasing from 4 to 6 % to now 9 to 12 % of battle-related injuries making the rate of vascular injury approximately six times that reported in prior conflicts [8–10]. The increased incidence of vascular injury may have several explanations, including an increased awareness of and attention to recording such injuries. Undoubtedly, the effectiveness of tourniquets and other damage control measures, use of body armor, strategic forward placement of surgical assets, and rapid evacuation to definitive care also allow the treatment of vascular injuries that would have been

A. Dua et al. (eds.), *Clinical Review of Vascular Trauma*,
DOI 10.1007/978-3-642-39100-2_22, © Springer-Verlag Berlin Heidelberg 2014

fatal in past wars. New diagnostic modalities like computed tomography angiography (CTA) may also account for a rise in the observed rate of civilian lower extremity vascular injuries [11]. The contemporary rate of vascular injury underscores the importance of high-quality sustainment training in order to maintain a competent vascular skillset for trauma surgeons. From that standpoint, producing endovascular competent trauma surgeons will likely become a major focus of acute care surgery training programs in the near future [5].

22.3 Diagnosis

Injury to the femoral and popliteal arteries is by far the most common vascular injury pattern encountered in modern combat. In a published series of 497 casualties with 523 combat-related vascular injuries, Dua and colleagues reported that 43 % involved femoral and popliteal vessels [12]. These injuries can often be masked by deep soft tissue injury and fractures. When actively bleeding, the optimal management of extremity vascular injury requires early recognition and treatment of hemorrhagic shock. The goal is to achieve hemostasis, restore normal physiology, and perform a successful vascular reconstruction as early as possible. Blood products should be rapidly transfused within minutes of admission with an emergency release of four units of type O packed red blood cells (PRBCs) and four units of thawed AB plasma sent on demand from the blood bank. Unstable patients with more than one bleeding body cavity or mangled extremity are considered "in extremis" and should trigger a massive transfusion protocol.

Recognizing the need for vascular reconstruction at the time of the trauma admission is crucial as progressive ischemic burden can result in ultimate graft failure and subsequent limb loss. The injured extremity should be evaluated for pulses, sensory or motor deficits, and the presence of a bruit or thrill. Lower extremity arterial vascular injuries usually involve long-bone fractures and large soft tissue wounds that can make the diagnosis by physical exam easy and accurate.

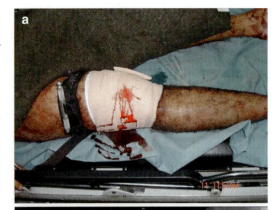

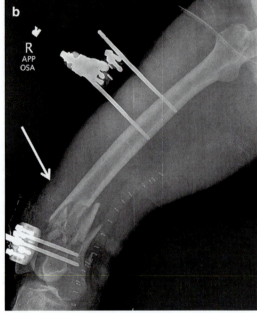

Fig. 22.1 A Special Operations Forces Tactical Tourniquet (SOFTT) controls hemorrhage from a popliteal artery injury (**a**), coupled with a plain radiograph showing a fracture of the supracondylar femur (**b**, *white arrow*), a pattern highly suggestive of a vascular injury (From Fox and Starnes [22])

Radiographs provide accurate clues that extremity vascular injuries exist. Supracondylar femur and tibial plateau fractures are frequently associated with injuries to the distal femoral and popliteal artery (Fig. 22.1). Deformed extremities are straightened and the onset of additional hemorrhage is controlled with direct pressure, gauze packing, hemostatic dressings, or tourniquets. Alternatively, in stable patients, without active bleeding, prehospital tourniquets should

Fig. 22.2 The combat application tourniquet (CAT) is carefully loosened to evaluate a popliteal vascular injury. The Emergency Medical Tourniquet (EMT) was applied above the narrow field tourniquets. A medial approach is preferred (*black line*) (Courtesy of COL (ret). John F. Kragh, Jr, MD, San Antonio, TX; From Fox and Starnes [22])

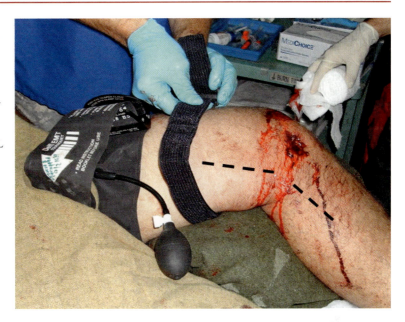

be carefully loosened to determine the degree, if any, of vascular injury (Fig. 22.2). A Doppler assessment is done to confirm the absence of pedal pulses and to perform an ankle-brachial index (ABI) when possible. A patient assessment when done in concert with an orthopedic surgeon will facilitate the necessary discussion regarding the sequence of the operation and preferred techniques for external fixation that best aid in the anticipated vascular exposure. Important information to relay to the entire operative team should include ideal patient positioning, the need for a shunt prior to fixation, the plan for vein harvesting in a contralateral extremity, and the desire for a C-arm or arteriography. Penetrating injuries without signs of arterial involvement such as a pulse deficit, expanding hematoma, bruit, or thrill generally do not require an arteriogram unless the ABI is <0.9. Obvious vessel injuries should be explored or managed with catheter-based techniques without further diagnostic studies.

Color-flow duplex (CFD) ultrasonography is an accurate noninvasive screening adjunct that can complement or sometimes be substituted for an arteriogram. This study can usually be obtained rapidly and used to detect occlusion, intimal flaps, and luminal defects. Bandages, open wounds, and orthopedic hardware may limit the utility of CFD in a trauma setting. CFD is highly operator dependent and has led many to prefer CTA as a noninvasive alternative of choice. Although ionizing radiation and nephrotoxicity are obvious disadvantages, these rapid multiplanar acquisitions allow for high-resolution three-dimensional reconstructions that can be superior to a catheter-based arteriogram. CTA has the advantage of imaging multiple extremities and the surrounding soft tissue simultaneously. CTA is also useful in surgical planning; however when an endovascular intervention is anticipated, the volume frequency and type of contrast agent to be administered should be discussed [11].

22.4 Operative Management

The first goal of the emergency operation is to control hemorrhage with close hemodynamic monitoring and judicious replacement of fresh warm blood products in equal ratios. The patient should have broad antibiotic coverage and be positioned supine on a fluoroscopic table with at least one uninjured limb prepped for a vein harvest.

Proximal control of hemorrhage is often accomplished by firm digital occlusion using an assistant's gloved hand prepped directly into the

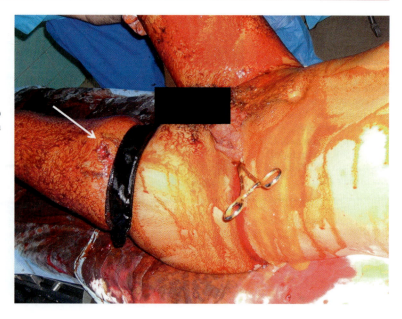

Fig. 22.3 Hemorrhage from a proximal left femoral artery gunshot wound is aptly controlled with a left retroperitoneal exposure and proximal clamping of the external iliac artery. The entrance wound (*white arrow*) is in the proximal lateral thigh

bleeding wound bed with Betadine spray. This is followed by careful dissection proximal and distal to the site of injury. Balloon catheters may also tamponade hemorrhage when a tourniquet or manual pressure is not effective, but blind insertion of surgical instruments can be unproductive, or harmful, and is discouraged. Tourniquets are left in place until the anesthetist has sufficient time to resuscitate the patient. Proximal thigh injuries are best managed by division of the inguinal ligament or by the retroperitoneal approach with clamp control of the external iliac artery (Fig. 22.3). The medial approach is preferred over the posterior approach for femoropopliteal injuries. The approach in relation to the knee joint is directed by the level of the wound; however total division of muscular attachments at the knee is sometimes required to control hemorrhage of transected arteries and veins. Although often thrombosed at the time, the injured vessels must be found and ligated because they will rebleed later after the patient is resuscitated. Retrograde advancement of a Fogarty catheter inserted from an uninjured distal site can also be used to locate the transected artery in a horrific wound that is no longer bleeding. A single bleeding tibial vessel can be ligated; however injury to the tibioperoneal trunk or multiple

vessels should be repaired. Associated nerve, bone, and soft tissue injury are the essential determinants of limb salvage. When making a decision to amputate or salvage an extremity, consider the patients' condition, extent of injury, and willingness to commit the patient to the necessary definitive orthopedic care and physical rehabilitation. No one situation or scoring system can replace the surgical judgment developed by an experienced team.

A primary end to end repair is preferred when lateral sutures cannot repair the injured vessel. Advantages of this repair include a single anastomosis and use of autologous tissue. Dividing nearby geniculate branches may gain some length in noncalcified vessels, but this repair should be both expedient and free of tension. Complete debridement of any disrupted tissue is an essential step of the repair, and sacrifices made to avoid an interposition conduit should be avoided.

If an interposition graft repair is required, the complexity and additional operative time required for vein harvest and interposition grafting should be appreciated, and the final operative plan and estimated time should be communicated early to the operative team. Saphenous vein taken from an uninjured limb including the arm is the

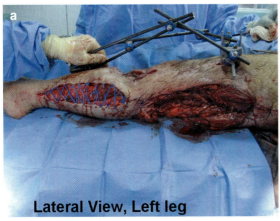

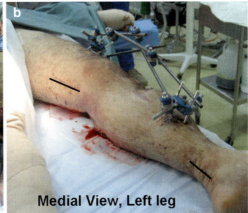

Fig. 22.4 A lower extremity fragment wound resulting in severe destruction of the popliteal and tibial vessels (**a**) was reconstructed with an above-knee popliteal to posterior tibial artery bypass using a reversed saphenous vein graft. Knee-spanning external fixation for this tibial plateau fracture can be applied quickly to stabilize the limb and permit excellent surgical exposure (*black line*) out of the injured region (**b**) (From Fox and Starnes [22])

preferred conduit for the reconstruction of lower extremity vascular injuries. However, in the author's experience expanded polytetrafluoroethylene (ePTFE) prosthetic grafts placed in larger vessels with good muscle coverage have been used successfully. Systemic anticoagulation is generally avoided for trauma except for an isolated vascular injury in a non-coagulopathic patient without extensive soft tissue damage.

Ballistic injuries transmit kinetic energy and result in intimal damage well beyond the transected arterial segment. Therefore, one should carefully open vessels longitudinally and inspect the quality of the luminal surface and the arterial inflow relative to the mean arterial pressure. When necessary, a Fogarty embolectomy catheter should be carefully advanced as tourniquets and limited heparin dosing easily result in thrombus accumulation. Special precautions should include routine flushing of the graft, and native artery with heparinized saline to dislodge fibrin strands, and platelet debris. This is best done with a solution of Papaverine and warm heparinized saline. A well-spatulated four-quadrant, heel-to-toe anastomosis is the easiest method to teach and perform in difficult situations. Small Heifetz clips or bulldog clamps can also minimize potential clamp injuries of small vessels. There is documented value in repair of concomitant venous

injuries to avoid the potential for early limb loss from venous hypertension or long-term disability from chronic edema. With combined arterial and venous injuries, arterial repair should precede venous repair to minimize further ischemic burden, unless the vein repair requires very little effort.

Shotgun or fragment injury produces large cavitary wounds; with severe disruption of the skin and loss of underlying muscle, it may be difficult to achieve suitable graft coverage. Greer and colleagues reported on The Walter Reed Army experience with combat-related graft ruptures of which 70 % were in the femoropopliteal region. A significant factor was the degree of muscle coverage in the face of a contaminated wound. Therefore, when confronted with this situation, a longer vein graft tunneled completely around the zone of injury should be chosen over a shorter inadequately covered vein interposition conduit [13]. External fixation positioning should not impede the planned operative exposure. Tunneling grafts and preservation of skin bridges are therefore important matters to discuss before fasciotomy incisions are made (Fig. 22.4). Devitalized tissue is excised and irrigated under low pressure, with careful evaluation of muscle tissue for viability. Injured nerve tissue should be tagged at both ends with

Fig. 22.5 Negative pressure (vacuum) therapy has facilitated earlier closure of fasciotomy surgical sites (**a**) and other deep cavitary wounds of the lower extremity. A vacuum seal can be easily obtained despite the use of orthopedic hardware in this child (**b**)

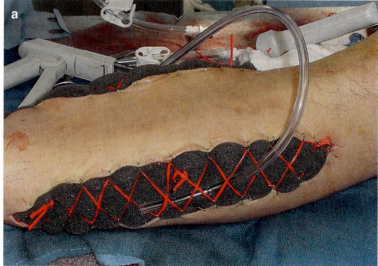

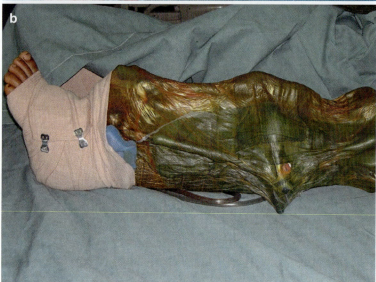

monofilament suture. A lengthy and meticulous debridement at the outset is not usually necessary as these wounds look much better in a few days after subsequent washouts and vacuum dressings. Always maintain a low threshold for performing a four-compartment fasciotomy. This is usually performed first and the length of the incision may vary with the clinical scenario but an incomplete fasciotomy can be catastrophic. The application of vessel loops to prevent skin retraction and the use of negative pressure dressings

have made primary closure more successful and eliminated the need for routine split-thickness skin grafts (Fig. 22.5).

22.5 Temporary Vascular Shunts

Temporary vascular shunts are effective damage control techniques that allow for delayed reconstruction and should be compared with the consequences of simple ligation. Temporary vascular

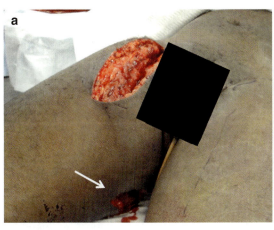
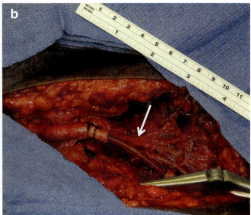

Fig. 22.6 A gunshot wound (*white arrow*, **a**) transected the right femoral artery (**b**). Flow was restored with a 14 French Argyle shunt (*white arrow*). The patient was transported to a facility that could perform a reversed saphenous interposition graft

shunts allow for perfusion during temporary delays needed for extremity fixation, patient transport, addressing more life-threatening injuries, or assessment of revascularization options including during vein harvest. Several high-quality papers have advanced its use during the wars in Iraq and Afghanistan. At the 2006 meeting of the Eastern Association for the Surgery of Trauma, the Air Force demonstrated that shunts placed in proximal vascular injuries have acceptable (86 %) patency, and failure of distal shunts did not decrease limb viability [14]. In 2007, Taller and colleagues reported successful shunting with 96 % patency among casualties evacuated from a remote Navy Echelon II – Forward Resuscitative Surgical Suite (FRSS) based in the western province of Iraq. The mean shunt time was 5 h 48 min (range, 3:40–10:49), and the authors meticulously documented the time from shunt placement to casualty presentation at the level 3 surgical facilities in Baghdad or Balad, Iraq. These authors also validated the earlier experience of a US Navy forward surgical unit and concluded that complex combat injuries to proximal extremity vessels should be routinely shunted at forward-deployed Echelon II facilities as part of the resuscitative, damage control process [15].

In 2009, Gifford and colleagues published an outcome analysis study. Data were collected from the Joint Theater Trauma Registry (JTTR). The study compared 64 shunted US casualties sustaining extremity vascular injury to 61 who were not shunted. After propensity score adjustment, there was a nonsignificant trend toward reduced risk of amputation in patients treated with temporary vascular shunts. This trend was greatest in patients with severely injured limbs. The authors concluded that temporary vascular shunting used as a damage control adjunct in management of wartime extremity vascular injury does not lead to worse outcomes [16]. Analyses from all available publications suggest that temporary vascular shunting is an effective technique to facilitate patient transfer and is preferable to prolonged reconstruction efforts in remote less capable locations. The author prefers an Argyle (Covidien, Mansfield, MA) sterile 6 in. straight shunt from a disposable kit containing four different sizes (8–14 French). The shunt is carefully inserted to avoid further intimal injury and secured with silastic vessel loops or silk sutures (Fig. 22.6). A continuous wave Doppler is used to confirm flow, and the vessel is definitively debrided at the time of reconstruction.

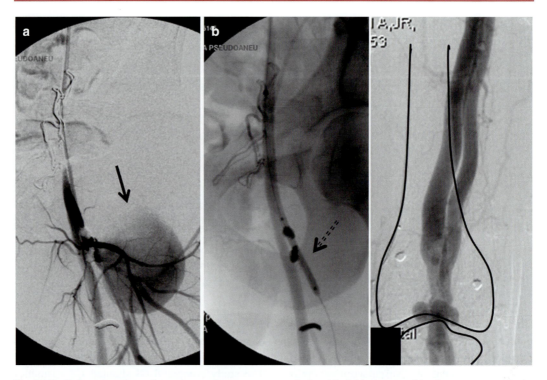

Fig. 22.7 Catheter-based arteriograms are necessary to detect occult vascular injuries after fragment wounds. A large left profunda femoral artery false aneurysm (*solid black arrow*, **a**) is controlled by transfemoral balloon occlusion (*dash black arrow*, **b**) prior to open repair. An early venous phase is pathognomonic of an arteriovenous fistula (**c**) seen in the popliteal region (*black lines* outline the femur and tibial plateau)

22.6 Endovascular Management

The established effectiveness of endovascular therapies in the setting of acute trauma has led to a growing acceptance to treat specific patterns of injury. A variety of catheter-based techniques have been particularly successful for vascular injuries such as occlusion, dissection, arteriovenous fistulae (AVF), and false aneurysms of the lower extremity (Fig. 22.7). Specifically, balloon-assisted tamponade, coil embolization, and covered stent placement appear to be well suited for stable patients with less severe extremity injuries. Transcatheter embolization can be done by extruding hemostatic agents (Gelfoam) or stainless steel coils through a 5 French catheter into the target vessel. For an AVF, a suitably sized coil is placed into the feeding artery proximally and distally to the fistula site. False aneurysms can also be treated by coil-induced thrombotic occlusion or by endoluminal repair with covered

stent placement. Transected vessels are also repaired with covered stents provided that a wire can successfully traverse the injury. This may require retrograde passage of wires for a complex injury. Despite obvious advantages endografts continue to require long-term surveillance as potential complications render the long-term outcome uncertain at this time [17–20].

22.7 Completion Imaging

Static film arteriography has largely been replaced with portable C-arm units capable of digital subtraction angiography. Contrast arteriography is very useful for locating the injured vascular bed when there are diffuse fragmentation wounds to the extremity. Hand-injected contrast images using butterfly needles without special wires or catheters can be acquired quickly using the digital subtraction mode on a mobile

C-arm unit. Completion assessments following open repair or endovascular interventions consist of a combination of physical exam, the handheld Doppler and selective arteriography [21].

22.8 Postoperative Considerations

The early postoperative period is focused on patient warming, resuscitation, and hourly vascular checks that should be performed with a handheld continuous wave Doppler probe. Palpable pulses and sometimes normal ankle-brachial ratios (>0.9) may be delayed until an appropriate resuscitation and warming period has occurred. Patients should remain in the ICU for at least 24 h. Ward transfer follows cardiopulmonary and metabolic stability once the threat of early graft failure and postoperative coagulopathic bleeding has diminished. Soft tissue bleeding should be anticipated and the extremity wrapped in bulky gauze. A typical patient is returned to the operating room every 24–48 h for fixator adjustment, additional debridement, and negative pressure "vacuum" dressing changes. The assessment for the onset of compartment syndrome or evidence of an incomplete fasciotomy is essential; hence, hourly neurological checks should also be performed in the early postoperative period. Aspirin is favored for all vascular repairs, and antibiotics are continued for at least 24 h. Compression garments and leg elevation is encouraged to minimize edema [3].

Conclusion

The simultaneous management of peripheral vascular injuries in the pursuit of life and limb is very challenging. The decision to amputate or reconstruct an ischemic limb requires sound judgment that often comes with experience. These patients have significant transfusion requirements, and the resuscitation should not be separated from the surgery. Tibial vessels can be ligated when a Doppler signal is obtainable in the distal extremity. Systemic heparin is not necessary; however adequate intimal debridement and liberal flushing with

heparinized saline during the repair is essential. A well-covered interposed saphenous vein graft is a durable conduit and favored over prosthetic materials. Venous reconstruction should be performed when time permits. Completion arteriography is not usually necessary, but a pulse exam should be confirmed with a continuous wave Doppler signal and ABIs.

References

1. McArthur CS, Marin ML. Endovascular therapy for the treatment of arterial trauma. Mt Sinai J Med. 2004;71(1):4–11.
2. Porter JM, Ivatury RR, Nassoura ZE. Extending the horizons of "damage control" in unstable trauma patients beyond the abdomen and gastrointestinal tract. J Trauma. 1997;42(3):559–61.
3. Fox CJ, Perkins JG, Kragh Jr JF, Singh NN, Patel B, Ficke JR. Popliteal artery repair in massively transfused military trauma casualties: a pursuit to save life and limb. J Trauma. 2010;69(1 Suppl):S123–34.
4. Leininger BE, Rasmussen TE, Smith DL, Jenkins DH, Coppola C. Experience with wound VAC and delayed primary closure of contaminated soft tissue injuries in Iraq. J Trauma. 2006;61(1):1207–11.
5. Rasmussen TE, Dubose JJ, Asensio JA, et al. Tourniquets, vascular shunts, and endovascular technologies: esoteric or essential? A report from the 2011 AAST Military Liaison Panel. J Trauma Acute Care Surg. 2012;73(1):282–5.
6. Fox CJ, Patel B, Clouse WD. Update on wartime vascular injury. Perspect Vasc Surg Endovasc Ther. 2011;23(1):13–25.
7. Rich NM, Baugh JH, Hughes CW. Acute arterial injuries in Vietnam: 1,000 cases. J Trauma. 1970;10(5):359–69.
8. White JM, Stannard A, Burkhardt GE, Eastridge BJ, Blackbourne LH, Rasmussen TE. The epidemiology of vascular injury in the wars in Iraq and Afghanistan. Ann Surg. 2011;253(6):1184–9.
9. Fox CJ, Gillespie DL, O'Donnell SD, et al. Contemporary management of wartime vascular trauma. J Vasc Surg. 2005;41(4):638–44.
10. Woodward EB, Clouse WD, Eliason JL, et al. Penetrating femoropopliteal injury during modern warfare: experience of the Balad Vascular Registry. J Vasc Surg. 2008;47(6):1259–64.
11. White PW, Gillespie DL, Feuerstein IM, et al. Sixty-four slice multidetector computed tomographic angiography in the evaluation of vascular trauma. J Trauma. 2010;68(1):96–102.
12. Dua A, Patel B, Kragh Jr JF, Holcomb JB, Fox CJ. Long-term follow-up and amputation-free survival in 497 casualties with combat-related vascular injuries and damage-control resuscitation. J Trauma Acute Care Surg. 2012;73(6):1517–24.

13. Greer LT, Patel B, Via KC, Bowman JN, Weber MA, Fox CJ. Management of secondary hemorrhage from early graft failure in military extremity wounds. J Trauma Acute Care Surg. 2012;73(4):818–24.

14. Rasmussen TE, Clouse WD, Jenkins DH, Peck MA, Eliason JL, Smith DL. The use of temporary vascular shunts as a damage control adjunct in the management of wartime vascular injury. J Trauma. 2006;61(1):8–12.

15. Taller J, Kamdar JP, Greene JA, et al. Temporary vascular shunts as initial treatment of proximal extremity vascular injuries during combat operations: the new standard of care at echelon II facilities? J Trauma. 2008;65(1):595–603.

16. Gifford SM, Aidinian G, Clouse WD, et al. Effect of temporary shunting on extremity vascular injury: an outcome analysis from the Global War on Terror vascular injury initiative. J Vasc Surg. 2009;50(3):549–55.

17. Starnes BW, Arthurs ZM. Endovascular management of vascular trauma. Perspect Vasc Surg Endovasc Ther. 2006;18(2):114–29.

18. Reuben BC, Whitten MG, Sarfati M, Kraiss LW. Increasing use of endovascular therapy in acute arterial injuries: analysis of the National Trauma Data Bank. J Vasc Surg. 2007;46(6):1222–6.

19. Rasmussen TE, Clouse WD, Peck MA, et al. Development and implementation of endovascular capabilities in wartime. J Trauma. 2008;64:1169–76.

20. Johnson III ON, Fox CJ, White P, et al. Physical exam and occult post-traumatic vascular lesions: implications for the evaluation and management of arterial injuries in modern warfare in the endovascular era. J Cardiovasc Surg (Torino). 2007;48(5):581–6.

21. Starnes BW, Beekley AC, Sebesta JA, Andersen CA, Rush Jr RM. Extremity vascular injuries on the battlefield: tips for surgeons deploying to war. J Trauma. 2006;60(2):432–42.

22. Fox CJ, Starnes BW. Vascular surgery on the modern battlefield. Surg Clin North Am. 2007; 87(5):1193–211, xi. Starnes BW, editor. Philadelphia: Elsevier.

Below-Knee Popliteal, Tibial, and Foot Injuries

23

John W. York and John F. Eidt

Contents

J.W. York, MD • J.F. Eidt, MD (✉)
Division of Vascular Surgery,
Greenville Health System,
University Medical Center,
Greenville, SC, USA
eidtjohnf @gmail.com

23.1   Introduction

Vascular injuries of the lower extremity pose some of the most challenging problems faced by vascular surgeons for a number of reasons. While these injuries are not typically life-threatening, the risk of limb loss in a young trauma patient amplifies the importance of making a complex series of correct clinical decisions with limited data under the pressure of time. The compressed anatomical relationships of the nerves, vessels, and bones of the lower leg make surgical repair challenging even for the most capable of vascular surgeons. In addition to focusing on the injured extremity, the vascular surgeon must remain wary of the balance between overly enthusiastic efforts to preserve the limb against the risk of death from associated injuries. The intent of this chapter is to review the epidemiology of lower leg vascular injuries, the optimum diagnostic strategies, the treatment options, and the pitfalls in management.

23.2   Incidence

Our understanding of the management of lower extremity vascular trauma has been derived in large part from wartime experience [1]. As recently as World War II, extremity vascular injuries were associated with amputation rates in excess of 70 % [2]. Armed with newly invented synthetic materials such as Dacron and improved surgical tools, surgeons during the

A. Dua et al. (eds.), *Clinical Review of Vascular Trauma*,
DOI 10.1007/978-3-642-39100-2_23, © Springer-Verlag Berlin Heidelberg 2014

Korean War began to experiment with repairing, rather than ligating, injured vessels with encouraging results [1]. Widespread application of modern limb salvage techniques dramatically reduced the amputation rate in Vietnam [3, 4]. Regrettably, the devastating effects of improvised explosive devices (IEDs) in Iraq and Afghanistan have resulted in a persistent need for amputation despite vast improvements in the delivery of battlefield care [3, 5]. Military surgeons have pioneered the use of intra-arterial shunts and mass transfusion protocols, techniques that are being rapidly adopted in the civilian theater [6–8].

The incidence of distal lower extremity vascular trauma in the civilian population is less well characterized than in the military due to the absence of uniform reporting requirements. The available evidence suggests that vascular trauma below the knee is related to the geographic setting with more penetrating wounds in the urban setting and a predominance of blunt injuries in the rural environment [9]. Based on data from the National Trauma Data Bank, the most commonly injured vessel in the lower extremity is the popliteal artery (35 %), followed in decreasing order by the superficial femoral artery (28 %), the common femoral artery (18 %), the posterior tibial artery (13 %), and the anterior tibial artery (9 %).

No data are available for injury to the peroneal artery due to the absence of an ICD-9 code [10]. Blunt vascular injuries exceed penetrating trauma in most civilian series consistent with recent evidence demonstrating a decrease in violent crime over the past 20 years.

A number of factors are predictive of outcomes in patients with extremity trauma including the location and number of injuries, the nature of the injury (blunt or penetrating), and, most notably, the severity of associated injuries to bone, nerve, and soft tissues. While the risk of mortality is increased with more proximal, penetrating injuries, the risk of limb loss is increased with more distal vascular injuries. In comparison to penetrating injuries, blunt injuries are associated with higher amputation rates due to a higher incidence of injuries to soft tissue, bone, and nerves [10, 11].

23.3 Anatomy

A clear understanding of arterial anatomy is essential to the accurate diagnosis and optimum treatment of lower leg vascular injury (Fig. 23.1). Vascular reconstructions below the knee are particularly challenging due to the small size of the vessels and the difficulty of surgical exposure.

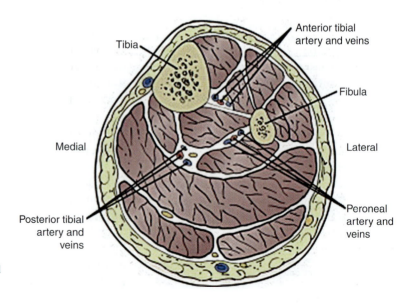

Fig. 23.1 Cross-sectional anatomy of the infrapopliteal arterial system

The three major arteries in the lower leg originate from the popliteal artery, but the configuration of these vessels may be quite variable. In the most common pattern, the infrageniculate popliteal artery bifurcates into the anterior tibial artery (AT) and the tibioperoneal trunk (TPT). The AT penetrates the interosseous membrane and courses longitudinally through the anterior compartment of the leg and becomes the dorsalis pedis (DP) artery as it crosses the ankle joint. In approximately 5 % of patients, the AT arises from the popliteal artery proximal to the knee joint and may be serendipitously preserved in the setting of injuries to the distal popliteal and proximal tibial vessels. The DP divides into five branches on the foot: the lateral tarsal, medial tarsal, first dorsal metatarsal, arcuate, and deep plantar branches. The TPT is a short artery, typically 4–6 cm in length though it may be nonexistent in some patients who have a true "trifurcation." The TPT divides into the peroneal artery and the posterior tibial (PT) artery. The PT is usually the largest of the three vessels and terminates below the ankle into the medial and lateral plantar arteries. Angiographically, the peroneal artery is easily distinguished from the AT and PT by its more central location between the tibia and fibula and by multiple branches. The peroneal artery is closely applied to the inner surface of the interosseous membrane in the deep posterior compartment and is the most difficult to expose of the three major arteries below the knee. The peroneal typically terminates in an inverted "Y" just proximal to the ankle joint providing critical collateral connections to the DP and PT.

The PT is easily approached through a longitudinal incision in the skin and deep fascia approximately 2–3 cm posterior to the tibia. The PT is immediately visible on the surface of the tibialis posterior muscle after incision of the deep fascia. The peroneal artery is deeper in the leg. It can be approached though a medial incision like the PT or can be exposed from a lateral approach after segmental resection of the fibula. The lateral approach to the peroneal is particularly appealing in the setting of significant soft tissue injury on the medial leg that could limit coverage of an arterial repair. The anterior tibial artery is exposed through a longitudinal incision in the skin and deep fascia approximately 2 cm lateral to the tibia. In most traumatic vascular injuries, the surgeon must make a decision whether to expose the injured vessels through traumatic skin lacerations or use more conventional incisions.

In making clinical decisions regarding the need for surgical intervention in lower leg trauma, it is critical to understand the redundancy of the blood supply to the foot. It may not always be necessary, and sometimes unwise, to reconstruct an isolated tibial artery injury in the absence of distal ischemia. In most cases, a single patent tibial artery is sufficient for distal perfusion of the foot and preservation of normal function. In the absence of hemorrhage, distal ischemia, or need for debridement of devitalized tissue, nonoperative management may be appropriate in selected patients. Non-emergent treatment of an intimal flap, arteriovenous fistula, or pseudoaneurysm can be undertaken electively.

23.4 Mechanism of Injury

Most penetrating injuries are due to gunshots, shotguns, and stabbing. Stab wounds usually result in isolated vascular injuries to both arteries and veins that can be treated by primary repair. In comparison to stab wounds, the extent of soft tissue damage, including vascular injury, is related both to the caliber and velocity of gunshots. High-velocity, military-style weapons may cause extensive damage well beyond the actual tract of the missile. In the assessment of vascular injury, the surgeon must be aware of the potential for vascular damage that is remote from the point of penetration. Shotgun wounds are notable for the inaccuracy of physical examination in detecting arterial injury, for more extensive soft tissue damage, and for the possibility of multiple vessel injuries.

Blunt arterial injuries may result from direct crushing, stretching, or laceration due to bony fragments. Blunt arterial injuries are often difficult to repair without vein graft interposition or bypass due to injury to a longer segment of arterial wall or delamination of the arterial wall with retraction of the intima. Both blunt and penetrating injuries that do not result in occlusion may result in pseudoaneurysm or arteriovenous fistula, which should be considered when planning follow-up surveillance. Regardless of the mechanism of injury, two principles govern operative repair: debride all nonviable vessels and complete the vascular repair without tension.

23.5 Clinical Assessment

The initial evaluation and resuscitation of trauma patients follows Advanced Trauma and Life Support (ATLS) protocols. Many patients with vascular injuries below the knee have other significant systemic injuries that must be evaluated and treated. This necessitates direct and clear communication between the vascular surgeon, the trauma surgeon, and other specialists. The vascular surgeon must be cognizant of systemic injuries in order to properly prioritize treatment of the injured extremity. It is particularly important to establish the presence of central nervous system injuries that might preclude anticoagulation. In addition, major vascular injuries in the chest, abdomen, or pelvis invariably take precedence over extremity vascular injuries.

Following establishment of a stable airway, control of obvious bleeding, and initial resuscitation, a detailed examination of the extremities can be performed during the secondary survey (Fig. 23.2). For both blunt and penetrating injuries, the extremity examination is focused around four functional components: bone, nerve, soft tissue, and vessels. Injury to three of these four functional elements constitutes a "mangled extremity" [12]. The clinician should note the presence of limb deformity or instability suggesting an underling fracture. The extent of skin loss

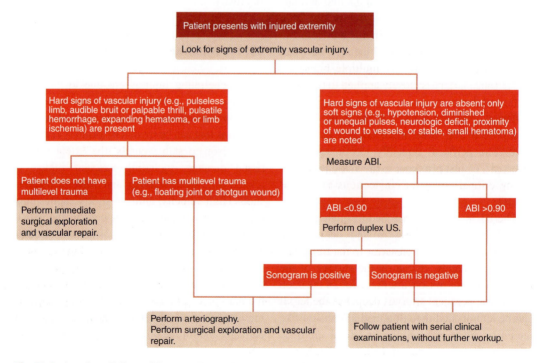

Fig. 23.2 American College of Surgeons Lower Extremity Vascular Injury Algorithm

---

Signs of traumatic vascular injury

Hard signs

- Observed pulsatile bleeding

- Arterial thrill by manual palpation

- Bruit auscultated over or near an area of arterial injury
- Absent distal pulse

- Visible expanding hematoma

Soft signs

- Significant hemorrhage by history

- Neurologic abnormality

- Diminished pulse compared with contralateral extremity
- Proximity of bony injury or penetrating wound

Fig. 23.3 Clinical indicators of vascular injury

or soft tissue injury is noted. Neurological evaluation of the extremity is usually limited to basic motor and sensory function. The sciatic nerve supplies the muscles of the lower leg after it divides into the tibial nerve and the peroneal nerve. The tibial nerve supplies the muscles of the posterior compartment and the skin of the medial hind foot. Injury to the peroneal nerve results in the inability to dorsiflex the foot. The deep peroneal nerve courses through the anterior compartment and provides motor innervation to anterior compartment and sensation to the first and second toes. The muscles of the lateral compartment are supplied by the superficial peroneal nerve which also provides sensation to the skin of the anterolateral foot. The femoral nerve provides cutaneous branches to the anterior thigh, muscular branches to the pectineus, sartorius, the quadriceps femoris, and the vastus group of muscles.

It is critical to perform a complete initial examination of the vascular system during the secondary survey in order to identify potentially lethal injuries and to repeat the exam at frequent intervals in order to detect significant changes. The presence, asymmetry, or absence of all peripheral pulses should be recorded in addition to the color and temperature of the extremity. Bruits and thrills in areas of suspected arterial injury may indicate the presence of significant stenosis, arteriovenous fistulae or pseudoaneurysm. The compartments of the affected extremity should be assessed subjectively for excessive pressure in comparison to the uninjured leg and measured objectively as necessary. Hematomas should be assessed for pulsatility or expansion. Distended superficial veins or excessive extremity edema may indicate proximal venous obstruction or the presence of arteriovenous communications.

The evaluation of vascular injuries utilizes a group of clinical indicators commonly referred to as "hard" and "soft" signs (Fig. 23.3). The hard signs of vascular injury include observed pulsatile bleeding; absent distal pulse; expanding hematoma; audible bruit; palpable thrill; or a cold, pale, or mottled extremity. The sensitivity of any hard sign is nearly 100 % in the detection of significant vascular injury [13]. In the absence of other higher-priority, life-threatening injuries, the presence of a hard sign of vascular injury typically indicates the need for emergency surgical treatment. In a patient with obvious extremity bleeding, the patient should be taken directly to the operating room for immediate exploration. In a patient with limb ischemia, expeditious vascular imaging, optimally performed in the operating room, prior to surgical exploration may be preferable to blind surgical exposure, particularly in patients with multiple sites of suspected injury. Recent experimental evidence suggests that the duration of limb ischemia is related to the magnitude of detrimental systemic effects following reperfusion, further emphasizing the need to avoid excessive delay in attempts to obtain preoperative imaging [14]. As previously discussed, in a patient without clinical signs of overt ischemia, the absence of an isolated pedal pulse may warrant nonoperative management particularly in the setting of other significant nonvascular injuries. Elective vascular imaging with color flow Doppler and CT-, MR-, or catheter angiography to rule out significant intimal flap, pseudoaneurysm, or arteriovenous fistula is appropriate in stable patients without ischemia if a nonoperative approach is elected.

The "soft" signs of vascular injury include a history of pulsatile bleeding, diminished pulse compared to the contralateral uninjured extremity, proximity of bony fragment or penetrating wounds adjacent to arterial structures, and isolated neurologic deficit of the injured extremity. The specificity of "soft signs" for the detection of significant arterial injury is less than 5 %.

As an adjunct to the physical examination, the ankle-brachial index (ABI) may aid assessing the presence and severity of vascular injury. The ABI is the ratio of the highest blood pressure detected by continuous wave Doppler at the level of the ankle of the injured lower extremity divided by the highest blood pressure in an uninjured upper extremity. Both upper and lower extremity blood pressure measurements are performed using the Doppler rather than a stethoscope. The ABI may be performed at the bedside with only a manual blood pressure cuff and a continuous wave Doppler and does not require advanced imaging equipment or a certified vascular technologist.

The accuracy of Doppler-derived ABI in patients with lower extremity vascular injuries has been reported with both penetrating and blunt lower extremity trauma. Lynch and Johansen examined the sensitivity and specificity of ABI measurements in trauma patients with suspected lower extremity vascular injury [15]. In this series of 100 consecutive injured limbs that were evaluated by Doppler-derived ABI and contrast angiography, an ABI of less than 0.9 was 87 % sensitive and 97 % specific for the detection arterial injury. From these data the authors suggested that in the absence of

hard signs of arterial injury, an ABI is an acceptable alternative to angiography particularly if there is an anticipated period of continued observation [16].

The use of ABI has also been applied to the evaluation of patients with blunt vascular injuries of the lower extremity associated with fractures and dislocations. A controlled trial that included 75 consecutive patients with knee dislocations that were believed to be at high risk for vascular injury was performed to determine the diagnostic accuracy of ABI [17]. The negative predictive value of a Doppler-derived ABI greater than 0.9 was 100 %. Of the 30 % of patients with an ABI less than 0.9, 70 % had an injury that was diagnosed by angiography, 50 % of which required repair. This study again demonstrates the value of a simple, noninvasive diagnostic test that provides important objective information that can be performed rapidly at the bedside [17].

Despite the obvious advantages of Doppler-derived ABI in the trauma setting, there are several situations and patient characteristics that may render the ABI inaccurate. Injuries to non-axial lower extremity arteries such as the profunda femoris or the peroneal artery may exist despite a normal ABI. Also, a nonobstructive intimal flap, an arteriovenous fistula, or a pseudoaneurysm may not be associated with a decrease in the ABI. In these situations a heightened clinical suspicion based on mechanism of injury and anatomic location of injury is instrumental in pursuing further diagnostic testing (Fig. 23.4).

23.6 Diagnostic Imaging

23.6.1 Selective Contrast Angiography

Mandatory surgical exploration of "proximity" extremity wounds was largely abandoned in the 1970s in favor of less invasive vascular

Fig. 23.4 Diagnostic algorithm for lower extremity vascular injury

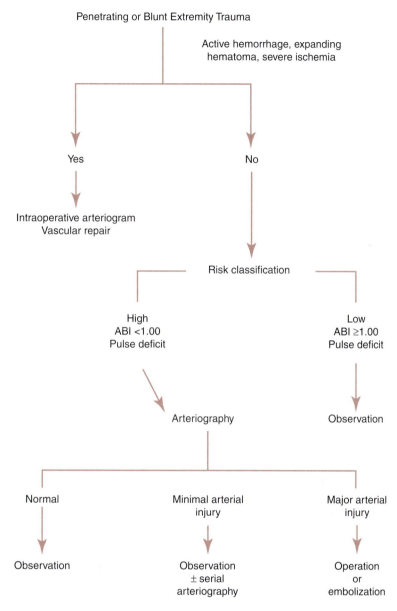

Penetrating or Blunt Extremity Trauma

Active hemorrhage, expanding hematoma, severe ischemia

Yes

No

Intraoperative arteriogram
Vascular repair

Risk classification

High
ABI <1.00
Pulse deficit

Low
ABI ≥1.00
Pulse deficit

Arteriography

Observation

Normal

Minimal arterial
injury

Major arterial
injury

Observation

Observation
± serial
arteriography

Operation
or
embolization

imaging [18]. Angiography has a sensitivity of >95 % and specificity of >90 % in detecting arterial injury [19]. In addition, diagnostic angiography- and combined with catheter-based intervention has emerged as a valuable treatment option in certain situations such as active hemor-

rhage, pseudoaneurysm, occlusion, and AV fistula in both blunt and penetrating injuries. On the other hand, angiography is invasive and has many well-recognized complications including puncture site complications, contrast nephropathy, allergic reactions, and remote vessel injury.

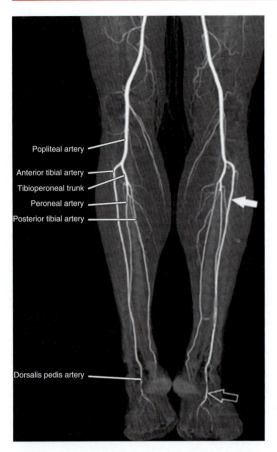

Popliteal artery

Anterior tibial artery

Tibioperoneal trunk

Peroneal artery

Posterior tibial artery

Dorsalis pedis artery

Fig. 23.5 CTA imaging of normal infrapopliteal arteries. The *solid arrow* indicates a dominant anterior tibial artery and the *open arrow* shows the dorsalis pedis artery at the ankle

23.6.2 Computed Tomographic Angiography

Multi-slice helical computed tomographic angiography (CTA) has been increasingly used in the evaluation of lower extremity vascular injuries in major trauma centers [20]. Major improvements in CT technology and its widespread availability have resulted in considerable reduction in the use of catheter-based angiography in the evaluation of extremity trauma (Fig. 23.5). CTA provides a rapid, noninvasive diagnostic tool that provides three-dimensional information regarding arterial injury as well as other soft tissue and bone injuries in the same anatomic region. The sensitivity and specificity of CTA for extremity vascular trauma has been demonstrated to be in excess of 95 % for both penetrating and blunt injuries to large proximal vessels [21].

Despite widespread use in the evaluation of trauma patients, there are a number of disadvantages associated with CTA that must be considered in evaluating potential injuries to the small arteries of the lower leg. Errors in timing and dose of the contrast bolus may result in inadequate visualization of the tibial vessels. Spasm associated with shock and hypothermia may further limit the adequate visualization of the distal vasculature. In addition, care must be taken to provide continuous monitoring of ventilation and hemodynamics during transport and transfer since the patient may be relatively inaccessible in the event of sudden clinical deterioration. Despite these disadvantages, CTA continues to gain widespread use in the evaluation of vascular extremity trauma.

23.6.3 Duplex Ultrasonography

Duplex ultrasonography (DUS) combines color flow Doppler ultrasound with conventional ultrasound to render high resolution imaging of vascular structures. The combination of the two modalities allows for the identification and imaging of specific arterial and venous structures. Duplex ultrasonography has been shown to be a reliable method of diagnosis in patients with potential vascular injuries and has been incorporated into a variety of trauma protocols. Sensitivity and specificity of duplex ultrasound in the evaluation of extremity vascular injury have been reported as high as 95 % with overall accuracy between 96 and 98 % [22, 23].

There are several advantages that make DUS an attractive option for evaluating vascular injury. It is noninvasive and painless, can be performed in the trauma resuscitation area, and is easily repeated. It provides information regarding the character of arterial flow, identification of active hemorrhage, dissection, pseudoaneurysm, and AV fistula. In addition, duplex ultrasound has the benefit of allowing interrogation of the venous system which frequently harbors occult injury [24].

Despite the aforementioned advantages of DUS, there are several important disadvantages and clinical situations where it may not be appropriate. DUS is highly operator dependent and may not be immediately available depending on local resources. It may not be possible to perform a complete arterial evaluation of an injured lower extremity due to overlying bandages or external fixation. Lastly, the inability of the patient to cooperate with the study due to pain, open wounds, or impaired state may limit the effectiveness of DUS. If any of these situations negatively impacts the performance of the DUS, then alternative imaging will be required.

23.7 Initial Management

Management can be organized by indication: hemorrhage, ischemia, and proximity. For patients with hemorrhage from extremity vascular injury, immediate surgical exploration is indicated. For patients with other hard signs of vascular injury, expeditious transfer to an operating room for image-directed surgical repair is appropriate. In the patient with soft signs of arterial injury or an abnormal ABI <0.9, additional imaging to identify arterial injury is recommended. In the setting of ischemia, despite the widely published recommendation that blood flow must be restored within 6 h of injury to avoid permanent ischemic injury, there is no absolute time limit beyond which vascular repair is absolutely contraindicated [25]. The degree of clinical ischemia is dependent on a number of factors in addition to the absolute duration of warm ischemia including the adequacy of collateral circulation, the presence of simultaneous venous obstruction, and overall hemodynamic stability. The vascular surgeon must take these factors into consideration in determining the optimal timing of surgical intervention.

Special discussion of the patient with suspected vascular injury in the association with fracture or dislocation is warranted. In the patient with a displaced fracture, the pulse and ABI should be determined both before and after orthopedic manipulation. If orthopedic manipu-

lation preserves or restores a normal palpable pulse and ABI, additional imaging is probably unnecessary. If orthopedic manipulation is not accompanied by preservation or prompt restoration of normal distal perfusion, then additional vascular management is based on the severity and duration of ischemia. Direct communication between the orthopedic and vascular surgeon is critical in this setting to determine the optimal sequence of operative events. In most cases in the absence of profound ischemia (e.g., audible but abnormal Doppler signal at the foot), the orthopedic procedure should be completed prior to vascular reconstruction. If external fixation is selected, the orthopedic and vascular teams must coordinate the location of the orthopedic hardware to allow surgical exposure of the vascular injury. This usually entails placement of orthopedic hardware along the lateral aspect of the lower leg to allow medial exposure of the tibial vessels. Fracture fixation prior to vascular repair has the benefit of providing superior stability of the vascular repair and assures that the vascular reconstruction will not be compromised when the fracture is distracted and realigned.

Early restoration of blood flow prior to orthopedic fixation is appropriate in patients with profound ischemia (absence of Doppler signal and significant motor/sensory deficit) particularly if the period of warm ischemia will exceed 4–6 h. In selected cases, an intraluminal shunt can be used to temporarily restore arterial flow during orthopedic manipulation. The technique of emergency vascular shunting is relatively straightforward. We prefer to use an outlying (30 cm) Sundt shunt that is designed with conical shoulders at each end to prevent dislodgement. We prefer to secure the shunt in place with umbilical tape tourniquets or large "vessel loops" which are nearly universally available. Flow through the shunt should be demonstrated with Doppler. Venous shunts are usually unnecessary and occasionally meddlesome. In general, we recommend formal vascular repair immediately after the orthopedic procedure is completed although prolonged use of a temporary shunt for more than 24 h has been reported.

23.8 Operative Preparation

The operating team should be prepared for unanticipated events. Special instruments for arterial repair including fluoroscopy should be available. The patient should be positioned on a table that is suitable for fluoroscopic imaging. The room should be arranged to accommodate additional equipment including cell saver and imaging equipment. Preoperative antibiotics with gram-positive coverage should be administered prior to skin incision. Additional gram-negative coverage should be administered if there are associated fractures. The injured lower extremity should be draped and prepped widely taking into consideration a proximal point that may be required to obtain arterial control or provide inflow for bypass. The contralateral leg should also be prepped into the field in the event that the contralateral greater saphenous vein (GSV) or deep femoral vein is required for arterial reconstruction.

23.8.1 Surgical Treatment

The initial step in surgical management is to obtain proximal control prior to exposure of the arterial injury. In general, proximal control should be established as close to the injury as possible without risking hemorrhage due to inadvertent entry into the injury site. Initial proximal control at the level of the common femoral artery will usually prevent life-threatening exsanguination from an extremity vascular injury, but will not provide sufficient hemostasis to allow completion of the arterial repair. The above-knee popliteal artery is exposed through a medial incision and retraction of the sartorius and vastus medialis muscles. For more distal injuries, proximal control of the below-knee popliteal artery is appropriate. Exposure is obtained through an 8–10 cm incision located a fingerbreadth behind the tibia followed by posterior retraction of the medial head of the gastrocnemius. The popliteal vein should be retracted toward the table to expose the artery and to avoid injury to the tibial nerve. Temporary proximal control using an extremity tourniquet is an acceptable alternative. The tourniquet should be deflated when conventional vascular control is obtained.

In the absence of a contraindication such as intracranial hemorrhage, extensive soft tissue injury, or intra-abdominal solid organ fracture, we prefer to administer systemic intravenous heparin (50 units/kg) during the period of vascular occlusion. Local instillation of dilute heparinized saline (1 unit/cc) into the inflow and outflow vessels is a satisfactory alternative if the risk of systemic anticoagulation is thought to be excessive. In either case, the surgeon should be prepared to use a Fogarty embolectomy catheter at the completion of the procedure to assure complete clearance of thrombus from the runoff.

Once proximal control is obtained, the area of injury can be directly exposed. Care should be taken to avoid overly aggressive dissection to prevent iatrogenic vascular injury. The following principles apply to all vascular injuries below the knee:

1. Vascular repairs should be tension-free. With the exception of the popliteal artery, primary repair is not usually possible for injuries that require resection of even very short vessel segments. Interposition vein graft should be considered if there is any concern that the reconstruction will be under excessive tension.
2. Debride all devitalized tissue. This is particularly important for arteries that have been crushed or injured by high-velocity bullets. To the degree possible, it is best to resect all injured artery until normal endothelium is visualized.
3. The completed arterial repair should replicate, as much as feasible, normal arterial anatomy. It is axiomatic that the arterial repair should not be stenotic, but it is equally important to avoid an excessively patulous repair that simulates the flow through an aneurysm. An overly large patch or a poor-size match between a small artery and larger vein can create turbulent flow patterns that increase the risk of thrombosis.
4. Adequate exposure is critical to performing a satisfactory vascular repair, and the surgeon is encouraged to extend the incision as needed.
5. Interrupted sutures reduce the risk of creating a stenotic repair due to "purse-stringing" a running suture.
6. Completion angiography is recommended.

23.8.1.1 Popliteal Artery and Vein

Injury to the popliteal artery up to 1 cm in length can usually be primarily repaired using fine monofilament suture (5-0 or 6-0 polypropylene). Loss of more than a centimeter in length usually requires an interposition graft. While synthetic grafts may be occasionally appropriate to avoid the delay associated with vein harvest, they are vulnerable to infection and are associated with inferior long-term patency in comparison to autogenous conduit.

Ligation of the popliteal vein may be associated with significant symptoms of venous obstruction [2]. In the setting of simple laceration, primary repair is easily accomplished, adds only minutes to the operation, and has the potential to preserve normal venous hemodynamics. More complex popliteal vein procedures including bypass are associated with a substantial risk of thrombosis. Ligation of the popliteal vein should almost always be an indication for four-compartment fasciotomy.

23.8.1.2 Tibial Vessels

Simple ligation of isolated injury to the PT, AT, or peroneal artery is usually well tolerated. We prefer to preserve at least two patent tibial vessels at the completion of the procedure even though viability of the foot is almost always assured if even one distal pulse can be established [26, 27]. If the patient is hemodynamically stable and vascular reconstruction will not unduly delay surgical treatment of other urgent injures (e.g., orthopedic), then we prefer to repair even isolated injuries to the AT or PT. Isolated injury to the peroneal artery is usually best treated by ligation. In extensive injuries to the lower leg that interrupt all three tibial vessels, flow in at least one tibial vessel should be restored.

The type of arterial repair is determined by the extent of arterial injury discovered at the time of exploration (Fig. 23.6). Focal lacerations, such as those seen most commonly in penetrating

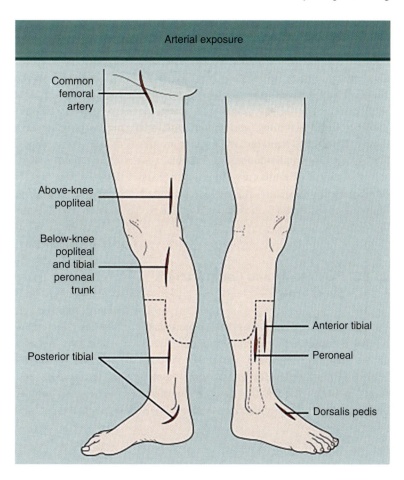

Fig. 23.6 Common incisions for infrapopliteal arterial exposure

injuries, without extensive arterial loss of length can generally be repaired either primarily or with the use of vein patch angioplasty.

In the setting of a longer arterial injury that precludes tension-free primary repair, vein graft interposition or bypass is recommended. The arterial anastomosis should be performed under magnification with fine polypropylene sutures. Completion angiography should be performed in the operating room to evaluate the reconstruction and confirm the adequacy distal perfusion.

23.8.2 Intravascular Shunts

Intravascular shunts have become a popular means of re-establishing temporary distal arterial flow in extremity vascular injuries primarily as a result of wartime trauma experience. Shunts have been shown to be an excellent means of providing distal perfusion following battlefield injury when there is an anticipated delay in definitive vascular repair and reperfusion [7]. Shunts placed in the proximal arteries above the knee have higher patency than shunts placed in the smaller arteries below the knee (86 % vs. 12 %). There appears to be a positive relationship between arterial and venous shunt use and the need for fasciotomy and amputation, but these data included a mixture of vascular injuries [28]. Due to the small diameter of the tibial vessels, the benefit of temporary shunting in distal infrapopliteal vascular injuries is limited. Shunting is discussed in a dedicated chapter of this textbook.

23.8.3 Fasciotomy and Compartment Syndrome

Decompression of compartmental hypertension has been recognized as an important component of the treatment of lower extremity vascular injuries. The lower leg consists of four compartments including the anterior, lateral, superficial posterior, and deep posterior compartments.

Reperfusion may result in rapid tissue swelling that initially obstructs venous outflow and eventually compromises arterial inflow. The risk of compartment syndrome is related to the duration and severity of ischemia, presence of venous outflow obstruction, extent of direct soft tissue trauma, as well as overall hemodynamic instability. Peripheral nerves are particularly sensitive to increased compartment pressures. Four-compartment fasciotomy should be considered in most cases of extremity vascular trauma with a period of prolonged ischemia, particularly in patients with venous outflow obstruction. The most common consequence of untreated compartment syndrome is peripheral nerve palsy resulting in an insensate limb as well as possible paralysis. Muscle necrosis can occur in severe cases of delayed decompression.

The indications for prophylactic fasciotomy (absence of compartment syndrome) in lower extremity injury include profound ischemia of greater than 4–6 h duration, combined arterial and venous injury, prolonged shock, venous ligation, and extensive soft tissue and skeletal injury (Fig. 23.7).

There are two options for performing four-compartment fasciotomy: one-incision and the two-incision techniques. The goal of both techniques is to incise the investing fascia of each muscle compartment of the lower leg to lower intracompartmental pressure both immediately and for future possible swelling. The one-incision technique is performed through a single 15–20 cm incision over the anterior compartment. The fascia over the anterior and lateral compartments is exposed and incised longitudinally to completely decompress both compartments. The posterior superficial compartment is entered just posterior to the fibula. The deep posterior compartment requires that the soleus muscle be released from the bony attachment.

The two-incision technique of fasciotomy is performed through medial and lateral incisions on the lower leg (Fig. 23.7). The anterior and lateral compartments are decompressed through the lateral incision, and the posterior

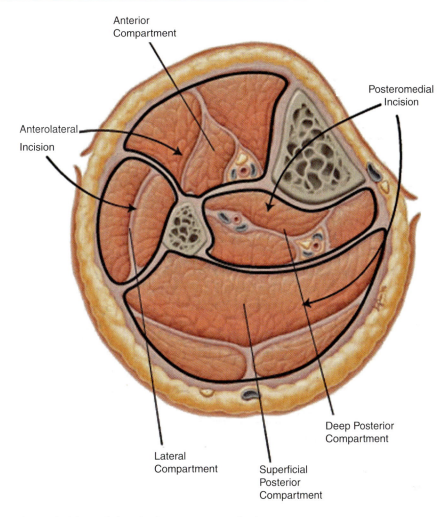

Fig. 23.7 The two-incision technique for four-compartment fasciotomy

superficial and deep compartments are entered through the medial incision. Details on fasciotomy can be found in the dedicated chapter in this textbook.

23.8.4 Endovascular Treatment

Endovascular treatment of vascular injuries has gained wide acceptance for a variety of injuries such as blunt aortic injuries, pelvis venous injuries, and control of hemorrhage in vascular beds that are difficult to expose. The use of endovas-

cular techniques in the treatment of vascular injuries below the knee is generally limited to coil embolization of nonessential arteries for hemorrhage and exclusion of pseudoaneurysms, and AV fistulas. Endografts are generally not appropriate in the small vessels below the knee. Recanalization of acutely occluded distal arteries is possible, but the potential scenarios in which this would be applicable are limited. This limitation is due in part to the nature of distal vascular injuries most of which are highly accessible for surgical approach. Further, there are very few options available for covered stents in the diameter range suitable for infrapopliteal artery treatment. Other possible applications of an endovascular adjunct are to establish proximal control using a catheter-directed intraluminal balloon and coil embolization of a feeder vessel prior to orthopedic repair of an adjacent fracture.

Access to the infrapopliteal arteries may be accomplished through a variety of access points in the arterial tree. The arterial cannulation site can be any patent vessel that is in continuity with the site of planned intervention. However, the access must be within the available delivery lengths of the endovascular devices necessary to successfully treat the arterial injury. Common access sites for treatment of infrapopliteal injuries include retrograde cannulation of the contralateral common femoral artery and an "up and over" approach to the opposite lower extremity, antegrade cannulation of the ipsilateral common femoral artery, and retrograde access through the pedal arteries at the ankle.

Retrograde and antegrade femoral access is commonly achieved by direct single-wall arterial puncture technique. In obese patients or those with hypotension in whom femoral pulses are not easily palpable, ultrasound guidance is recommended to avoid additional arterial injury. Following successful access to the contralateral CFA, a guide wire is passed across the bifurcation followed by a crossover sheath. Antegrade puncture of the ipsilateral CFA must be planned carefully, as inadvertent direct puncture of the SFA or PFA may increase the risk of puncture site occlusive complications.

23.8.5 Tibiopedal Retrograde Access

Tibiopedal retrograde access (TRA) has gained favor in the endovascular suite as an alternative technique to cross lower extremity atherosclerotic occlusions with a wire. In this procedure, traditional access is initially obtained from the common femoral artery either ipsilateral or contralateral to an infrainguinal occlusion. Antegrade attempts to cross the occluded arterial segment may be unsuccessful due to fibrosis or

calcification. Subintimal techniques for crossing these occlusions from may be limited by severe arterial wall calcification, perforation, or extension of the subintimal plane too distal (beyond important collaterals). Reentry devices are valuable in the femoropopliteal artery, but none exist for tibial use. Consequently, retrograde techniques provide an alternative access to the vessel.

There are several methods to achieve retrograde access to the tibial arteries. The most basic approach involves a single proximal access site (either ipsilateral or contralateral common femoral artery) with catheter advanced to the infrainguinal region [28–31]. This first strategy requires a patent tibial artery and good collateral distal to the occluded tibial artery. A small catheter (2.4–2.8 Fr) is passed over a 0.014 in. flexible wire down the patent tibial artery, through the collateral, and then retrograde to the distal aspect of the tibial occlusion. Once the wire traverses the occlusion, then it can be brought out the sheath in a retrograde direction. Intervention can then proceed from the proximal access site over the externalized retrograde wire. A catheter could also be advanced through the occlusion over the retrograde wire before it is removed with antegrade replacement of the wire through the distally placed catheter.

The second strategy involves using two access sites, one from the common femoral artery and one from the distal tibial artery. The proximal access enables contrast injection for direct visualization of the tibial artery at the time of puncture. The distal puncture can also be performed after "road mapping" or using ultrasound guidance. After puncture, a 0.014 or 0.018 in. wire is advanced retrograde. A small dilator, sheath, or catheter can support the wire. After crossing the occlusion, the wire can be externalized through the proximal access with a snare or direct delivery of the wire into the sheath or catheter. Usually the largest, most accessible tibial artery is chosen, such as the anterior tibial artery or posterior tibial artery. The peroneal artery is accessed least frequently.

The third strategy utilizes a technique of dual balloon inflation and can be utilized in patients in which the occlusion cannot be crossed despite dual access. Small balloons (~2 mm diameter) disrupt the membrane between the two subintimal channels creating a communication enabling wire traversal and subsequent treatment of the occlusion.

Even with very experienced physicians, complications from TRA include arterial occlusion, dissection, and perforation. Radiation exposure of the operator's hands can be very significant since cannulation of the artery rarely is successful with one pass of the needle. The distal tibial artery can be further traumatized from sheath insertion, removal of winged balloons, or atheromatous embolization. The greatest challenge might be achieving hemostasis of the tibial artery puncture site after the intervention. Often just hand pressure is held over the site, but other options include use of a radial artery hemostatic band over the puncture site, inflation of a blood pressure cuff over the puncture site, and inflation of a small balloon delivered from a proximal sheath and inflated at the puncture site after sheath removal [29, 31].

Once access has been obtained to the vascular territory that has been injured, there are multiple options available. The treatment of acute hemorrhage or AV fistula may be accomplished by precise placement of appropriately sized coils, gel foam, or glue to cause thrombosis of the target vessel. Flow-limiting dissections can be treated by angioplasty and stent placement stabilizing the intraluminal septum to restore unimpeded distal flow, and pseudoaneurysms may be effectively treated with stent placement with or without trans-stent coil embolization of the pseudoaneurysm cavity. Each of these techniques requires advanced endovascular skills which should only be attempted by well-trained, experienced vascular specialists.

23.8.6 Primary Amputation

One of the most challenging decisions facing a surgeon is whether to perform a primary amputation after extremity trauma. There are a variety of assessment tools designed to quantitatively predict the viability of a severely injured lower extremity such as the Mangled Extremity Severity Score (MESS) [32]. This scoring system assigns values based on the severity of skeletal or soft tissue injury, limb ischemia, shock, and patient age. In a small study, a MESS score of 7 or greater accurately predicted limb loss in almost 100 % of patients. Unfortunately, there is not a scoring system that reliably contributes to the decision to perform primary amputation [32]. While such evaluation tools like MESS are helpful in the development of an organized assessment, the predictive value has been suspect in accurately predicting limb function outcomes except for those with very severe extremity injuries, and MESS should never be utilized as the sole deciding factor in amputation. Most vascular injuries below the knee are not isolated injuries. Long bone fractures, nerve injuries, and soft tissue injuries are commonly encountered as a result of both penetrating and blunt injuries. Input from vascular surgeons, trauma surgeons, plastic surgeons, and orthopedic surgeons is essential to provide the best possible assessment of viability of the injured extremity.

A warm ischemia time of greater than 6 h has long been felt to be the threshold for limb viability, beyond which there is an assumed increased incidence of limb loss. This time frame was established as the result of canine studies of hind limb ischemia by Miller et al. dating back to 1949 [33]. In this model, limb salvage decreased as ischemia time increased. Limb salvage for ischemia time less than 6 h was 90 %; for 12–24 h, the limb salvage rate was 50 %; and for greater than 24 h, the limb salvage rate was a less than 20 %. While these ischemic times are useful as a guide to management, strict reliance on these data should be avoided when contemplating primary amputation. The decision should be made based on a comprehensive evaluation of the degree of distal perfusion following vascular repair, the anticipated nerve deficit, and the perceived functional outcome following recovery. Re-establishment of perfusion to the distal extremity can be accomplished in most cases, but

.W. York and J.F. Eidt

the major determinants of functionality are the degree of nerve deficit as well as the extent of bone and soft tissue defect. In the event of a fixed insensate foot secondary to prolonged nerve ischemia or tissue loss to the degree that there is no potential for functional weight bearing and ambulation, serious consideration should be given to primary amputation.

23.8.7 Postoperative Management

Following vascular repair, patients should be monitored closely in an ICU acute care setting in order to monitor hemodynamic status, and perform serial vascular examinations with Doppler interrogation of distal perfusion to assess patency. The injured lower extremity should be maintained in an elevated position (>30°) if possible to decrease edema. This positioning is especially important in patients with open fasciotomy wounds as it decreases edema and soft tissue volume that can improve the chances of delayed primary closure.

Patients must also be carefully monitored for evidence of reperfusion injury following restoration of arterial flow to ischemic tissue. Release of oxygen free radicals and other products of cellular lysis may lead to metabolic acidosis, hypotension, cardiac arrhythmia, renal failure, multi-system organ failure, and death. Prompt administration of oxygen free radical scavengers such as mannitol, sodium bicarbonate, and heparin has been advocated to reduce the impact

of toxic radicals formed during periods of tissue anoxia. Prophylactic administration of mannitol and sodium bicarbonate is recommended prior to reperfusion of ischemia tissue.

23.8.8 Outcomes

The outcomes in terms of mortality and limb loss in infrapopliteal vascular trauma are based on the extent of associated nerve, bone, and soft tissue injuries (Fig. 23.8). In a recent report vascular injuries below the knee with less than two of these associated tissue injuries resulted in no amputations. However, if all three associated tissue injuries were present, limb loss was 54 % [34].

Proximal lower extremity vascular injuries have a higher mortality rate but decreased rate of limb loss, while distal lower arterial injuries have a lower mortality rate but increased frequency of amputation [35]. From the injury mechanism standpoint, popliteal or tibial injuries are twice as likely to require amputations if sustained secondary to blunt injury emphasizing that concomitant tissue injury significantly affects outcome of limb salvage [35].

23.8.9 Pitfalls and Pearls

The successful management of patients with extremity vascular injuries requires careful attention to the detail, meticulous technique, and

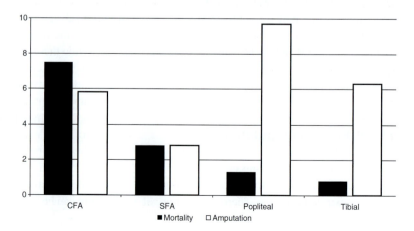

Fig. 23.8 Mortality and amputation rates (percentages) by most proximal vessel injured

seasoned judgment. Even the most capable of vascular surgeons has struggled to avoid the pitfalls that stand in the way of achieving the ideal clinical result for each patient. The most common challenges that face the surgeon can be divided into the evaluation, treatment, and posttreatment phases.

It is critical to obtain a detailed history of the events leading to the vascular injury. The description of the accident scene by the EMTs, such as the presence and quantity of blood, may provide important clues to the presence of an arterial injury. A history of vascular disease or peripheral intervention may have a significant impact on the selection of treatment options. A history of alcohol use may warrant prophylaxis against delirium tremens. Vasoactive drug injection (e.g., amphetamines) may complicate vascular repairs. In addition, the vascular surgeon must be wary of life-threatening nonvascular injuries (e.g., brain, abdominal solid organ, or cardiac) that may take priority over extremity injuries.

The physical exam should focus on identification of signs of vascular injury as well as assessment of other complicating systemic injuries. All peripheral pulses should be palpated and recorded along with any sensory or motor deficits before (and after) every orthopedic manipulation. Extremity deformity should be assessed. The ABI can serve as an important adjunct to the physical exam. While a normal ABI (>0.9) does not eliminate the possibility of a vascular injury, an abnormal ABI should generally be followed by appropriate imaging to define the presence and significance of vascular injuries. In patients with critical limb ischemia, the decision to further delay revascularization by obtaining vascular imaging in a radiology suite must be weighed against the harm of prolonged ischemia. Contrast angiography performed intraoperatively at the time of surgical exploration represents the most efficient method of evaluating the suspect arterial tree. CTA on the other hand allows evaluation of proximal extremity vessels as well as orthopedic and soft tissue injuries. CTA, and Imaging of the arteries below the knee may be inadequate due to timing of the contrast bolus. Ultrasound may be useful to evaluate isolated injuries and to detect simultaneous deep vein thrombosis but is often not available at night or weekends and may be limited by hematoma, orthopedic hardware, and patient cooperation.

The most important decision that the surgeon faces is the decision for surgical intervention. In many cases, a viable extremity even in the presence of a known vascular injury may be best treated without immediate surgery. The surgeon must weigh the risk of intervention against the risk of acute limb loss and/or the likelihood of long-term limb dysfunction. In the presence of a solitary pulse palpable in either the dorsalis pedis or posterior tibial artery and normal ABI, most injuries to isolated tribal vessels are best treated conservatively. Most pseudoaneurysms and arteriovenous connections can be treated electively.

In the operating room, the surgeon should prepare for the worst-case scenario rather than reacting after the fact. Most injured patients should be placed in the supine position, and both lower extremities including the groins should be draped to ensure availability of autogenous conduit (e.g., deep femoral or saphenous vein) and/or access sites for percutaneous angiography and intervention. One exception to this rule is isolated blunt injury to the popliteal artery. In patients with posterior dislocation of the knee, the injury to the popliteal artery (and vein) is almost invariably limited to the segment of the artery directly adjacent to the joint line. Many surgeons prefer to expose the popliteal artery through an S-shaped posterior incision after harvesting saphenous vein with the patient in the supine position. Injuries that involve the infrapopliteal trifurcation (origin of anterior tibial artery, tibioperoneal trunk, and origins of peroneal and posterior tibial artery) are notoriously difficult to expose due to the likelihood of concomitant venous and bone injury. There is a rich plexus of short, wide veins that must usually be divided to expose the proximal trifurcation. Use of a thigh-high pneumatic tourniquet can dramatically reduce the risk of blood loss in this sitting and decrease the chance of iatrogenic venous injury.

Meticulous attention to atraumatic vascular technique is critical in the management of distal extremity injury. Care should be taken to limit the handling of all injured blood vessels and veins with particular emphasis on avoiding direct injury to the endothelium. Fine interrupted sutures may be preferable to running sutures which can create circumferential stenosis if excessive tension is used during the anastomosis or tying the knot. Interrupted sutures also simplify the anastomosis in the setting of substantial size mismatch. Arteries in young healthy patients are more likely to spasm than atherosclerotic arteries in older patients. In addition, in most patients with isolated vascular trauma, systemic heparinization is appropriate. If there are concomitant injuries that preclude the safe use of systemic anticoagulation, liberal use of local heparin flush is usually effective in preventing thrombosis during the vascular repair. It is important to remember that while most vascular patients are on aspirin or other antiplatelet agents, the same is uncommon in trauma patients. Platelet aggregation at the site of vascular suture lines can result in vexing thrombosis. Some surgeons prefer to administer dextran to reduce the risk of platelet aggregation. It is useful to forward flush and back bleed inflow and outflow vessels vigorously, followed by irrigation with heparinized saline immediately before restoring flow.

In assessing the severity of the arterial injury, the surgeon must decide between primary repair and interposition grafting. One of the most common errors is persisting in attempts to perform a primary repair when a short interposition graft would be better. In most cases, the injured artery should be completely excised or bypassed rather than persisting in futile efforts at primary repair that risk thrombosis or disruption related to excessive tension on the arterial repair. Most surgeons prefer to use autogenous tissue for vascular repair in the setting of gross contamination because of the risk of synthetic graft infection. Synthetic grafts may be appropriate in the absence of suitable autogenous conduit (rare) or for expediency (common).

The adequacy of distal perfusion must be assessed after the arterial repair. A palpable pulse may not be immediately detected following restoration of arterial flow, but the Doppler signal should be significantly improved. On-table angiography to confirm the patency of the repair as well as distal runoff is strongly recommended. Distal embolism frequently accompanies proximal arterial injuries. Simple catheter thrombectomy is usually highly effective in retrieving fresh thrombus, but it should be noted that overly aggressive use of balloon thrombectomy can induce significant endothelial injury. Balloon trauma can result in severe vasospasm acutely and may be associated with intimal hyperplasia within the first few months following vascular repair.

Four-compartment fasciotomy should be considered in all patients with significant warm ischemia time prior to revascularization and in patients with concomitant venous injuries. Postoperatively the injured extremity should be elevated to reduce edema. Pulses and Doppler signals should be checked frequently during the first few hours to assure the durability of the repair. DVT prophylaxis should be employed. Prophylactic antibiotics should be used as in other vascular cases. Long-term follow-up should be arranged.

Conclusion

Vascular injuries below the knee present a difficult challenge to vascular surgeons due to the complex nature of injuries in this anatomic region. A multidisciplinary approach is vital in management as there are commonly associated nerve, bone, and soft tissue injuries all of which affect outcomes. There are several principles in the management of these injuries: (1) control of hemorrhage; (2) assess whether the injured limb is salvageable; (3) assess extent of vascular injury and degree of distal perfusion; (4) reassess distal perfusion following reduction of displaced fractures; (5) reconstruct or ligate injured arteries, if bleeding; and (6) recognize, prevent, and treat compartment syndrome and reperfusion injury.

References

1. Rich NM, Rhee P. An historical tour of vascular injury management: from its inception to the new millennium. Surg Clin North Am. 2001;81:1199–215.
2. Rich NM, Hobson RW, Collins Jr GJ, Andersen CA. The effect of acute popliteal venous interruption. Ann Surg. 1976;183:365–8.
3. Fox CJ, Gillespie DL, O'Donnell SD, Rasmussen TE, Goff JM, Johnson CA, et al. Contemporary management of wartime vascular trauma. J Vasc Surg. 2005;41:638–44.
4. Rich NM, Baugh JH, Hughes CW. Acute arterial injuries in Vietnam: 1,000 cases. J Trauma Acute Care Surg. 1970;10:359–69.
5. Markov NP, DuBose JJ, Scott D, Propper BW, Clouse WD, Thompson B, et al. Anatomic distribution and mortality of arterial injury in the wars in Afghanistan and Iraq with comparison to a civilian benchmark. J Vasc Surg. 2012;56:728–36.
6. Rasmussen TE, Clouse WD, Jenkins DH, Peck MA, Eliason JL, Smith DL. The use of temporary vascular shunts as a damage control adjunct in the management of wartime vascular injury. J Trauma Acute Care Surg. 2006;61:8–15.
7. Rasmussen TE, DuBose JJ, Asensio JA, Feliciano DV, Fox CJ, Nuñez TC, et al. Tourniquets, vascular shunts, and endovascular technologies: esoteric or essential? A report from the 2011 AAST Military Liaison Panel. J Trauma Acute Care Surg. 2012;73:282–5.
8. Starnes BW, Beekley AC, Sebesta JA, Andersen CA, Rush RMJ. Extremity vascular injuries on the battlefield: tips for surgeons deploying to war. J Trauma Acute Care Surg. 2006;60:432–42. doi:10.1097/01.ta.0000197628.55757.de.
9. Oller DW, Rutledge R, Clancy T, Cunningham P, Thomason M, Meredith W, et al. Vascular injuries in a rural state: a review of 978 patients from a state trauma registry. J Trauma. 1992;32:740–5; discussion 745–6.
10. Kauvar D, Sarfati M, Kraiss L. National trauma database analysis of mortality and limb loss in isolated lower extremity vascular trauma. J Vasc Surg. 2011;53:1598–603.
11. Moniz M, Ombrellaro M, Stevens S, Freeman M, Diamond D, Goldman M. Concomitant orthopedic and vascular injuries as predictors for limb loss in blunt lower extremity trauma. Am Surg. 1997;63:24–8.
12. de Mestral C, Sharma S, Haas B, Gomez D, Nathens AB. A contemporary analysis of the management of the mangled lower extremity. J Trauma Acute Care Surg. 2013;74:597–603. doi:10.1097/TA.0b013e31827a05e3.
13. Frykberg ER, Dennis JW, Bishop K, Laneve L, Alexander RH. The reliability of physical examination in the evaluation of penetrating extremity trauma for vascular injury: results at one year. J Trauma. 1991;31:502–11.
14. Percival TJ, Rasmussen TE. Reperfusion strategies in the management of extremity vascular injury with ischaemia. Br J Surg. 2012;99:66–74.
15. Lynch K, Johansen K. Can Doppler pressure measurement replace "exclusion" arteriography in the diagnosis of occult extremity arterial trauma. Ann Surg. 1991;214:737.
16. Johansen K, Lynch K, Paum M, Copass M. Non-invasive vascular tests reliably exclude occult arterial trauma in injured extremities. J Trauma. 1991;31:515–9.
17. Vogel T, Furkovich G. Injuries to the peripheral blood vessels. In: Soba WW, editor. ACS general surgery principles and practice. 6th ed. New York: WebMD Professional Publishing; 2007. p. 1400.
18. Kendall RW, Taylor DC, Salvian AJ, O'Brien PJ. The role of arteriography in assessing vascular injuries associated with dislocations of the knee. J Trauma. 1993;35:875–8.
19. Fox N, Rajani RR, Bokhari F, Chiu WC, Kerwin A, Seamon MJ, et al. Evaluation and management of penetrating lower extremity arterial trauma: an Eastern Association for the Surgery of Trauma practice management guideline. J Trauma Acute Care Surg. 2012;73:S315–20.
20. Peng PD, Spain DA, Tataria M, Hellinger JC, Rubin GD, Brundage SI. CT angiography effectively evaluates extremity vascular trauma. Am Surg. 2008;74:103–7.
21. Soto JA, Múnera F, Morales C, Lopera JE, Holguín D, Guarín O, et al. Focal arterial injuries of the proximal extremities: helical CT arteriography as the initial method of diagnosis1. Radiology. 2001;218:188–94.
22. Bynoe RP, Miles WS, Bell RM, Greenwold DR, Sessions G, Haynes JL, et al. Noninvasive diagnosis of vascular trauma by duplex ultrasonography. J Vasc Surg. 1991;14:346–52.
23. Kuzniec S, Kauffman P, Molnár LJ, Aun R, Puech-Leão P. Diagnosis of limbs and neck arterial trauma using duplex ultrasonography. Cardiovasc Surg. 1998;6:358–66.
24. Gagne PJ, Cone JB, McFarland D, Troillett R, Bitzer LG, Vitti MJ, et al. Proximity penetrating extremity trauma: the role of duplex ultrasound in the detection of occult venous injuries. J Trauma Acute Care Surg. 1995;39:1157–63.
25. Menzoian JO, Doyle JE, LoGerfo FW, Cantelmo N, Weitzman AF, Sequiera JC. Evaluation and management of vascular injuries of the extremities. Arch Surg. 1983;118:93–5.
26. Scalea TM, DuBose J, Moore EE, West M, Moore FA, McIntyre R, et al. Western Trauma Association critical decisions in trauma: management of the mangled extremity. J Trauma Acute Care Surg. 2012;72:86–93. doi:10.1097/TA.0b013e318241ed70.
27. Shah DM, Corson JD, Karmody AM, Fortune JB, Leather RP. Optimal management of tibial arterial trauma. J Trauma. 1988;28:228–34.

28. Montero-Baker M, Schmidt A, Bräunlich S, Ulrich M, Thieme M, Biamino G, et al. Retrograde approach for complex popliteal and tibioperoneal occlusions. J Endovasc Ther. 2008;15:594–604.
29. Fusaro M, Tashani A, Mollichelli N, Medda M, Inglese L, Biondi-Zoccai GG. Retrograde pedal artery access for below-the-knee percutaneous revascularisation. J Cardiovasc Med. 2007;8:216–8.
30. Rogers RK, Dattilo PB, Garcia JA, Tsai T, Casserly IP. Retrograde approach to recanalization of complex tibial disease. Catheter Cardiovasc Interv. 2011;77:915–25.
31. Zhuang K, Tan S, Tay K. The "SAFARI" technique using retrograde access via peroneal artery access. Cardiovasc Intervent Radiol. 2012;35:927–31.
32. Johansen K, Daines M, Howey T, Helfet D, Hansen ST. Objective criteria accurately predict amputation following lower extremity trauma. J Trauma. 1990;30:568–72; discussion 572–3.
33. Miller HH, Welch CS. Quantitative studies on the time factor in arterial injuries. Ann Surg. 1949;130:318–438.
34. Whitman GR, McCroskey BL, Moore EE, Pearce WH, Moore FA. Traumatic popliteal and trifurcation vascular injuries: determinants of functional limb salvage. Am J Surg. 1987;154:681–4.
35. Kauvar DS, Sarfati MR, Kraiss LW. National trauma databank analysis of mortality and limb loss in isolated lower extremity vascular trauma. J Vasc Surg. 2011;53(6):1598–603.

subsequent to reperfusion secondary to the release of breakdown products from injured cells. Cell and tissue edema develops, resulting in an increase in pressure within the compartment which is limited by its fascial encasement. It is also theorized that reperfusion can result in the development of venous thrombosis secondary to procoagulant release from necrotic tissue. This thrombosis then spreads from the necrotic tissue to the marginal zones of perfusion, leading to further muscle necrosis, release of inflammatory mediators, and propagation of the cycle of increased pressure and necrosis [9]. The amount of pressure increases, and the duration of its presence affects the amount of tissue injury which occurs. Canine models have demonstrated that prolonged elevation of pressures, as well as the degree of pressure elevation within the compartment contributed to decreased nerve conduction velocities, consistent with the effects of ischemia [10].

Recognition of compartment syndrome is the first crucial step in treatment of the affected extremity. The longer the diagnosis of compartment syndrome goes unrecognized, and the compartment pressure is allowed to rise, the more significant the nerve and muscle damage and subsequent necrosis. If discovered early in its course, significant tissue damage can be prevented. Treatment of compartment syndrome requires fasciotomy of the affected compartments. Prophylactic fasciotomies should also be considered in the setting of significant ischemia (greater than 4–6 h), in the setting of combined orthopedic and vascular injuries, or in a patient with whom there is significant concern for the development of compartment syndrome, where monitoring of the compartment may be difficult [2]. The most common locations for development of compartment syndrome are the calf and forearm, though compartment syndrome can develop in the thigh, foot, and hand as well [11]. Lower extremity fasciotomy begins with recognition that there are four compartments which require decompression: anterior, lateral, superficial posterior, and deep posterior. The anterior compartment is most often affected and, with ischemia to the superficial peroneal nerve, results in the

classically described paresthesias in the web space between the first and second toes. Although there are a variety of techniques in performing fasciotomy of the lower extremity, the gold standard is a two-incision, four-compartment fasciotomy. The anterior and lateral compartments are released from an anterior lateral incision. The medial incision will decompress the deep posterior and superficial posterior muscle compartments [12]. Release of the fascia overlying the muscles of affected compartments will reveal a bulging of the affected muscles which should be evaluated for necrosis and debrided as indicated. Skin incisions are left open, with the use of either a negative pressure dressing or moist gauze dressings, with a goal of delayed primary closure once the edema has resolved. If the patient is unable to undergo delayed primary closure, a split thickness skin graft is often used for closure.

Fasciotomy is not a benign procedure, with postoperative complications including infection, nerve injury, chronic pain, and disfiguring wounds. Despite this, failure to perform fasciotomy when needed is perhaps the most feared complication. Eight hours after onset of total ischemia, irreversible muscle and peripheral nerve damage exists [13]. Patients who require revision of fasciotomies or performance of delayed fasciotomies were associated with higher rates of muscle excision, amputation, and mortality. Casualties from the Iraq and Afghanistan campaigns, who underwent delayed fasciotomy, were shown to have had twice the rate of amputation and a threefold increase in mortality. Increase in myonecrosis puts the patient at increased risk of infection as well as increased risk of acute kidney injury from rhabdomyolysis [14].

24.3 Medical Management Considerations in Blunt Thoracic Aortic Injury

Blunt thoracic aortic injury (BTAI) is the second leading cause of death from blunt trauma after head injury [15]. BTAIs have been associated with falls from heights, auto vs. pedestrian accidents, and motorcycle crashes. By far, however, the most common cause of blunt thoracic aortic injury is motor vehicle crashes, which account for more than 70 % of such injuries. The incidence of BTAI increases with age and is rarely seen in the pediatric population [16]. The overall incidence of patients with these injuries who survive to receive hospital care is less than 0.5 % [17], while the actual incidence of BTAI is much higher [18]. In fact, an autopsy study of 304 deaths from traffic accidents in Los Angeles County found that 33 % of patients had a rupture of the thoracic aorta. Eighty percent of these deaths occurred at the scene, and only 20 % reached the hospital prior to death [19]. For those who survive to reach hospital care, prompt diagnosis and aggressive management of blood pressure are critical in preventing free rupture of the previously contained aortic rupture. The most common location for aortic injury is the medial aspect of the lumen, just distal to the left subclavian artery, often referred to as the aortic isthmus. Injury to the aortic isthmus is found in about 93 % of hospital admissions with BTAI and 80 % of autopsy studies [18]. In terms of the injury type, the most common is creation of a false aneurysm (58 %), aortic dissection (25 %), and intimal tear (20 %) [17].

Although CT angiography is now the gold standard in diagnosing BTAI with both a sensitivity and negative predictive value approaching 100 %, there are classically described findings on initial chest x-ray which may increase the suspicions of the care team [20]. These findings include a widened mediastinum, obliteration of the aortic knob, loss of perivertebral pleural stripe, depression of the left mainstem bronchus, deviation of a nasogastric tube to the right, a left apical pleural hematoma ("apical cap"), and a massive left hemothorax. The presence of fractures of the clavicle, upper ribs, scapula, or sternum are markers for increased risk of BTAI [18].

Patients with active extravasation from an aortic injury require immediate operation. Starnes et al. demonstrated that hypotension at the time of presentation to the emergency department, loss of vital signs prior to arrival, as well as rupture as the type of injury were predictive of death secondary to BTAI [21]. Most patients who survive to hospital care have a contained aortic injury. The goal in management of these patients is preventing free rupture via aggressive blood pressure control. Ninety percent of ruptures will occur within the first 24 h of injury [18]. Because of this, immediate repair of all aortic injuries was the standard of care for many years. Recent studies have demonstrated that with strict blood pressure control, the majority of these injuries could be repaired in a delayed fashion [22, 23]. With blood pressure control, the risk of rupture is 1.5 %/h; without control of blood pressure, the risk remains at 12 % [24]. In 2007 the results of the American Association for the Surgery of Trauma prospective study demonstrated a significantly higher mortality in the early repair group vs. delayed repair with an adjusted odds ratio of 7.78, 95 % CI 1.69–35.7, $p = 0.008$. This study also confirmed prior studies which demonstrated that despite lower mortality, delayed repair was associated with significantly longer ICU and hospital length of stay [25].

The medical management of BTAI is derived primarily from the management of nontraumatic aortic dissections. The goals of antihypertensive therapy in the management of aortic injury are to prevent further dissection or free rupture of the injury. This frequently is referred to as anti-impulse control, which is lessening the pulsatile load, or aortic stress (dP/dT), in order to slow the propagation of the injury and prevent rupture [26]. Propagation of aortic injury is thought to be not only secondary to elevated blood pressure itself, but on the velocity of the left ventricular contraction [26]. For this reason, optimal therapy is considered to consist of a beta-blocker, with the addition of a vasodilator for refractory hypertension. Contraindications to medical management in addition to evidence of free rupture include impaired perfusion to the gastrointestinal tract or legs and the inability to control hypertension despite medical treatment [27]. Goals for therapy are a heart rate of 55–65 beats per minute and systolic blood pressure 100–120 mmHg, or as low as the patient can tolerate [28].

The foundation of anti-impulse therapy begins with the use of beta-blockers. Esmolol is the preferred drug as it has rapid onset and a short half-life, making it easily titratable. Its onset of action is less than 60 s, and short half-life contributes to duration of action between 10 and 20 min. Esmolol is a pure β1 receptor blocker, which, in addition to decreasing blood pressure through an inotropic effect, has a chronotropic effect of decreased heart rate [29]. Labetalol has a longer half-life than esmolol and therefore has a longer duration of action. It has a slower onset of action, 2–5 min, but longer duration of action, peaking at 5–15 min and lasting 2–4 h. Labetalol blocks both α and β receptors, thereby affecting blood pressure and contractility. Although labetalol does have a negative chronotropic effect secondary to the blocking of β receptors, it does not decrease the heart rate as substantially as esmolol, making labetalol a better choice for patients who present with lower heart rates [29]. Propranolol and metoprolol are beta-blockers which are not recommended in the acute phase of treatment. They have a longer duration of action (6–8 h), and there is no way to quickly reverse the beta-blockade should the patient go into shock. These are good choices of treatment in the subacute phase when they can be given as additional boluses as the patient is transitioned to oral regimens [29].

Vasodilators are good adjuncts to beta-blocker therapy when multidrug therapy is required for blood pressure control. Sodium nitroprusside is a potent vasodilator of both the arterial and venous systems. It has a long history of use in management of hypertensive crisis and aortic dissection. It has a rapid onset of action and a half-life of 3–4 min. It does however require close monitoring and requires frequent dose adjustments. Nitroprusside also increases intracranial pressure and in the trauma population is often contraindicated for this reason. It has also been associated with coronary steal, decreased oxygen circulation, and reflex tachycardia. For these reasons and the risk of cyanide toxicity, nitroprusside should only be used as a medication of last resort [28].

In lieu of nitroprusside, many advocate for the use of fenoldopam. Fenoldopam is a dopamine-1 agonist and selective arteriolar/renal dilator. It has a rapid onset and short duration of action (half-life 5 min). It has been shown to increase creatinine clearance and does not exhibit coronary steal. Fenoldopam can however produce reflex tachycardia and EKG changes including nonspecific T-wave changes. After long-term infusion, it produces a mild tolerance [28].

Nicardipine is a dihydropyridine calcium channel blocker. It causes relaxation of the arterial smooth muscle resulting in peripheral vasodilation and resultant blood pressure reduction. Nicardipine causes cerebral and coronary vasodilation with minimal negative inotropic or chronotropic effect and has been shown in cardiac surgery patients to have little effect on ventricular preload or cardiac output. It is easily and rapidly titratable, and it has minimal effect on the atrioventricular nodal conduction. Oxygen delivery to the cells is maintained, and there is no effect on oxygen requirements. An added benefit is that nicardipine is metabolized by the liver and is therefore safe to use in patients with renal insufficiency. As a calcium channel blocker, it is also useful in patients with COPD and asthma where β-blockade may be contraindicated [28].

Non-dihydropyridines such as verapamil or diltiazem have fallen out of favor over the last several years. The non-dihydropyridine group functions via strong chronotropic and inotropic effects, with minimal effect on the systemic blood pressure. It is the large effect on decreasing cardiac contractility which has made them a less commonly used class of drugs in the treatment of hypertension in the face of blunt thoracic aortic injury [28, 29].

24.4 Critical Care Management of Blunt Cerebrovascular Injury

Blunt carotid injury (BCI) and blunt vertebral injuries have been collectively referred to as blunt cerebrovascular injuries (BCVI). Over the last two decades, significant advances in screening, diagnosis, and treatment of BCVI have occurred. Initial estimates predicted blunt carotid artery injury-associated mortality rates of 23 %, with 48 % of those survivors have significant permanent, severe neurologic sequela [30]. Advancements in the field of BCVI can largely be attributed to the institution of screening programs and resultant increase in diagnosis of initially asymptomatic patients. Initial estimates of suggested BCI rates of 0.1 % of blunt trauma victims admitted to trauma centers. With increased detection as a result of screening programs, the incidence has now been estimated between 0.4 and 1 % of all blunt trauma admissions [30].

Significant investigation has been put forth into the development of screening programs in the detection of BCVI. Early detection of injuries, while the patient remains asymptomatic, provides a window for intervention in hopes of preventing the subsequent morbidity and mortality associated with the occurrence of a stroke. Trauma patients who present with arterial hemorrhage from the neck, mouth, nose, or ears; large or expanding cervical hematomas; cervical bruits in a patient less than 50 years old; and focal or lateralizing neurologic defects including hemiparesis, transient ischemic attack, Horner's syndrome, oculosympathetic paresis, or vertebrobasilar insufficiency, or evidence of cerebral infarction on CT or MRI are presumed to have a BCVI until proved otherwise [30]. There is evidence to suggest that stroke rates are significantly lower in patients treated for BCVI, when compared with those untreated [31–33]. Furthermore, when screening is limited to the at-risk population, screening and treatment have been demonstrated to be cost effective [34]. The identification of a high-risk group prompting screening has gone through much debate and evolution over the last decade. Fundamental mechanisms associated with carotid artery injury include cervical hyperextension or hyperflexion with rotation and stretching of the carotid artery over the lateral articular processes of the cervical vertebral bodies C1–C3, direct cervical trauma, intraoral trauma, and basilar skull fracture involving the carotid canal [35, 36]. The vertebral artery is associated with cervical spine injuries, especially subluxations and fractures of the foramen transversarium [37]. Further analyses have suggested the following as high-risk factors for BCVI which

should prompt screening: injury mechanism compatible with severe cervical hyperextension with rotation or hyperflexion; Lefort II or III midface fractures; basilar skull fracture involving the carotid canal; closed head injury consistent with diffuse axonal injury with Glasgow Coma Scale score less than 6; cervical vertebral body or transverse foramen fracture, subluxation, or ligamentous injury at any level, or any C1–C3 level fracture; near-hanging resulting in cerebral anoxia; or seatbelt or other clothesline-type injury associated with significant pain, swelling, or altered mental status [38]. Cothren et al. studied 244 patients, with a 34 % positive screening yield. In patients who were initially asymptomatic, but had contraindications to antithrombotic therapy, there was a 21 % rate of ischemic neurologic events, compared to 0.5 % in those who were asymptomatic and treated with heparin or antiplatelet agents [39]. This data has been used to justify the screening of asymptomatic patients who are at high risk because of associated injuries or mechanisms of injuries as discussed above.

The manner in which patients are screened has also evolved over the last decade with the associated advances in technology. Four-vessel cerebral arteriography has been considered the gold standard for diagnosis of BCVI. It is, however, invasive, with associated risk of complication, and is resource intensive. While the initial comparisons with 4-slice computed tomography revealed disappointing results, the widespread adoption of 16-slice CT scanners has demonstrated superior results. CT angiography has demonstrated 100 % sensitivity for carotid injury and 96 % sensitivity for vertebral artery injury [40]. Other studies have suggested a relatively high false-positive rate, suggesting that 16-slice CTA may be oversensitive. Cerebral arteriography is still warranted in the setting of high clinical suspicion and a normal CTA to definitively exclude an injury [41].

Management strategies for blunt cerebrovascular injuries include observation, surgical repair, antithrombotic drugs, and endovascular strategy. Secondary to the high morbidity and mortality associated historically with untreated

Table 24.1 Blunt carotid and vertebral arterial injury grading scale (Biffl et al. [42])

Injury grade	Description
I	Luminal irregularity or dissection with <25 % luminal narrowing
II	Dissection or intramural hematoma with ≥25 % luminal narrowing, intraluminal thrombus, or raised intimal flap
III	Pseudoaneurysm
IV	Occlusion
V	Transection with free extravasation

BCVI, namely, ischemic and thrombotic cerebrovascular accidents, observation should only be employed as a method of treatment when there are contraindications to alternate therapies [41]. The treatment of choice for a given patient is determined by the location and grade of the injury (Table 24.1) as well as the patient symptomatology [39]. Surgical management is limited for BCVI. Grade I injuries are associated with a low stroke risk, which cannot justify surgical repair. Repair is often considered for higher-grade injuries; however, the anatomical location of most injuries in relation to the skull base makes surgical access difficult [41]. Because of these reasons, nonsurgical management is currently the mainstay of treatment for BCVI. That being said, if there is a Grade II–V injury which is surgically accessible, operative repair should be considered [30]. Initial studies in the treatment of BCVI demonstrated improved neurologic outcomes in symptomatic patients and stroke prevention in asymptomatic patients with anticoagulation via heparin. Protocols for heparin therapy have been modified over time to minimize the risk of bleeding in the patient population which often has multisystem trauma. Current recommendations include initiation of heparin drip without bolus, at 10 units/kg/h with a goal partial thromboplastin time of 40–50 s [41, 42]. More recent reports including large cohorts of patients suggest that systemic heparinization and antiplatelet therapy (clopidogrel 75 mg daily or aspirin 325 mg daily) have equivalent efficacy in the prevention of stroke [43, 44]. To date there are no randomized control trials proving superiority of either anticoagulation or antiplatelet therapy, though many choose to initially treat with heparinization when multiple surgical procedure with high risk of bleeding are indicated for the patients other associated injuries. It is also important in patients with concomitant traumatic brain injuries that the decision regarding anticoagulation and antiplatelet therapy be discussed in conjunction with the neurosurgery teams, in order to balance the risk of potential stroke with the risk of intracranial hemorrhage. Although they were unable to demonstrate statistical significance, a large study from the Denver group suggests that heparin may be a superior therapy to antiplatelet therapy in stroke prevention and in improvement of neurological symptoms following cerebral ischemia [41]. Grade V injuries are associated with high mortality and require immediate attempts at obtaining control, through surgical repair if accessible, or via endovascular means if inaccessible.

Follow-up imaging in the case of BCVI has proven to be instrumental in the treatment of such injuries both in terms of evaluating for progression of the injury and resolution. Most authors recommend repeat CT angiography in 7–10 days, or with any deterioration in neurologic status. Follow-up imaging resulted in a change of therapy for 65 % of grade I injuries and 51 % of grade II injuries [41]. In a follow-up study, Cothren et al. repeated imaging at 10 days after the initial diagnosis of BCVI was made, which demonstrated a healing rate of 46 % when treated with aspirin and/or clopidogrel, 43 % for aspirin, and 39 % for heparin. Alternatively, injury progression rates for BCVIs were 10 % for aspirin, 12 % for heparin, and 15 % for aspirin and/or clopidogrel. Approximately half of all grade I BCVIs fully healed, whereas less than 10 % of grade II, III, or IV injuries healed in same time period [34, 39].

In the case of progressive vessel narrowing, or enlargement of pseudoaneurysm, the use of endovascular stenting has been employed in an effort to maintain patency of the vessel [41]. Initial studies suggested a 17 % incidence of stent-related complications, including a 45 % occlusion rate, initially suggesting that the risk of endovascular stenting outweighs the benefits [34, 39].

Subsequent studies however reported good safety and patency results, though their application of stents also include antiplatelet therapy [33]. Continued studies are required to determine the true efficacy of stents in the acute setting.

Patients who continue to demonstrate injury after the follow-up imaging are recommended to continue long-term antithrombotic therapy, as stroke has been reported as long as 14 years after injury. To date, the therapy of choice and duration of treatment have not been determined [41]. Warfarin was initially recommended for long-term anticoagulation; however, with demonstrated efficacy of antiplatelet therapy, this is now the preferred treatment [42]. Recommendations for antiplatelet therapy are derived from knowledge gained with cardiac stents and percutaneous interventions. Dual therapy (aspirin with clopidogrel) is indicated for cardiac indications; however, only single-agent therapy is recommended for stroke prevention secondary to the increased bleeding risk, and no demonstrated benefit in mortality [43–45]. More studies are necessary to determine the optimal therapy in the management of BCVI. Aspirin is the current therapy of choice in treatment of BCVI in patients with persistent lesions when acute bleeding risks from associated injuries have resolved.

24.5   Venous Thromboembolism Prophylaxis

Multisystem trauma patients have a significant risk of developing deep venous thrombosis (DVT). Without prophylaxis, the rates of DVT may exceed 50 % in high-risk patients. After major trauma the risk of pulmonary embolism ranges from 0.4 to 50 % [46]. In trauma patients there is level I evidence supporting DVT prophylaxis with LMWH or LDUH as soon as resuscitation is complete and the bleeding risk acceptable [47]. The challenge in clinical decision making centers around the timing of initiation of prophylaxis based on assessment of bleeding risk. Reasonable concern exists regarding the appropriate time to begin prophylaxis, specifically in patients suffering from high-risk injuries

including intracranial hemorrhage (ICH), blunt solid organ injury, and spinal cord injury. Mechanical prophylaxis, in the form of intermittent compression pumps, is recommended instead of or as an adjunct to pharmacologic prophylaxis, depending on the bleeding risk and the VTE risk for the given patient [48].

Few studies exist which evaluate the failure of nonoperative management (NOM) of blunt solid organ injuries in patients treated with LMWH. Alejandro et al. found no change in the failure of NOM and no increase in blood transfusion requirements for patients with blunt splenic trauma who received early (≤48 h) and late (>48 h) prophylaxis [49]. Eberle et al. studied failure of NOM in patients with splenic, liver, and kidney injuries treated with early and late administration of LMWH. They found no differences in the failure rates or PE/DVT rates between early (≤3 days) and late (>3 days) administration of LMWH. A smaller study of 22 patients with solid organ injury receiving LMWH within the first 24 h found that 0 of 10 patients with liver injures, and 2 of 12 patients with splenic injuries receiving LMWH failed NOM [50]. Limitations of this study, and others assessing the management of blunt trauma, include failure to document specific risks for failure of NOM including contrast extravasation, pseudoaneurysm, or large hemoperitoneum. Further studies are necessary to assess organ-specific failure rates. Studies are ongoing, though seem to indicate that prophylactic LMWH is safely administered between 48 and 72 h, in patients who have demonstrated cessation of acute bleeding.

Perhaps more worrisome than solid organ bleeding is that of worsening intracranial hemorrhage in patients with traumatic brain injury. Patients with brain injury are especially at risk for venous thromboembolism (VTE) compared to the general trauma population [51]. Reported rates of progression of hemorrhage after LMWH range from 1.46 to 14.5 %, depending on exclusion criteria [52]. Although Kwiatt et al. present a higher progression rate than other studies secondary to broad inclusion criteria, they also concluded that the timing for initiation of LMWH did not alter the rebleed rate, when comparing

LMWH administered at ≤48 h, >48 h, and after 7 days [52]. Although not standardized, the majority of studies assessing the timing of initiation of VTE prophylaxis in patients with intracranial hemorrhage suggest documentation of stable head CT, which are monitored every 24 h after admission until stability is documented. These decisions are often made in conjunction with neurosurgical specialists and tend to start 24 h after documentation of stable CT head findings [53]. Following a similar protocol Dudley et al. demonstrated a low incidence of VTE (7.3 %), and 0.4 % symptomatic rebleed rate, when LMWH was started 48–72 h after initial trauma, provided stability of intracranial hemorrhage was documented [54]. Further studies are needed to evaluate the rates of progression, as well as rates of VTE in this population to better determine the safety and efficacy.

Determining the appropriate timing for initiation of chemoprophylaxis for VTE often requires a multidisciplinary evaluation in the polytrauma patient. Clinicians should take into consideration the patients' clinical risk factors relative to specific organ injured and presence of risk factors for bleeding. This should be weighed against the known relative increase in VTE in the trauma population and associated morbidity and mortality.

24.6 Antiplatelet Therapy

Cardiovascular disease, including acute coronary syndrome, remains the leading cause of death in industrialized countries, despite evolving therapeutic targets [55]. Platelets serve as a major therapeutic target, as the use of antiplatelet therapy allows for the inhibition of platelet aggregation [56]. Research is ongoing into the effect of such irreversible platelet inhibitors, without adequate reversal agents in the trauma population. Within the first 24 h after injury, posttraumatic intracranial hemorrhage increased in more than half of patients with traumatic brain injuries. Exacerbation secondary to inhibition of platelet activity is most likely to occur during this time period, and withdrawal of antiplatelet agents must be considered [57]. However, cessation of medication will not have an immediate impact on bleeding as the effect of the antiplatelet agents is not rapidly reversed. Cessation of antiplatelet therapy is also not without risk. After coronary stent placement, the risk of thrombosis is increased 30-fold if clopidogrel is discontinued within the first 30 days [58]. Stopping clopidogrel within the first 6 months of stent placement is an independent determinant of stent thrombosis [59]. At the same time, it is recognized that there is an increased risk of bleeding in patients on antiplatelet therapy. The risk of stent thrombosis must be carefully weighed against the risk of worsening intracranial hemorrhage. Bridging therapy with heparin was shown to be ineffective in reducing cardiac events after cessation of antiplatelet therapy [60]. In a review of 1,236 patients hospitalized for acute coronary syndrome, 4.1 % of cases were secondary to withdrawal of antiplatelet therapy, with a mean delay of 10 ± 1.9 days [61]. The rate of delayed intracranial hemorrhage is found in approximately 1–1.4 % of patients on antiplatelet therapy [62].

Wong et al. performed a retrospective case-controlled study comparing patients with traumatic brain injury who were receiving clopidogrel, aspirin, or warfarin compared to a control group. The results demonstrated a 14.7-fold increase in mortality in patients on clopidogrel [63]. Although the studies assessing morbidity and mortality are limited, primarily related to small sample size and retrospective nature, concern exists that patients on antiplatelet therapy are at a higher risk of mortality and morbidity following traumatic brain injury. Subsequent studies may also benefit from measurement of platelet function, rather than absolute presence of absence of medication as it related to bleeding risk. Nonetheless, extreme caution and liberal use of CT imaging should be employed in patients treated with antiplatelet therapy. No evidence exists at this time regarding the timing for resuming antiplatelet therapy in patients with multisystem trauma. Care should be taken in patients with closed-space injuries, where delay in recognition of delayed bleed can be catastrophic. This risk of surgical or traumatic bleeding must closely be balanced with the risk of stent thrombosis. Patient history, including timing of stent placement, type of stent, and reason for initiation of antiplatelet therapy, although often unavailable in the acute traumatic setting, is of significant value in this decision-making process. Further studies are ongoing in this evolving arena.

References

1. Feliciano DV, Cruse PA, Spjut-Patrinely V, Burch J, Mattox KL. Fasciotomy after trauma to the extremities. Am J Surg. 1988;156(6):533–6.
2. Percival TJ, White JM, Ricci MA. Compartment syndrome in the setting of vascular injury. Perspect Vasc Surg Endovasc Ther. 2011;23(2):119–24.
3. Tremblay LB, Feliciano DV, Rozycki GS. Secondary extremity compartment syndrome. J Trauma. 2002;53:833–7.
4. Mattox KL, Moore EE, Feliciano DV. Trauma. 7th ed. Chicago: McGraw-Hill Professional; 2013. p. 819–21.
5. Uliasz A, Ishida JT, Fleming JK, Yamamoto LG. Comparing the methods of measuring compartment pressures in acute compartment syndrome. Am J Emerg Med. 2003;21:143–5.
6. Hargens AR, Schmidt DA, Evans KL, et al. Quantitation of skeletal-muscle necrosis in a model of compartment syndrome. J Bone Joint Surg Am. 1981;63:631–6.
7. Kosir R, Moore FA, Selby JH, et al. Acute lower extremity compartment syndrome (ALECS) screening protocol in critically ill trauma patients. J Trauma. 2007;63:268–75.
8. Ricci MA, Graham AM, Corbisiero R, Baffour R, Mohamed F, Symes JF. Are free radical scavengers beneficial in the treatment of compartment syndrome after acute arterial ischemia? J Vasc Surg. 1989;9:244–50.
9. Blaisdell FW. The pathophysiology of skeletal muscle ischemia and the reperfusion syndrome: a review. Cardiovasc Surg. 2002;10:620–30.
10. Ricci MA, Corbisiero RM, Mohamed F, Graham AM, Symes JF. Replication of the compartment syndrome in a canine model: experimental evaluation of treatment. J Invest Surg. 1990;3:129–40.
11. Hope MJ, McQueen MM. Acute compartment syndrome in the absence of fracture. J Orthop Trauma. 2004;18:220–4.
12. Fildes J. Advanced surgical skills for exposure in trauma. 1st ed. Chicago: American College of Surgeons; 2010. p. 28–36.
13. Whitesides TE, Heckman MM. Acute compartment syndrome: update on diagnosis and treatment. J Am Acad Orthop Surg. 1996;4:209–18.
14. Finkelstein JA, Hunter GA, Hu RW. Lower limb compartment syndrome: course after delayed fasciotomy. J Trauma. 1996;40:342–4.
15. Clancy TV, Gary MJ, Covington DL, Brinker CC, Blackman D. A statewide analysis of level I and II trauma centers for patients with major injuries. J Trauma. 2001;51:346–51.
16. Demetriades D, Murray J, Martin M, et al. Pedestrians injured by automobiles: relationship of age to injury type and severity. J Am Coll Surg. 2004;199:382–7.
17. Demetriades D, Velmahos GC, Scalea TM, et al. Operative repair or endovascular stent graft in blunt traumatic thoracic aortic injuries: results of an American Association for the Surgery of Trauma multicenter study. J Trauma. 2008;64:561–70.
18. Demetriades D. Blunt thoracic aortic injuries: crossing the Rubicon. J Am Coll Surg. 2012;214(3):247–59.
19. Teixeira PG, Inaba K, Barmpara G, et al. Blunt thoracic aortic injuries: an autopsy study. J Trauma. 2011;70:197–202.
20. Mirvis SE, Shanmuganathan K. Diagnosis of blunt traumatic aortic injury 2007: still a nemesis. Eur J Radiol. 2007;64:27–40.
21. Starnes BW, Lundgren RS, Gunn M, Quade S, Hatsukami TS, Tran NT, Mokadam N, Aldea G. A new classification scheme for treating blunt aortic injury. J Vasc Surg. 2012;55(1):47–54.
22. Fabian TC, Davis KA, Gavant ML, et al. Prospective study of blunt aortic injury and helical CT is diagnostic and antihypertensive therapy reduces rupture. Am Surg. 1998;227:666–77.
23. Mattox KL, Wall MH. Historical review of blunt injury to the thoracic aorta. Chest Surg Clin N Am. 2000;10:167–82.
24. Hemmila MR, Arbabi S, Rowe SA, et al. Delayed repair for blunt thoracic aortic injury: is it really equivalent to early repair? J Trauma. 2004;56:13–23.
25. Demetriades D, Velmahos GC, Scalea TM, et al. Blunt traumatic thoracic aortic injuries: early or delayed repair- results of an American Association for the Surgery of Trauma prospective study. J Trauma. 2009;66(4):967–73.
26. Varon J, Marik PE. The diagnosis and management of hypertensive crisis. Chest. 2000;118:214–27.
27. Golledge J, Eagle K. Acute aortic dissection. Lancet. 2008;372:55–66.
28. Khoynezhad A, Prestis K. Managing emergency hypertension in aortic dissection and aortic aneurysm surgery. J Card Surg. 2006;21:S3–7.
29. White A, Broder J, Mando-Vandrick J, et al. Acute aortic emergencies – part 2: aortic dissections. Adv Emerg Nurs J. 2013;35:28–52.
30. Biffl WL, Cothren CC, Moore EE, et al. Western trauma association critical decisions in trauma: screening for and treatment of blunt cerebrovascular injuries. J Trauma. 2009;67:1150–3.
31. Biffl WL, Hr. Ray CE, Moore EE, et al. The unrecognized epidemic of blunt carotid arterial injuries: the importance of routine follow-up arteriography. Ann Surg. 2000;235:699–707.
32. Miller PR, Fabian TC, Croce MA, et al. Prospective screening for blunt cerebrovascular injuries: analysis

of diagnostic modalities and outcomes. Ann Surg. 2002;236:386–95.

33. Edwards NM, Fabian TC, Claridge JA, et al. Antithrombotic therapy and endovascular stents are effective treatment for blunt carotid injuries: results from long-term follow-up. J Am Coll Surg. 2007;204:1007–15.

34. Cothren CC, Moore EE, Ray Jr CE, et al. Screening for blunt cerebrovascular injuries is cost effective. Am J Surg. 2005;190:845–9.

35. Crissey MM, Bernstein EF. Delayed presentation of carotid intimal tear following blunt craniocervical trauma. Surgery. 1974;75:543–9.

36. Zelenock GB, Kazmers A, Whitehouse Jr WM, et al. Extracranial internal carotid artery dissections: non-iatrogenic traumatic lesions. Arch Surg. 1982; 117:425–30.

37. Biffl WL, Moore EE, Elliott JP, et al. The devastating potential of blunt vertebral arterial injuries. Ann Surg. 2000;231:672–81.

38. Biffl WL, Moore EE, Ryu RK, et al. The unrecognized epidemic of blunt carotid arterial injuries: early diagnosis improves neurologic outcome. Ann Surg. 1998;228:462–70.

39. Cothren CC, Moore EE, Ray Jr CE, et al. Carotid artery stents for blunt cerebrovascular injury: risks exceed benefits. Arch Surg. 2005;140:480–6.

40. Eastman AL, Chason DP, Perez CL, McAnulty AL, et al. Computed tomographic angiography for the diagnosis of blunt cervical vascular injury: is it ready for primetime? J Trauma. 2006;60:925–9.

41. Biffl WL, Ray Jr CE, Moore EE, et al. Treatment related outcomes from blunt cerebrovascular injuries: the importance of routine follow-up arteriography. Ann Surg. 2002;235:699–707.

42. Biffl WL, Moore EE, Offner PJ, et al. Blunt carotid arterial injuries: implications of a new grading scale. J Trauma. 1999;47:845–53.

43. Fabian TC, Patton Jr JH, Croce MA, et al. Blunt carotid injury: importance of early diagnosis and anticoagulant therapy. Ann Surg. 1996;223:513–25.

44. Cothren CC, Moore EE, Biffl WL, et al. Anticoagulation is the gold standard therapy for blunt carotid injuries to reduce stroke rate. Arch Surg. 2004;139:540–6.

45. Hermosillo AJ, Spinler SA. Aspirin, clopidogrel, and warfarin: is the combination appropriate and effective or inappropriate and too dangerous. Ann Pharmocother. 2008;42:790–805.

46. Eberle B, Schnuriger B, Inaba K, et al. Thromboembolic prophylaxis with low-molecular-weight heparin in patients with blunt solid abdominal organ injuries undergoing nonoperative management: current practice and outcomes. J Trauma. 2011;70:141–7.

47. Geerts WH, Jay RM, Code KI, et al. A comparison of low-dose heparin with low-molecular-weight heparin as prophylaxis against venous thromboembolism after major trauma. N Engl J Med. 1996;334:701–7.

48. Guyatt GH, Akl EA, Crowther M, et al. American College of Chest Physicians Antithrombotic Therapy and Prevention of Thrombosis Panel CHEST guidelines. 2012. http://journal.publications.chestnet.org/issue.aspx?journalid=99&issueid=23443&direction=P.

49. Alejandro KV, Acosta JA, Rodriguez PA. Bleeding manifestations after early use of low-molecular weight heparins in blunt splenic injuries. Am Surg. 2003;60:1006–9.

50. Norwood SH, McAuley CE, Berne JD, et al. A potentially expanded role for enoxaparin in preventing venous thromboembolism in high risk blunt trauma patient. J Am Coll Surg. 2001;192:161–7.

51. Knudson MM, Ikossi DG, Khaw L, et al. Thromboembolism after trauma: an analysis of 1602 episodes from the American College of Surgeons National Trauma Data Bank. Ann Surg. 2004;240: 490–8.

52. Kwiatt ME, Patel MS, Ross SE, et al. Is low-molecular weight heparin safe for venous thromboembolism prophylaxis in patients with traumatic brain injury? A Western Trauma Association multicenter study. J Trauma Acute Care Surg. 2011;73:625–8.

53. Saadeh BS, Gohil K, Bill C, et al. Chemical venous thromboembolic prophylaxis is safe and effective for patients with traumatic brain injury when started 24 hours after the absence of hemorrhage progression on head CT. J Trauma Acute Care Surg. 2012;73: 426–30.

54. Dudley RR, Ishtiaque A, Bonnici A, et al. Early venous thromboembolic event prophylaxis in traumatic brain injury with low-molecular-weight heparin: risks and benefits. J Neurotrauma. 2010;27: 2165–72.

55. Lopes RD. Antiplatelet agents in cardiovascular disease. J Thromb Thrombolysis. 2011;31:306–9.

56. Benyon C, et al. Clinical review: traumatic brain injury patients receiving antiplatelet medication. Crit Care. 2012;16:228–35.

57. Narayan RK, Maas AIR, Servadei F, et al. Progression of traumatic intracerebral hemorrhage: a prospective observational study. J Neurotrauma. 2008;25: 629–39.

58. Moussa ID, Colombo A. Antiplatelet therapy discontinuation following drug eluting stent placement: dangers, reasons, and management recommendations. Catheter Cardiovasc Interv. 2009;74: 1047–54.

59. Airoldi F, Colombo A, Morici N, et al. Incidence and predictors of drug-eluting stent thrombosis during and after discontinuation of thienopyridine treatment. Circulation. 2007;116:745–54.

60. Vincenzi MN, Meislitzer T, Heitzinger B, et al. Coronary artery stenting and non-cardiac surgery. A prospective outcome study. Br J Anaesth. 2006;96: 686–93.

61. Ferraris VA, Ferraris SP, Moliterno DJ, Camp P, Walenga JM, Messmore HL, Jeske WP, Edwards FH, Royston D, Shahian DM, Peterson E, Bridges CR, Despotis G, Society of Thoracic Surgeons. The Society of Thoracic Surgeons practice guideline series: aspirin and other antiplatelet agents during

operative coronary revascularization. Ann Thorac Surg. 2005;79(4):1454–61.

62. Peck KA, Sise CB, Shackford SR, Sise MJ, Calvo RY, Sack DI, Walker SB, Schechter MS. Delayed intracranial hemorrhage after blunt trauma: are patients on preinjury anticoagulants and prescription antiplatelet agents at risk? J Trauma. 2011;71(6):1600–4.

63. Wong DK, Lurie F, Wong LL. The effects of clopidogrel on elderly traumatic brain injured patients. J Trauma. 2008;65:1303–8.

Peripheral Vascular Neurologic Injuries

25

Jessica R. Stark and Daniel H. Kim

Contents

J.R. Stark, MD (✉) • D.H. Kim, MD
Department of Neurosurgery,
University of Texas Medical School at Houston,
Houston, TX, USA
jessica.r.stark@uth.tmc.edu

25.1   Anatomy and Physiology

Peripheral nerves provide the final motor pathway for impulses to the trunk and extremities as well as that for sympathetic fibers. Axons also provide afferent pathways for position sense, pressure, touch, temperature perception, and pain. These axons are extensions of the central nervous system and have an active axoplasmic flow. The majority of nerve volume is composed of connective tissues and not axons and their myelin covering. These connective tissue layers, including the endoneurium, perineurium, interfascicular epineurium, and epineurium, and their attendant fibroblasts respond to serious injury with a proliferative and disorganized pattern. Thus, despite a rich and forgiving blood supply and a substantial neuronal ability to reform axons, serious injury to a nerve results in poor spontaneous recovery [1].

If the axons are divided by injury, Wallerian degeneration occurs. This is a process that takes several weeks to complete and includes the gradual dissolution of axoplasm and myelin distal to an injury and their gradual phagocytosis. Peripheral nerves have a basal lamina provided by Schwann cells that surrounds the axons, while the central nervous system (CNS) does not. The basal lamina, although destroyed at the injury site, survives proximal and distal to it [2, 3]. In the distal stump of an injured nerve, the lamina surrounds deposits of degenerating myelin and axoplasmic debris, which are gradually phagocytized [4–6]. As the neurites grow

A. Dua et al. (eds.), *Clinical Review of Vascular Trauma*,
DOI 10.1007/978-3-642-39100-2_25, © Springer-Verlag Berlin Heidelberg 2014

distally, the basal lamina tends to resist the expanding force of the growing neurite and channels its advance within the sheath to reach the "guidance system of the distal stump." Trophic factors help to attract the new neurite; however, the growing neurite can be sometimes blocked or deflected. The fiber is then forced to change pathways or divide many times by the disorganized proliferation of the endoneurial and interfascicular epineurial connective tissues in response to injury [7–9]. This can result in distal stump axons of fine caliber and poor myelination, and axons may not reach their former sites of innervation.

25.2 Basic Nerve Responses to Injury

The cell body, which is located in the anterior horn of the spinal cord, the posterior root ganglion, or in the autonomic ganglion, undergoes chromatolysis when an axon is interrupted [10]. When neuronal chromatolysis is regenerative in nature, the cytoplasm increases in volume, primarily due to an increase in ribonucleic acid (RNA) and associated enzymes [11]. RNA changes from large particles to submicroscopic particles, which results in an apparent loss of Nissl substance. From 4 days after injury until a peak is reached at 20 days, the amount of RNA and its metabolic rate increases [12]. RNA provides the polypeptides and proteins necessary for replenishment of axoplasm.

There are three basic ways in which nerve fibers can respond to trauma: neurapraxia, axonotmesis, and neurotmesis. In neurapraxia, there is a block in conduction of the impulse down the nerve fiber and recovery takes place without Wallerian degeneration. This is probably a biochemical lesion due to a concussion or shock-like injury to the fiber [8, 9]. In the case of the whole nerve, neurapraxia is brought about by compression or by relatively mild, blunt blows, including some low-velocity missile injuries close to the nerve. Thus, injury where there is potential for compression or stretch can produce some element of neurapraxia [13]. Peroneal paralysis due to a prolonged cross-legged position is a classic

example of neurapraxic injury. Segmental demyelination of some fibers may occur, and other fibers may actually undergo axonotmesis, producing occasional fibrillations in muscles; however, the overwhelming picture is one of normal axons without Wallerian degeneration [14, 15]. Such an injury selectively affects the larger fibers serving muscle contraction, touch, and position sense while sparing the fine fibers subserving pain and sweating. Thus, these injuries usually have an element of pain. Since connective tissue elements as well as most of the microscopic anatomy of the axons and its coverings are preserved, recovery is assured but may take a few days to weeks.

Axonotmesis involves the loss of the relative continuity of the axon and its covering but the connective tissue framework is preserved, thus causing Wallerian degeneration to occur [16]. Axonotmesis is usually the result of a more severe crush or contusion injury. There is usually an element of retrograde proximal degeneration of the axon, and this loss must first be overcome when regeneration occurs. The regenerative fibers must first cross the injury site and then regenerate down the distal stump. The neurite tip progresses down the distal stump at an average rate of a millimeter per day and moves faster if closer to the CNS and slower if at a very distal site [17, 18].

A more severe contusion, stretch, or laceration produces neurotmesis, and axons and connective tissues lose their continuity. Denervational changes recorded by electromyography (EMG) are the same as those seen with axonotmetic injury; however, reversal of these changes and recovery are unlikely because regenerating axons become mixed in a swirl with regenerating fibroblasts and collagen, producing a disorganized repair site or neuroma [19]. Regenerating axons may not function effectively even after reaching distal end organs unless they arrive close to their original site [20]. When denervated, the structure of muscle begins to change histologically by the third week after injury. The muscle fibers kink and their cross-striations decrease [21]. Atrophy or shrinkage of the muscle mass becomes evident within a few weeks and will persist unless reinnervation occurs [22].

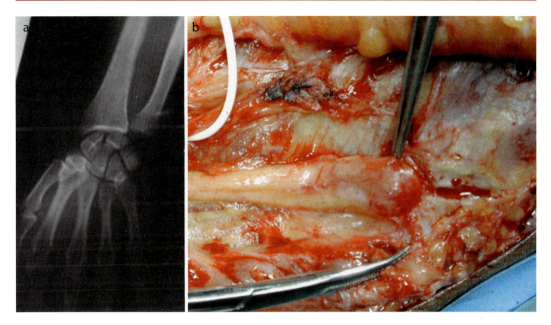

Fig. 25.1 Sharp laceration due to glass to the ulnar nerve

25.3 Mechanisms and Pathology of Injury

25.3.1 Transection

Soft tissue lacerations have the potential to injure nerves, but the nerve is sharply severed in only 30 % of cases [23]. Acute sharp nerve injuries are favorable lesions for early repair. Intraneural damage due to soft tissue laceration without direct nerve laceration results in injuries of variable severity due to contusive and stretching mechanisms [24]. Almost 15 % of nerve injuries associated with a potentially transecting mechanism actually leave the nerve in partial continuity [25]. Loss of function results from a variable amount of neurotmesis, axonotmesis, and neurapraxia, but the nerve or a portion of it is still in continuity [26]. With time, this bruised and stretched segment of nerve thickens. Depending on the severity of internal disruption, a neuroma in continuity may form. This can be found even though functional loss distal to the soft tissue laceration is complete.

If a nerve is partially transected, the injury to those cut fibers is by definition neurotmetic; however, the fibers not directly transected have a variable degree of injury. Functional loss can be mild and incomplete to severe and total. In humans, the partially transected portion of the nerve seldom regenerates well enough to restore function. In sharp transection, the amount of proximal and distal neuroma formation is much less than with contusive or blunt transection (Fig. 25.1). Blunt transection is associated with an acute ragged tear of the epineurium and an irregular, longitudinal extent of damage to a segment of the nerve (Fig. 25.2). Bruising and hemorrhage can extend for several centimeters up and down either stump. With time, sizable proximal and distal neuromas develop. Retraction and proliferative scars around the stumps are often more severe than those seen with sharp transection [27].

25.3.2 Lesions in Continuity

The most severe nerve injuries do not transect or distract nerves but leave them in gross continuity. Lesions in continuity can be either focal or diffuse and may even have skipped areas of damage, depending on the mechanism of injury. In most cases, the entire cross section of the nerve has a

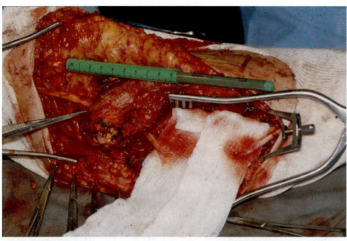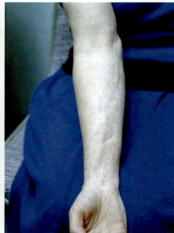

Fig. 25.2 Blunt laceration due to chain saw to the median nerve

similar extent of internal damage [28]. In some cases, one or more fascicles may be partially or completely spared, with clinic examination showing partial neurological deficits. Effective spontaneous regeneration depends on minimal connective tissue damage. Predicting which lesions in continuity will recover adequate distal function spontaneously is difficult; however, the mechanism of injury can help determine this. A less severe compressive or contusive injury, a very mild stretch injury, or a gunshot wound (GSW) is more likely to spare some internal connective tissue architecture and permit a structured axonal regenerative response. Those injuries resulting from more contusive and stretching forces associated with high-speed land, water, and air accidents are less likely to regenerate in a fashion leading to useful distal function. Despite these generalizations, it is difficult to predict outcome; therefore, most lesions of continuity are followed clinically and reevaluated at intervals for several months before surgical repair is undertaken [25, 29].

25.3.3 Stretch, Traction, and Contusion

Blunt forces imparted to nerves remain by far the most common mechanisms underlying nerve injury [30]. Normally, the nerve can withstand moderate stretch forces given its elastin and collagen-rich perineurial layer, which endows tensile strength, and its excellent ability to glide during physiologic motion [31]. Even an 8 % stretch can lead to a disturbance in intraneural circulation and blood-nerve barrier function, while stretch beyond 10–20 % results in structural failure [32, 33]. Such forces can occasionally distract a nerve, pulling it totally apart or more commonly leaving it in continuity but with considerable internal damage. If distracted by substantial forces, the nerve is frayed, and both stumps are damaged over many centimeters. Retraction and scar around both stumps are severe. Mechanisms responsible for a relatively mild degree of stretch may be associated with fractures or to a lesser degree from surgical retraction [34]. More commonly, traction forces are sufficient to tear apart intraneural connective tissue structure as well as disconnect axons [35]. The stretch mechanism is also responsible for segments of damage to a nerve displaced by high-velocity missiles, especially with GSWs [36].

Brachial plexus injury is a common disorder resulting from a stretch mechanism. Stretch or traction injuries to the plexus most commonly result from extremes of movement at the shoulder joint, with or without actual dislocation or fracture of the humerus or clavicle. Typically, either upper or lower elements of the plexus may

Fig. 25.3 Sciatic nerve injury by gunshot wound

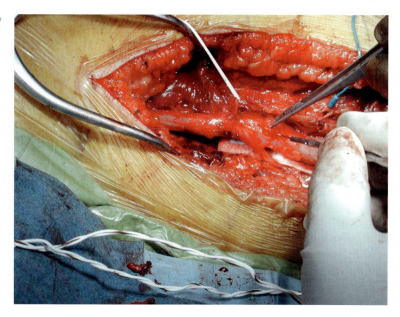

suffer the predominant injury; however, with severe traction forces, all elements may be involved in addition to the phrenic nerve and even subclavian vessels. The stretched elements may be left in continuity and have a mixture of neurapraxia and axonotmesis. Most traction injuries do not cause avulsion but cause a severe degree of internal disruption. Traction along the axis of the brachial plexus can tear their roots out of the spinal cord. Other common injuries occur during the birth process, such as Erb's palsy, which involves the upper and middle trunk from forcible depression of the shoulder. Klumpke paralysis involves damage to the lower trunk, roots, or spinal nerves from hyperabduction of the arm. The important point with stretch injuries is that although some may improve, many do not require operative reconstruction [1].

25.3.4 Gunshot Wounds

A frequent source of contusion and stretch injury to nerves are GSWs. In the majority of cases, nerves injured by GSWs are left in physical continuity (Fig. 25.3) [37]. In 85 % of missile injuries, there is not a direct strike to the nerve, but nerve injury may be as severe as in a direct hit [38]. As the missile approaches the nerve, the nerve explodes away from its trajectory and then implodes back as the missile passes by [39]. These dual acute stretching forces as well as contusive forces can result in a neurapraxic block in conduction, axonotmesis, neurotmesis, or a mixture. If missiles transect or partially lacerate a nerve, the lesion is a blunt and not a sharp injury. The nerve end tends to be shredded and irregular, with hemorrhagic contusive changes in both stumps [40]. Subsequently, a bulbous proximal neuroma and less-swollen distal neuroma form as with other blunt transecting mechanisms like fan blades, propellers, and chain saws. Because it takes time to determine the extent of tissue damage, a delay in exploration and repair is usually indicated [41].

25.3.5 Compression

Compression of nerve fibers appears to produce alterations in paranodal myelination, axonal thinning, and segmental demyelination. The degree of recovery after compression or ischemic injury may be accurately predicted in some clinical situations. Most palsies associated with unconsciousness due to anesthesia or poor positioning or pressure during operations as well as those related to improper application of plaster casts carry a good prognosis for spontaneous recovery [42]. Sometimes the compression or crushing injury has been severe or prolonged enough to cause damage that is irreversible unless an operative procedure is done. The brachial plexus, ulnar, sciatic, and peroneal nerves are the most commonly affected.

25.3.6 Compartment Syndrome

Volkmann contracture, a serious complication of undetected compartment syndrome, can occur from severe swelling and hemorrhage into the anterior compartment of the forearm or prolonged ischemia from brachial artery injury, which results in diffuse segmental damage to the median nerve and volar forearm muscles [43]. This type of ischemia is frequently associated with supracondylar fracture of the humerus and dislocation of the elbow; however, blunt trauma can result in enough swelling to compress nerves. Ischemia of a sufficient magnitude to produce Volkmann's contracture results in severe endoneurial scarring over so long a segment of the median nerve that spontaneous regeneration is unlikely. In addition to the median nerve, the radial and even occasionally the ulnar nerve may be involved because of a severely swollen elbow and forearm. Compression of the median nerve must be immediately relieved by operation. Similarly, anterior compartment syndrome of the leg results in progressive peroneal palsy or foot drop, often from a fracture of the tibia or fibula. Compartment pressures can be directly measured if needed, as is discussed elsewhere. If the difference between arterial pressure and tissue pressure is less than 40 mmHg, or the compartment pressure is greater than 30 mmHg, ischemic infarction is likely to occur.

25.3.7 Electrical and Thermal Injury

Electrical injury by passage of a large current through a peripheral nerve usually results from accidental contact of the extremity with a high-tension wire [44]. Conservative management of the nerve injury with early orthopedic reconstruction seems to have the best outcome [45]. Prognosis with low-voltage injuries is excellent but variable with high-voltage injuries [45]. Histologically, electrical injury causes necrosis with subsequent replacement with connective tissue. Though uncommon, thermal injury can result in neural damage from a transient neurapraxia to severe neurotmesis with extensive necrosis. Direct injury or secondary damage from constrictive fibrosis can affect long lengths of nerves, often necessitating nerve grafts.

25.4 Clinical Evaluation and Testing

Detailed history and thorough physical examination are essential for evaluation of nerve injuries. Before a lesion to a peripheral nerve can be ruled out, it is necessary to assess that the most distal portion of that nerve is functioning [46, 47]. For the upper limb, gross innervation can be confirmed by having the patient make a five-fingered cone with the tips of the fingers and then extending the thumb [48, 49]. The intact ulnar nerve bunches the fingers into a cone and the opponens pollicis muscle, which is innervated by the median nerve, brings the thumb to the fingers. The radial nerve extends the thumb. Similarly for the lower extremity, if the great toe can be extended, the peroneal nerve is intact, and if the great toe can be flexed, the tibial nerve is intact.

Sensory and autonomic function testing is equally important. The median and ulnar nerves can be tested by pinprick over the palmar surface of the distal phalanx of the index finger and little finger, respectively; however, the radial nerve has no reliable autonomous zone for testing. The tibial nerve can be tested by stimuli to the heel, and the peroneal nerve can be tested by stimuli to the dorsum of the foot in the web space of the first toe. The presence of Tinel's sign, i.e., percussion on a distal nerve causing paresthesias, provides some evidence favoring axonal regeneration, though it does not predict the quantity or quality of the new fibers [1].

Electromyography is valuable in localizing nerve lesions. There are three phases to EMG. The first is a brief burst of electrical activity in response to needle placement in the muscle. The second is flat line reflecting the muscle at rest. The third is an electrical response to muscle contraction or nerve stimulation. With serious denervation, there is loss or severe reduction in Phase I, with spontaneous firing of rapid biphasic, low-amplitude sharp waves or fibrillations in Phase II. In Phase III there is either no evoked muscle action potential or a poorly formed one [1].

Myelography is an important test for supraclavicular brachial plexus injuries as well as lumbosacral stretch injuries [50–53]. If a meningocele is present, this suggests an avulsed nerve root or severe internal damage. Presence of a meningocele indicates that there was enough force to produce an arachnoid tear. Computed tomography (CT) scans are useful for stretch injuries, and magnetic resonance imaging (MRI) can confirm degeneration of a nerve.

25.5 Operative Care

External neurolysis involves cleaning the nerve of investing tissues, thereby freeing up the nerve in a full circumferential fashion. After neurolysis has been completed, the nerve should be assessed to determine whether further intervention is needed. Stimulating and recording electrodes are placed on the nerve proximal to the lesion, which should produce a recordable nerve action potential (NAP). The electrodes are then moved distally, and if there is a NAP below the level of intervention, this suggests that the time interval since injury is less than 9 months, making recovery likely with external neurolysis alone [1].

Internal neurolysis involves careful splitting of a nerve into its individual fascicles. An indication for internal neurolysis is an injury that is more severe to one portion of a nerve than another that requires a split or partial repair despite the presence of a transmitted NAP across the lesion. Other indications include severe neuropathic pain for which conservative medical management has failed [1].

If a nerve has been transected or if a short gap exists following the resection of a lesion in continuity, an end-to-end epineurial repair can be performed. The proximal and distal ends are debrided, the stumps are mobilized, and a tension-free repair is performed. The limb needs to be immobilized for several weeks in order to prevent any tension on the repair. At times, the length of the resected nerve is too long for direct repair and a graft is needed. Most grafts are fashioned from the sural nerve, although cutaneous nerves of the forearm can also be used [1].

Nerve transfer is the substitution of a functioning, expendable nerve or part of a nerve with a nonfunctioning nerve. Transfers are indicated for preganglionic injuries in which nerve grafting would not be possible, but with the success rate of transfers, surgeons are now using transfers rather than grafts for postganglionic injuries [1].

25.6 Brachial Plexus

The brachial plexus originates from the C5 to T1 spinal nerve roots and branches into three trunks, followed by the anterior and posterior divisions and the three cords (medial, lateral, and posterior) (Fig. 25.4). The nerves, their innervated muscles, and impact from injury are detailed in Table 25.1. Suprascapular nerve injury is common in athletes who receive repetitive trauma from shoulder depression and abduction or in stretch injuries from humeral or midshaft clavicular fractures [54].

A very proximal injury to the C5 nerve root results in paralysis of the rhomboids, deltoid, and supraspinatus and weakens the serratus anterior and infraspinatus. The biceps and brachialis may display partial weakness due to dual supply with C5 and C6. Sensory loss may also be present over the cap of the shoulder. C6 injuries may impact on biceps, brachialis, supinator, and brachioradialis, a strong flexor of the elbow. The latissimus dorsi, another adductor of the arm, is weak or paralyzed with proximal C6 lesions. With an upper trunk lesion (C5–6), the posture of the upper extremity and hand is that of Erb's palsy, with paralysis of supraspinatus, infraspinatus,

Fig. 25.4 The five regions of the brachial plexus and their relation to the anterior tubercles, clavicle, and coronoid process

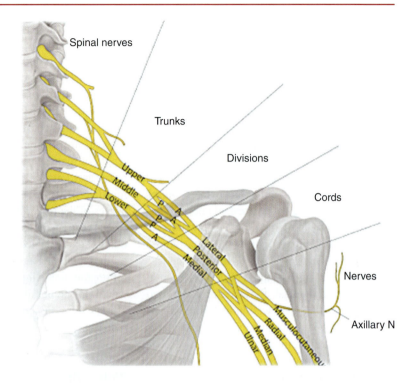

Table 25.1 Nerve root and muscle innervations

Nerve	Root/origin	Muscle innervated	Result if injured
Dorsal scapular	C5	Rhomboid	Some winging of the scapula; awkward shoulder abduction
Long thoracic	C5–7	Serratus anterior	Severe winging of scapula
Suprascapular	Upper trunk plexus	Supraspinatus; infraspinatus	Difficulty with initial abduction/external rotation
Axillary	Posterior cord plexus	Deltoid	Difficulty with abduction beyond 30°
Thoracodorsal	C6–8	Latissimus dorsi	Difficulty with shoulder adduction

deltoid, latissimus dorsi, biceps/brachialis, brachioradialis, and supinator [1].

The middle trunk is formed by the C7 nerve root and supplies most of the triceps, which extends to the forearm. Fibers from the middle trunk may also provide input to the extensor carpi radialis and sometimes to the extensor carpi ulnaris, which dorsiflex the wrist. A proximal C7 nerve injury can result in loss of fibers to the lateral cord, which supplies the pronator teres as well as wrist and finger flexors. Isolated C7 injuries result in paresis and not paralysis as they contribute predominately to muscles supplied by one or more other roots.

The lower trunk includes the C8 and T1 nerve roots. Finger and thumb extensors as well as flexors and intrinsics primarily receive input from C8. Loss results in weakness or paralysis of extensors to the thumb, forefinger, and long finger. Sensory loss may result in ulnar distribution involving the ring and little finger. T1 supplies the hand intrinsics, especially the abductor digiti minimi and opponens digiti minimi. Sensory loss may occur with lesions here as well as in the ulnar distribution. With injury to the lower trunk, a complete loss of all hand intrinsics, including those in the ulnar and median distribution, occurs as well as variable degrees of finger and wrist flexor loss [1].

With brachial plexus injuries, electromyographic studies as well as plain radiographs can be helpful for evaluations of fractures in the area.

Concomitant vascular injuries may be assessed with angiography or venography. Myelography can be helpful if nerve root avulsion is in question. CT and MRI are good studies for ruling out tumors and may be able to replace myelography and other studies in the future for determining nerve damage.

Sharp injury with laceration to the tissues surrounding the brachial plexus has the potential to transect a portion of the plexus. The presence of Tinel's sign elicited by tapping the supraclavicular area can be quite useful in differentiating between spinal nerve transection or rupture and root avulsion [55]. A positive Tinel's sign, which is perceived by the patient as tingling in an anesthetic arm or hand, usually indicates transection or rupture rather than avulsion. An early repair of clean stab wounds involving C5–7 can be expected to yield a return of function close to normal levels; however similar early repair to C8–T1 results in only some recovery of hand function that is far from normal. Primary repair within 72 h is advised for sharply transected plexus elements, whereas delayed repair is reserved for blunt transections or injuries in continuity [56].

The most common injury to the brachial plexus is caused by stretch/contusion, usually secondary to motor vehicle accidents [57, 58]. Regardless of the mechanism of injury, a conservative nonsurgical approach has predominated historically. C5–6 distribution stretches have a relatively low incidence of avulsion, may recover spontaneously, and may be associated with severe damage to C7. These injuries are excellent candidates for direct repair, aided by neurotization, with very good results. C5–7 distribution stretches have more roots avulsed than C5–6 stretches and spontaneous recovery occurs less often. There is a variable loss of finger and wrist movement; nonetheless, some of these lesions are candidates for direct repair with acceptable results. Although some regain usable shoulder and arm function with C5–T1 direct repair, results overall are not as good. Graft repair from a single root, often C5, is frequently augmented with neurotization. Complications from repair include risk of phrenic nerve paralysis and pneumothorax.

Gunshot wounds are the second largest mechanism of injury to the brachial plexus following stretch/contusion. GSWs most commonly cause lesions in continuity, though transection and vascular injures occur as well. The best outcomes typically occur with upper trunk and lateral and posterior cord lesions, but recovery occurs with some C7 to middle trunk and medial cord to median nerve repairs.

25.7 Radial Nerve

The radial nerve has major contributions from the C6 to C8 nerve roots and is the major outflow of the posterior cord distal to the origin of subscapular, thoracodorsal, and axillary nerves. Innervated muscles include the triceps, anconeus, brachioradialis, extensor carpi radialis longus (ECRL), extensor carpi radialis brevis (ECRB), and through its continuation, the extensor carpi ulnaris, supinator, extensor digitorum communis, extensor digiti minimi, abductor pollicis longus, extensor pollicis longus and brevis, and extensor indicis muscles. A key clinical point in assessing the level of nerve injury is whether the patient's latissimus dorsi muscle, innervated by the thoracodorsal nerve, and the deltoid muscle, innervated by the axillary nerve, are functioning. If both are clinically active, then the lesion spares the posterior cord and involves the radial nerve more distally. Few radial nerve injuries involve the triceps as triceps innervation is very proximal. Injury to the radial nerve at the mid-arm level from a humeral fracture is the most common mechanism of injury [59, 60].

Other mechanisms of injury at this level include GSW, contusion, simple compression or stretch without fracture, injection injury, tumors, and entrapment. The hallmarks of injury at this level are loss of brachioradialis and more distal radial-innervated functions with sparing of triceps [61, 62]. This results in characteristic wrist drop and finger drop. The radial nerve can be injured more distally by accidental drug injection, distal humeral fracture, direct contusion, or GSW [60, 63]. An elbow-level radial nerve injury causes loss of function of the ECRL and

ECRB muscles. These injuries are most frequently associated with penetrating wounds, fractures, or dislocations of the elbow by cyst or tumor or Volkmann ischemic contractures [64]. Posterior interosseous nerve involvement seriously affects the function of more distal muscles but spares some supination provided by the biceps and exhibits weak wrist extension. The sensory territory of the radial nerve encompasses the dorsum of the hand and some of the wrist, though it may be small even with complete nerve injury due to overlap from the median and ulnar nerves [65]. The outcome of surgical repair of the radial nerve with or without tendon transfer is considered excellent [60, 66–68]. Despite favorable outcome with proper management of radial nerve injuries, recovery of the extensor communis and extensor pollicis longus muscles is difficult to obtain. Fortunately, tendon transfer to the extensor expansion of the digits is an excellent substitute.

25.8 Median Nerve

The median nerve provides important input to both forearm-level extrinsic and hand intrinsic muscles, especially to the thumb. It originates at the axillary level from the lateral cord, also called the sensory root, and medial cord, called the motor root. The course of the median nerve from its origin to destinations is straight. As a result, not much length can be gained from mobilization. This makes some period of immobilization after repair of the median nerve mandatory to avoid tension on the repair [69]. Median nerve injuries are often associated with ulnar nerve involvement. Injuries to the median nerve along the medial aspect of the arm are caused by glass, knife, or GSWs and iatrogenic injuries from vascular bypass or arteriovenous (AV) fistula construction for dialysis. A high median nerve palsy can be caused by compression due to hematoma or pseudoaneurysm or contusion of the nerve in the axilla or medial arm. Proximal median nerve injury results in sensory deficits as well as loss of function of the pronator teres and quadratus, palmaris longus, flexor carpi radialis, flexor

digitorum superficialis, flexor digitorum profundi, flexor pollicis longus, and lumbricals. In a patient with a high median nerve paralysis, wrist flexion is in an ulnar deviation because flexor carpi ulnaris is no longer opposed by flexor carpi radialis. Distal flexion of the thumb and pure abduction of the thumb is lost. At the elbow and proximal forearm, mechanisms of injury are the same as proximal injuries with a similar distribution of deficits, though function of the pronator teres may be spared.

Martin-Gruber anastomosis occurs when fibers destined for some of the ulnar-innervated intrinsics may travel in an elbow-level branch from the median to ulnar nerve or through the anterior interosseous nerve branch of the median nerve. Thus, injury to the proximal median nerve may be more severe than usual; however, injury to the proximal ulnar nerve would result in less hand intrinsic paralysis. Volkmann ischemic contracture is a devastating complication of a supracondylar fracture or elbow dislocation caused by severe blunt trauma. Here contusion or stretch of the brachial artery results in spasm or damage to the vessel, secondary ischemia, and possible infarct of the volar flexor compartment muscles [1]. Acute swelling secondary to a large contusive blow to the forearm can result in median nerve injury. Early fasciotomy and neurolysis of the median and often posterior interosseous nerve is necessary.

The anterior interosseous nerve innervates the flexor digitorum profundus, flexor pollicis longus, and pronator quadrates, and dysfunction results in loss of the pinch mechanism commonly known as the anterior interosseous nerve syndrome. This typically results from entrapment of the nerve following penetration or contusive injuries to the forearm [70]. At the middle or distal forearm, the median nerve can be injured in association with a fracture involving the radius or ulna [71]. Loss includes flexor pollicis longus, thenar intrinsic muscles, and lumbricals to the index and middle finger and sensory deficits to the dorsoradial aspect of thenar prominence. At the wrist level, injuries are usually from sharp mechanisms resulting in loss of intrinsic muscles and sensory distribution of the median nerve except for that of the palmar cutaneous branch, which takes off before the wrist. At the wrist level, patients can suffer injury to the nearby ulnar nerve and develop carpal tunnel syndrome from scar tissue. Dissections of the proximal median nerve can be associated with injury to the brachial artery on which it lies.

25.9   Ulnar Nerve

The ulnar nerve is important for coordinated hand function. It innervates the flexor carpi ulnaris, flexor digitorum profundus, abductor pollicis, flexor pollicis brevis, lumbricals, hypothenar, and all dorsal and palmar interosseous muscles. The ulnar nerve originates at the axillary level from the medial cord. The most proximal muscle innervated by the ulnar nerve is the flexor carpi ulnaris, which flexes the wrist in an ulnar direction. Injury proximal to the distal forearm-level branch of the dorsal cutaneous nerve results in rather complete ulnar sensory loss. Distal lesions can result in an ulnar claw in which the little and ring finger lumbricals have lost function and the fingers are pulled toward the palm due to unopposed flexor motion. The most common ulnar nerve lesion is entrapment at the elbow level usually from elbow fracture or dislocation, resulting in paresthesias in an ulnar distribution, particularly in the little and ring fingers (Fig. 25.5). Sensory symptoms typically develop before muscle weakness of the hand intrinsic and hypothenar muscles [1].

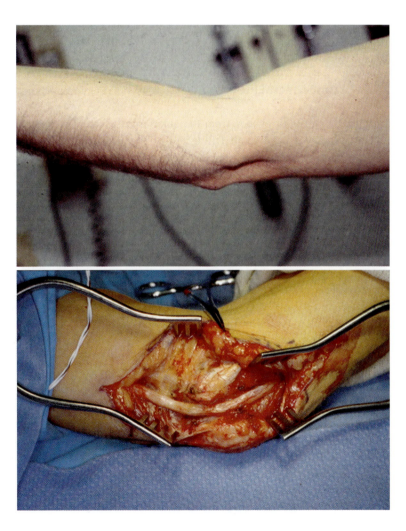

Fig. 25.5 Ulnar nerve entrapment at elbow level

There are three zones of entrapment at the wrist level. Zone I consists of the ulnar nerve in the proximal aspect of Guyon's canal where it is proximal to its bifurcation into the deep branch and superficial branches [72]. This is the most frequent site of spontaneous distal entrapment, but injury can also be due to wrist fractures and cysts [73, 74]. There is ulnar sensory loss, which spares the dorsal cutaneous branch, supplying the dorsum of the hand. Zone II comprises the deep motor branch, with entrapment typically resulting from palmar trauma, pressure, ganglion, or carpal synovitis [75, 76]. Weakness or paralysis occurs in the palmar and dorsal interosseous, little and ring finger lumbrical, and adductor pollicis and flexor pollicis brevis with intact sensation [77]. Zone III involves compression at the superficial branch level at the distal aspect of Guyon's canal, giving a pure sensory loss.

25.10 Lumbosacral Plexus

The lumbar plexus originates from the anterior primary rami of L1–L4, with L1, L2, and L4 splitting into upper and lower branches and the lower branch of L2, upper branch of L4, and entire L3 splitting into anterior and posterior divisions. The L1 upper branch divides into the iliohypogastric and ilioinguinal nerves. The L1 lower branch and L2 upper branch join to form the genitofemoral nerve. The anterior division of the L2 lower branch and both L3 and the L4 upper branches contribute to the obturator nerve. The posterior divisions of L2 and L3 divide into the small and large branch, with the small branch of each joining to form the lateral femoral cutaneous nerve and the large branch of each joining the L4 posterior division to form the femoral nerve. The sensory divisions are the central extensions of the dorsal root ganglia and do not regenerate after injury.

The iliohypogastric, ilioinguinal, and genitofemoral nerves are rarely injured from trauma but iatrogenic injuries from abdominal or pelvic surgeries can occur. The pelvic-level femoral nerve can be damaged due to a penetrating lower abdominal injury from GSWs, motorcycle handlebars, or stab wounds. Injury to the nerve at this level results in weakness of the iliacus, quadriceps, and sartorius muscles causing loss of hip flexion, hyperextension of the knee, and loss of knee jerk and sensory loss to the anteromedial thigh. The lateral femoral cutaneous nerve is usually affected by stretch injury, entrapment, or during removal of bone graft from the ilium. Injury results in the characteristic syndrome of meralgia paresthetica: tingling, burning pain in the lateral thigh, and frequent hyperesthesia so severe that the lateral thigh is easily irritated by clothing or touch. The obturator nerve can be injured as a result of lumbosacral injuries or a pelvic fracture, resulting in a mildly disturbed gait in which the leg is externally rotated and tends to swing outward when the patient walks [1].

The sacral plexus has contributions from the lumbosacral trunk formed by the lower branch of L4, the L5 anterior division, anterior division of S1, and portions of the anterior divisions of S2, S3, and S4. There are 12 named branches of the sacral plexus: (1) sciatic nerve consisting of peroneal and tibial divisions, (2) superior gluteal and (3) inferior gluteal nerves, (4) posterior femoral cutaneous nerve, (5) perforating cutaneous nerve, (6) nerve to the quadratus femoris and inferior gemellus, (7) nerve to the obturator internus and superior gemellus, (8) nerve to the piriformis, (9) nerve to the levator ani and coccygeus, (10) nerve to the sphincter ani muscles, (11) pelvic splanchnic nerves, and (12) pudendal nerve. The superior gluteal nerve supplies the gluteus medius and minimus muscles, which aid in the abduction and medial rotation of the thigh. With injury to the nerve, the leg tends to rest in an outwardly rotated position; therefore, when standing on the affected leg, the contralateral pelvis drops down. An injury to the inferior gluteal nerve that supplies the gluteus maximus results in weak extension of the hip. Patients have difficulty arising from a sitting position or climbing steps. The rest of the nerves have variable patterns of injury and are rare in isolation but occur more often with sacral plexus injuries [1].

Fig. 25.6 Stretch/contusion injury to the sciatic nerve

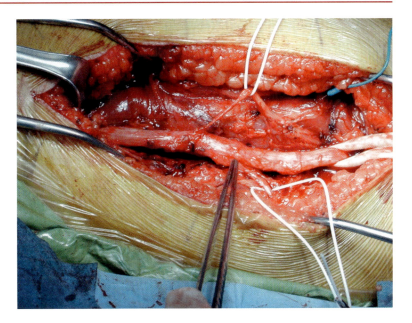

25.11 Sciatic Nerve

The sciatic and femoral nerves are the two major innervations for the lower extremity. Except at the pelvic level, both nerves are unlikely to be injured at the same time. If either nerve is injured alone, the ability to bear weight with the extremity continues despite some paresis. The sciatic nerve is formed from the anterior and posterior division of the L4–S2 spinal nerves and the anterior division of S3. The anterior divisions form the tibial nerve and the posterior divisions form the peroneal nerve. While one or more branches to the hamstring muscle arise from the sciatic nerve's tibial division, the lateral hamstring is supplied by the peroneal division of the sciatic nerve. Thus lateral hamstring weakness or paralysis accompanied by a foot drop likely represents a proximal peroneal division injury. A buttock-level sciatic nerve injury rarely involves the gluteus maximus and medius and rarely results in total paralysis of the hamstring muscle. A complete sciatic injury at this level results in loss of plantar and dorsiflexion, foot inversion and eversion, and toe flexion and extension. The peroneal division rather than the tibial division is often preferentially injured at a high proximal level possibly due to the peroneal nerve's lateral position, thus resulting in greater exposure to stretch/contusion during blunt trauma, such as fractures or hip dislocations (Fig. 25.6) [78].

25.12 Tibial Nerve

The tibial nerve arises from the medial half of the sciatic nerve, usually at the middle to distal one-third. The tibial nerve gives rise to branches to the gastrocnemius, plantaris, popliteus, tibialis, flexor digitorum longus, and flexor hallucis longus. The posterior tibial nerve gives rise to the calcaneal and lateral and medial plantar nerves, which provide sensory innervation to the heel and plantar aspects of the foot. Foot intrinsic muscle loss is not a serious sequel for tibial dysfunction but can result in clawing of the toes. Tibial repair at any level is always worthwhile provided there is a proven poor potential for spontaneous regeneration. This is in part because there is a great opportunity for recovery of plantar function and protective sensation to the sole of the foot can be regained. Ankle-level injuries involving the tibial or plantar nerves are often associated with fractures but can be caused by blunt contusions or GSWs [1].

25.13 Common Peroneal Nerve

The peroneal nerve innervates the anterior tibialis, extensor digitorum communis, extensor hallucis longus and brevis, and extensor digitorum longus and brevis muscles [79]. The common peroneal nerve (CPN) is superficial as it passes lateral to the surgical neck of the fibula, and it is at this point that the nerve is most susceptible to injury. The peroneal nerve is fixed proximally at the sciatic notch and fibular neck; thus, it is less able to accommodate stretch, which increases its propensity to injury [80]. Close to its origin, one or more branches leave to form the sural nerve, sometimes complimented by a branch from the tibial nerve. The sural nerve is the major sensory nerve of the lower extremity supplying the posterolateral distal one-third of the leg and dorsolateral side of the foot. Injuries to the sural nerve result in hypersensitivity to light touch or loss of sensation. Injury to the CPN causes weakness of the deep branch-innervated ankle and toe dorsiflexors and superficial branch-innervated ankle evertors. Tendon transfer or partial fusion of the ankle can sometimes ameliorate the foot drop seen with peroneal palsy. Injury to the deep branch also results in decreased sensation in the region between the great and second toes. Involvement of the superficial branch results in decreased sensation in the anterior-lateral calf and dorsum of the foot. The largest injury category for the peroneal nerve occurs at the knee level from stretch/contusion due to motor vehicle accidents or sports-related injuries, which are very difficult to manage [81, 82].

25.14 Femoral Nerve

The femoral nerve is one of the major outflows of the lumbar plexus supplying the iliacus, quadriceps, and sartorius muscles. The saphenous nerve arises from the anteromedial femoral nerve, supplying sensory innervation to the medial knee, medial leg, and instep region of the foot. Injury to the femoral nerve results in inability to extend the leg and sensory deficits in the previously mentioned regions. Injury is typically due to iatro-

genic causes, though pelvic and hip fractures, GSWs, and lacerations occur as well. Results after repair seem to be favorable [31, 83, 84].

Conclusion

Detailed history and physical examination is mandatory when nerve injury is suspected. Knowledge of the anatomy and innervations for the affected nerve is important in localization of lesions. There are many aspects to consider when it comes to nerve injuries and repair. The mechanism of injury as well as the involved nerve results in a wide variety of choices in treatment from conservative to early or late operative management. The type of procedure also varies by nerve injured and mechanism of injury. Electromyography can be helpful to determine the location of the lesion as well as progress of motor function over the recovery period. Post-injury follow-up and rehabilitation are important for recovery.

References

1. Kim DH, Midha R, et al. Nerve injuries: operative results for major nerve injuries, entrapments, and tumors. 2nd ed. Philadelphia: WB Saunders; 1995.
2. Hudson A, Morris J, Weddell G. An electron microscope study of regeneration in sutured rat sciatic nerves. Surg Forum. 1970;21:451–3.
3. Morris JH, Hudson AR, Weddell G. A study of degeneration and regeneration in the divided rat sciatic nerve based on electron microscopy. Z Zellforsch. 1972;124:76–203.
4. Ashbury A. The histogenesis of phagocytes during Wallerian degeneration procedures. Sixth international congress of neuropathology. Masson & Cia, Paris; 1970.
5. Pelligrino RG, Rithie JM, Spencer PS. The role of Schwann cell division in the clearance of nodal axolemma following nerve section in the car. J Physiol (Lond). 1982;334:68.
6. Waller A. Experiments on the section of the glossopharyngeal and hypoglossal nerves of the frog. Philos Trans R Soc Lond B Biol Sci. 1850;140:423–9.
7. Ramon Y, Cajal S. Degeneration and regeneration of the nervous system. Trans: May RM. New York: Oxford University Press; 1928.
8. Seddon H. Degeneration and regeneration. In: Seddon H, editor. Surgical disorders of the peripheral nerves. Edinburgh: E & S Livingston; 1972. p. 9–31.

9. Sunderland S. Nerve injuries and their repair: a critical appraisal. Edinburgh: Churchill Livingston; 1991.

10. Sears TA. Structural changes in motor neurons following axotomy. J Exp Biol. 1987;132:93–109.

11. Edstrom JE. Ribonucleic acid changes in motor neurons of frog during axon regeneration. J Neurochem. 1959;5:43–9.

12. Ducker TB, Kaufmann FC. Metabolic factors in the surgery of peripheral nerves. Clin Neurosurg. 1977; 24:406–24.

13. Rudge P, Ochoa J, Gilliatt RW. Acute peripheral nerve compression in the baboon. J Neurol Sci. 1974;23: 403–20.

14. Denny-Brown D, Brenner C. Lesion in peripheral nerve resulting from compression by spring clip. Arch Neurol Psychiatry. 1944;52:120.

15. Gilliatt RW, Ochoa J, Ridge P, et al. Cause of nerve damage in acute compression. Trans Am Neurol Assoc. 1974;99:71–574.

16. Ochoa J, Fowler TJ, Gilliatt RW. Anatomical changes in peripheral nerves compressed by a pneumatic tourniquet. J Anat. 1972;113:433–55.

17. Aitken JT, Thomas PK. Retrograde changes in fiber size following nerve section. J Anat. 1962;96:121–9.

18. Rydevik B, Lundborg G. Permeability of intraneural microvessels and perineurium following acute, graded experimental nerve compression. Scand J Plast Reconstr Surg. 1977;11:179–87.

19. Gilliatt R. Physical injury to peripheral nerves, physiological and electrodiagnostic aspects. Mayo Clin Proc. 1981;56:361–70.

20. Zalewski A. Effects of neuromuscular reinnervation on denervated skeletal muscle by axons of motor, sensory, and sympathetic neurons. Am J Physiol. 1970; 219:1675–9.

21. Sunderland S, Ray LJ. Denervation changes in muscle. J Neurol Neurosurg Psychiatry. 1950;13: 159–77.

22. Richardson PM. Neurotrophic factors in regeneration. Curr Opin Neurobiol. 1991;111:401–6.

23. Ducker TB, Garrison WB. Surgical aspects of peripheral nerve trauma. Curr Probl Surg. 1974;1:62.

24. Sunderland S. Nerve and nerve injuries. 1st ed. Baltimore: Williams & Wilkins; 1968.

25. Kline DG. Physiological and clinical factors contributing to the timing of nerve repair. Clin Neurosurg. 1977;24:425–55.

26. Seddon HJ. Three types of nerve injury. Brain. 1943; 66:238–88.

27. Ducker TB. Pathophysiology of peripheral nerve trauma. In: Omer GE, Spinner M, editors. Management of peripheral nerve problems. Philadelphia: WB Saunders; 1980.

28. Kline DG, Hudson AR. Acute injuries of peripheral nerves. In: Youmans J, editor. Neurological surgery. Philadelphia: WB Saunders; 1990.

29. Midha R, Kline DG. Evaluation of the neuroma in continuity. In: Omer GE, Spinner M, Van Beek AL, editors. Management of peripheral nerve problems. 2nd ed. Philadelphia: WB Saunders; 1998. p. 319–27.

30. Gentili F, Hudson AR, Midha R. Peripheral nerve injuries: types, causes, and grading. In: Wilkins RH, Rengachary SS, editors. Neurosurgery, vol. 3. 2nd ed. New York: McGraw-Hill; 1996. p. 3105–14.

31. Sunderland S. Nerves and nerve lesions. Edinburgh: Churchill Livingstone; 1978.

32. Lundborg G, Rydevik B. Effects of stretching the tibial nerve of rabbit. A preliminary study of the intraneural circulation and the barrier function of the perineurium. J Bone Joint Surg. 1973;55B:390–401.

33. Liu CT, Benda CE, Lewey FH. Tensile strength of human nerve: experimental physiological and histological study. Arch Neurol Psychiatry. 1948;59: 322–36.

34. Seletz E. Surgery of peripheral nerves. Springfield: Charles C Thomas; 1951. p. 119–37.

35. Speed JS, Knight RA. Peripheral nerve injuries. In: Campbell's operative orthopaedics, vol. 1. St. Louis: CV Mosby; 1956. p. 947–1014.

36. Omer GE. Nerve injuries associated with gunshot wounds of the extremities. In: Gelberman RH, editor. Operative nerve repair and reconstruction. Philadelphia: JB Lippincott; 1991. p. 655–70.

37. Kline DG. Civilian gunshot wounds to the brachial plexus. J Neurosurg. 1989;70:166–74.

38. Spurling RG, Woodhall B. Medical Department, United States Army, Surgery in World War II: neurosurgery, vol. 2. Washington, DC: US Government Printing Office; 1959.

39. Puckett WO, Grundfest H, McElroy W, et al. Damage to peripheral nerves due to high velocity missiles without direct hit. J Neurosurg. 1946;3:294–9.

40. Whitcomb BB. Techniques of peripheral nerve repair. In: Spurling RG, editor. Medical Department, United States Army, Surgery in World War II: neurosurgery, vol. 2, part 2: peripheral nerve injuries. Washington, DC: US Government Printing Office; 1959.

41. Kline DG, Hackett ER. Reappraisal and timing for exploration of civilians peripheral nerve injuries. Surgery. 1975;78:54–65.

42. Mackinnon SE, Dellon AL. Surgery of the peripheral nerve. New York: Thieme Medical Publishers; 1988.

43. Goldner JL, Goldner RD. Volkmann's ischemia and ischemic contractures. In: Jupiter JB, editor. Flynn's hand surgery. Baltimore: Williams and Wilkins; 1991.

44. Di Vincenti FC, Moncrief JA, Pruitt BA. Electrical injuries: a review of 65 cases. J Trauma. 1969;9: 497–507.

45. Grube BJ, Heimbach DM, Engrav LH, et al. Neurologic consequences of electrical burns. J Trauma. 1990;30:254–8.

46. Hudson A, Berry H, Mayfield F. Chronic injuries of peripheral nerves by entrapment. In: Youmans J, editor. Neurological surgery: a comprehensive reference guide to the diagnosis and management of neurosurgical problems. 2nd ed. Philadelphia: Saunders; 1982.

47. Kempe L. Operative neurosurgery, vol. 2. New York: Springer; 1970.

48. Medical Research Council, Nerve Injuries Committee. Aids to investigation of peripheral nerve injuries.

MRC war memorandum no. 7. London: His Majesty's Stationery Office; 1943.

49. Seddon HJ. Surgical disorders of peripheral nerves. Baltimore: Williams & Wilkins; 1972.

50. Carvalho GA, Nikkah G, Matthies C, et al. Diagnosis of root avulsions in traumatic brachial plexus injuries: value of computerized tomography, myelography, and magnetic resonance imaging. J Neurosurg. 1997;86: 69–76.

51. Leffert RD. Clinical diagnosis, testing, and electromyographic study in brachial plexus traction injuries. Clin Orthop Relat Res. 1988;237:24–31.

52. Murphey F, Hartung W, Kirklin JW. Myelographic demonstration of avulsing injury of brachial plexus. Am J Roentgenol. 1947;58:102–5.

53. Simard J, Sypert G. Closed traction avulsion injuries of the brachial plexus. Contemp Neurosurg. 1983;50: 1–6.

54. Yu JS, Fischer RA. Denervation atrophy caused by suprascapular nerve injury: MR findings. J Comput Assist Tomogr. 1997;21:302–3.

55. Landi A, Copeland S. Value of the Tinel sign in brachial plexus lesions. Ann R Coll Surg Engl. 1979;61: 470–1.

56. Kline DG, Judice DJ. Operative management of selected brachial plexus lesions. J Neurosurg. 1983; 58:631–49.

57. Davis DH, Onofrio BM, MacCarty CS. Brachial plexus injuries. Mayo Clin Proc. 1978;53:799–807.

58. Fletcher I. Traction lesions of the brachial plexus. Hand. 1969;1:129–36.

59. Holstein A, Lewis GB. Fractures of the humerus with radial nerve paralysis. J Bone Joint Surg. 1963;45A: 1382–6.

60. Jayendrahumar J. Radial nerve paralysis associated with fractures of the humerus. Clin Orthop. 1983;172: 171–5.

61. Pollock FH, Drake D, Bovill E, et al. Treatment of radial neuropathy associated with fracture of the humerus. J Bone Joint Surg. 1981;63A:239–43.

62. Seddon H. Nerve lesion complicating certain closed bone injuries. JAMA. 1947;135:191–4.

63. Ling CMS, Loong SC. Injection injury of the radial nerve. Injury. 1976;8:60–2.

64. Reid RL. Radial nerve palsy. Hand Clin. 1988;4: 179–82.

65. Savory WS. A case in which after the removal of several inches of the musculospiral nerve, the sensibility of that part of the skin of the hand which is supplied by it was retrained. Lancet. 1868;2:142.

66. Kettlekamp DB, Alexander H. Clinical review or radial nerve injury. J Trauma. 1967;7:424–32.

67. Nickolson OR, Seddon HJ. Nerve repair in civil practice. Br Med J. 1957;2:1065–71.

68. Zachary RB. Results of nerve suture. In: Seddon HJ, editor. Peripheral nerve injuries. Medical research council no 282. London: Her Majesty's Stationary Office; 1952.

69. Tarlov IM. How long should an extremity be immobilized after nerve suture? Ann Surg. 1947;126:336–76.

70. O'Brien MD, Upton ARM. Anterior interosseous nerve syndrome. J Neurol Neurosurg Psychiatry. 1972;35:531–6.

71. Abbott L, Saunders J. Injuries of the median nerve in fractures of the lower end of the radius. Surg Gynecol Obstet. 1933;57:507–11.

72. Forshell KP, Hagstrom P. Distal ulnar nerve compression caused by ganglion formation in the Loge de Guyon. Case report. Scand J Plast Reconstr Surg. 1975;9:77–9.

73. Brooks DM. Nerve compression by simple ganglia. J Bone Joint Surg Br. 1952;34:391–400.

74. Mallet BL, Zilkha KJ. Compression of the ulnar nerve at the wrist by a ganglion. Lancet. 1955;268:890–1.

75. Gelberman R. Ulnar tunnel syndrome. In: Gelberman R, editor. Operative nerve repair and reconstruction. Philadelphia: JB Lippincott; 1991.

76. Hunt J. Occupational neuritis of the deep palmar branch of the ulnar nerve. J Nerv Ment Dis. 1908;35: 673.

77. Shea JD, McClain EJ. Ulnar-nerve compression syndromes at and below the wrist. J Bone Joint Surg Am. 1969;51:1095–103.

78. Rizzoli H. Treatment of peripheral nerve injuries. In: Coates JB, Meirowsky AM, editors. Neurological surgery of trauma. Washington, DC: Office of the Surgeon General, Department of the Army; 1965.

79. Mackinnon SE, Dellon A. Other lower extremity nerve entrapments. In: Surgery of the peripheral nerve. New York: Thieme Medical Publishers; 1988.

80. Thoma A, Fawcett S, Ginty M, et al. Decompression of the common peroneal nerve: experience with 20 consecutive cases. Plast Reconstr Surg. 2001;107: 1183–9.

81. Highet WB, Holmes W. Traction injures to the lateral popliteal and traction injuries to peripheral nerves after suture. Br J Surg. 1943;30:212.

82. Nobel W. Peroneal palsy due to hematoma in the common peroneal nerve sheath after distal torsional fractures and inversion ankle sprains. J Bone Joint Surg Am. 1966;48:1484–95.

83. Osgaard O, Husby J. Femoral nerve repair with nerve autografts. Report of two cases. J Neurosurg. 1977;47: 751–4.

84. Rakolta GG, Omer Jr GE. Combat-sustained femoral nerve injuries. Surg Gynecol Obstet. 1969;128: 813–7.

Pediatric Vascular Injuries

26

Nathan P. Heinzerling and Thomas T. Sato

Contents

N.P. Heinzerling, MD • T.T. Sato, MD (✉)
Division of Pediatric Surgery, Children's Hospital
of Wisconsin, Milwaukee, WI, USA

Department of Surgery, Medical College
of Wisconsin, Milwaukee, WI, USA
e-mail: ttsato@chw.org

26.1   Introduction

Traumatic injuries remain the most common cause of death and disability among the pediatric population with an estimated 20,000 deaths each year [1]. However, vascular injuries in infants and children occur with a reported incidence rate of 0.6–1.4 % and are relatively uncommon [2, 3]. Due to the rarity of pediatric vascular injuries and the paucity of literature on the subject, evidence-based surgical management has been largely based on extrapolation of data from adult vascular injuries. Few studies have specifically focused on pediatric vascular trauma. Relevant pediatric literature is largely composed of anecdotal case studies and single-institution retrospective reviews. However, there are a number of clinically significant and age-specific issues encountered with pediatric vascular trauma. Anatomic differences between children and adults create variation in injury distribution and severity. In most children, there is less soft tissue, body fat, and connective tissue protecting internal organs and central vascular structures compared to adults. Neonates and infants are at risk for iatrogenic arterial injury from diagnostic and therapeutic procedures commonly performed at major pediatric centers. Younger children have relatively large heads, immature cervical muscles, and more compliant ligaments that predispose to torsion, shear, and vascular stretch injury.

Extremity fractures are common in children, either in isolation or in the constellation of multiple blunt injuries sustained in falls, motor

A. Dua et al. (eds.), *Clinical Review of Vascular Trauma*,
DOI 10.1007/978-3-642-39100-2_26, © Springer-Verlag Berlin Heidelberg 2014

vehicle crashes, and pedestrians struck by vehicles. Supracondylar fractures of the humerus in children have a significant rate of associated brachial artery injury. The pediatric thorax is more compliant and compressible, and significant injury may occur in the absence of rib fractures. Fortunately, thoracic aortic injury from blunt trauma is significantly less common in children than adults. Finally, energy is dispersed over a smaller surface area, causing a larger concentration of energy in any given anatomic region. Along with the social and psychological characteristics of children, these age-specific characteristics create differences in the patterns of pediatric vascular injuries and influence specific management strategies.

26.2 Epidemiology

Pediatric vascular injuries are relatively uncommon. A comparative, retrospective review of the National Trauma Data Bank from 2001 to 2006 demonstrated that of 251,787 injured children less than 16 years of age, 1,138 (0.6 %) had a reported vascular injury excluding digital vessel and unspecified injuries; this was significantly lower than the 1.6 % incidence rate found in the adult cohort 16 years of age and older ($p < 0.01$) [2]. Compared to adults, pediatric patients with vascular injuries had significantly lower Injury Severity Scores, fewer penetrating injuries, and fewer thoracic aortic injuries. Vascular injuries in children were also associated with lower overall mortality compared to adults (13.2 % versus 23.2 %, $p < 0.001$). However, pediatric vascular injuries remain significant in terms of morbidity and mortality. Contemporary overall mortality from truncal vascular injury in children 17 years old or less treated at an established level I pediatric trauma center in Houston remained 25 % [3]. Hemodynamic instability at presentation was associated with lower survival rates for thoracic, abdominal, and cervical vascular injuries in these children. Data from the National Pediatric Trauma Registry support an approximately 13 % crude mortality rate associated with vascular injuries, which significantly exceeds the 2.9 % overall mortality rate reported in the registry [4].

Table 26.1 Demographics and location of pediatric vascular injury ages 0–16 years from the National Trauma Data Bank (mean age 10.7 years old, $N = 1,138$)

	Number	Percent
Male	838	73.6
Penetrating mechanism	478	42.8
Upper extremity	406	35.7
Abdomen	275	24.2
Lower extremity	212	18.6
Chest	150	13.2
Neck	113	9.9

Adapted from Barmparas et al. [2]

These analyses do not include children with iatrogenic femoral arterial injury following cardiac catheterization or arterial line monitoring.

The four most common mechanisms of injury in adults and children are motor vehicle collisions, firearm injuries, stab wounds, and falls. Blunt traumatic mechanisms account for more than half of the vascular injuries observed in children. The most commonly injured vessels in children are in the upper extremity. Injury to the brachial artery should be suspected in a child presenting with a pulseless extremity associated with a supracondylar humerus fracture. When distal pulses remain absent following prompt humerus reduction, urgent diagnostic vascular evaluation is warranted. The second most common site of vascular injury in the pediatric patient is the abdomen and most commonly involves the inferior vena cava and iliac and renal vessels. The next most common sites of injury are the lower extremity, chest, and neck. Abdominal and thoracic aortic injury from blunt trauma is distinctly uncommon in children, although this may represent reporting bias of injuries to children surviving to emergency room admission (Table 26.1). These anatomic patterns of vascular injury are similar in several single-institution reviews of pediatric trauma patients [3–9].

26.3 Clinical Evaluation and Diagnostic Imaging

Successful assessment and management of pediatric vascular injury assumes expeditious provision of adequate airway, breathing, and circulation. The mechanism of injury is often useful when assessing for immediately life-threatening injuries. In particular, obvious blunt or penetrating torso injuries presenting with hypotension are associated with increased morbidity and mortality in children. Given the physiological reserve of children, it is important not to underestimate the severity of injury on the basis of adequate blood pressure alone. Tachycardia, tachypnea, cool extremities, and lethargy despite a relatively normal or measurable blood pressure are worrisome signs for impending cardiovascular collapse from hypovolemic shock in a child.

Initial assessment for possible truncal or peripheral vascular injury in a child relies on exquisite physical examination. Evidence for arterial injury is generally divided into hard and soft signs of injury, and this remains a useful clinical algorithm for determining further intervention in children. Hard signs of vascular injury include pulsatile bleeding from the wound(s), a rapidly expanding or pulsatile hematoma, evidence of an arteriovenous fistula, or signs of distal ischemia (pallor, pulselessness, poikilothermia, paresthesias, and pain). Importantly, many pediatric vascular injuries are associated with open extremity fractures and/or soft tissue injury, and therefore, the ability to rapidly assemble a multidisciplinary team with expertise in pediatric resuscitation, trauma, orthopedics, vascular surgery, plastic surgery/microvascular reconstruction, and radiology is imperative.

The presence of hard signs necessitates prompt intervention to control hemorrhage and attempts at restoration of vascular continuity. Soft signs of injury include persistent shock despite ongoing resuscitation, wound hematoma, diminished peripheral pulses, proximity of wound trajectory to major vessels, or evidence of injury to a nerve adjacent to a vessel. In hemodynamically normal children with suspected extremity vascular injury, the most appropriate next step is to determine the ankle brachial index (ABI). An ABI of less than 0.9 in a young adult or child greater than 1 year of age should prompt further diagnostic evaluation for vascular injury. A potential exception is in newborn infants discussed below.

Following resuscitation and clinical examination, diagnostic evaluation of hemodynamically normal children with clinical signs of vascular injury is indicated. Traditionally, biplanar angiography has been considered the gold standard imaging modality. However, similar to the adult experience, imaging techniques that are less invasive than conventional angiography are gaining wider acceptance. CT angiography is now emerging as one of the more valuable, adjunctive diagnostic tools for vascular injury in children given the nearly universal presence and immediate access to CT scan imaging at pediatric hospitals.

Prospective, systematic evaluation of imaging alternatives for pediatric vascular injuries has been challenging, in part, due to the infrequent nature of these injuries. The difficulty in determining the most appropriate diagnostic modality is underscored in a retrospective review of blunt carotid artery injury in the National Pediatric Trauma Registry, a multicenter national registry with 78 participating institutions [10]. This study demonstrated a blunt carotid injury rate of 0.03 % (15 of 57,659 pediatric blunt trauma patients). Recorded diagnostic imaging procedures included angiography, duplex ultrasonography, and magnetic resonance angiography. Unfortunately, definitive conclusions regarding the best imaging modality for these injuries could not be made because of the low incidence of pediatric vascular injuries and the variability in pediatric hospital-based imaging resources.

The utility of contrast-enhanced CT scan imaging was evaluated in a retrospective review of adults presenting with thoracic, abdominal, and/or pelvic trauma over a 30-month period. CT imaging was compared to conventional angiography for those patients undergoing angiography within 24 h of contrast-enhanced CT scan imaging [11]. A total of 63 traumatic torso injuries were evaluated in 48 patients (46 blunt with trauma, 2 with penetrating trauma). Contrast-enhanced CT scan imaging findings strongly correlated with angiographic findings; CT scan imaging was found to have 94.1 % sensitivity and 97.6 % negative predictive value for detection of ongoing hemorrhage within the torso and 92.6 % sensitivity for predicting need for surgical or endovascular intervention. Despite this retrospective study's limited sample size and lack of CT angiographic imaging technique, these findings demonstrate significant diagnostic utility using contrast-enhanced CT scan imaging for identification of torso vascular injuries requiring further intervention.

While there are no randomized comparisons of CT versus MR angiography in the diagnosis of pediatric traumatic vascular injuries, MR angiography is valuable in identification of intracerebral and cervical vascular injuries associated with traumatic brain injury. However, when MR angiography is compared to CT angiography, there are distinct advantages for CT angiography in children. These include more rapid imaging acquisition and decreased need for significant sedation and/or anesthesia. The results from several studies evaluating the use of CT angiography in adult vascular trauma have also provided the rationale for its use in children with possible cervical, torso, or extremity vascular injury [12, 13]. A retrospective series from a Level 1 Trauma Center at the University of Miami reviewed the use of CT angiography in 78 pediatric patients with suspected cervical or extremity vascular injuries caused by either blunt or penetrating trauma [14]. CT angiography was diagnostic for major vascular injury in 11 patients with penetrating trauma, giving rise to 100 % sensitivity, 93 % specificity, a positive predictive value of 85 %, and a negative predictive value of 100 %. For 8 patients with vascular injury from blunt trauma, CT angiography was 88 % sensitive and 100 % specific with a 100 % positive predictive value and 97 % negative predictive value. The accuracy of CT angiography to identify major vascular injury for either penetrating or blunt trauma in children less than 19 years of age exceeded 95 % in this report.

Similar to the adult experience, CT angiography appears to have comparable sensitivity and specificity to conventional contrast angiography in pediatric trauma. Additionally, greater resolution of injuries to adjacent structures is achieved with CT in comparison to angiography. The relative ease of access, shorter time to achieve diagnostic images, greater ability to simultaneously assess adjacent structures, and less invasive nature of CT angiography are compelling factors to consider when imaging is deemed necessary. Both conventional angiography and CT angiography share the risk of radiation exposure and contrast-induced nephropathy. However, controlling the scan pass frequency, x-ray tube current, peak voltage, pitch factor, and gantry rotation allows for reduction of radiation exposure [15]. Complications of conventional angiography in pediatric patients include issues related to sedation and difficulty with vascular access. Arterial access complications include hematoma, pseudoaneurysm and arteriovenous fistula formation, acute arterial thrombosis, and lower extremity limb-length discrepancy resulting from chronic femoral artery occlusion.

Finally, for pediatric extremity vascular injuries, duplex ultrasonography may be useful in initial evaluation and long-term follow-up. However, the use of duplex ultrasonography in the acute assessment of pediatric vascular injury has not been well studied, and its use is generally reflective of institutional availability and experience.

26.4 Specific Vascular Injuries in Children

The diagnosis and management of most vascular injuries in children follows all established guidelines for adults. A few unique clinical management issues in children and adolescents with vascular injury are more thoroughly discussed below.

26.4.1 Aortic Injuries

The incidence rate of aortic injuries in adults is well established and remains one of the most commonly reported causes of death at the scene of motor vehicle crashes. The incidence rate of traumatic aortic rupture in children is lower but continues to carry significant morbidity and mortality. The incidence of pediatric thoracic aortic injury ranges from 0.1 to 2.1 % with blunt mechanisms most common [1, 16]. A retrospective review from Seattle reported the most common cause of thoracic aorta injury in children was blunt trauma from car versus pedestrian (46 %) followed by motor vehicle crashes (38 %); none of the children with thoracic aortic injury from motor vehicle crashes were wearing seat belts [17]. Aortic disruption due to blunt trauma can be caused by either direct chest wall compression or sudden torsional and/or deceleration causing shear stress [18]. While the aortic arch is relatively fixed, the descending aorta is more mobile, causing the aortic isthmus to be the most common site of blunt aortic injury in both children and adults.

Signs associated with blunt injury to the thoracic aorta are similar in both adults and children. Suspicious findings on chest x-ray include widening of the mediastinum, loss of the aortic knob, presence of a left pleural cap, deviation of the trachea to the right, fracture of the first or second ribs, scapula fracture, depression of the left mainstem bronchus, obliteration of the aortopulmonary window, and deviation of the esophagus to the left. Given the relative compliance of the chest wall in younger patients, children may have blunt aortic injury without demonstrable rib, clavicular, or scapular fractures. Presence of these signs upon initial examination mandates further evaluation of the aorta. CT angiography has largely replaced conventional angiography as the primary modality used to diagnose pediatric aortic injury.

Management of pediatric traumatic aortic rupture requires modification of some perioperative and operative strategies. Due to the significant forces required to injure the aorta, these children are at high risk for other organ injuries, particularly the brain, solid organs, spine, and spinal cord. In the absence of significant traumatic brain injury, early use of beta-blockade and control of blood pressure is warranted. Operative repair with or without mechanical circulatory support remains the standard treatment for comparison [19]. In the presence of traumatic brain injury, the use of medications to reduce heart rate and blood pressure must be judiciously weighed against the need for maintaining adequate cerebral perfusion pressure. Most children with traumatic aortic rupture are adolescents that approximate adult

size; in younger children, the aorta is significantly smaller in caliber and is generally more fragile. Establishment of intraoperative cardiopulmonary bypass procedures in children may be technically challenging and requires size- and weight-specific cannulas, instrumentation, and surgeon experience. The use of femoral arterial and/or venous access for bypass may be limited by the diminutive caliber of these vessels in smaller children.

Access and use of size-specific aortic grafts in children must also consider future growth, and both short- and long-term follow up is essential. Children undergoing thoracic aortic repair for trauma should be followed by an experienced pediatric cardiologist to determine flow characteristics across the graft; if hemodynamically significant "pseudocoarctation" occurs across the graft during adolescence or adulthood, graft replacement is warranted. Finally, in the presence of traumatic brain injury or other associated injuries at risk for hemorrhage, strategies aimed at minimizing systemic anticoagulation during repair include using heparin-coated cardiopulmonary bypass circuits, utilization of aortic bypass techniques with intracorporeal shunts that do not require systemic heparin, and selective deployment of endovascular stent grafts.

The rationale for using endovascular stent grafts to treat pediatric aortic rupture reflects the successful use of stents in adult trauma victims and, in part, the experience with stent grafts to treat congenital aortic coarctation. A multicenter observational study conducted by the Congenital Cardiovascular Interventional Study Consortium (CCISC) evaluated 350 adult and pediatric patients undergoing stent placement, operative repair, or balloon angioplasty to treat aortic coarctation [20]. There was a significantly lower acute complication rate with stent placement compared with patients undergoing operative repair or balloon angioplasty. In this nonrandomized study, stents were placed in patients that were significantly older (mean age 16.6 years) and larger (mean bodyweight 55 kg) compared to patients undergoing operative repair or balloon angioplasty. Subgroup analysis of patients 6–12 years of age demonstrated that stenting had a lower overall acute complication rate (1.8 %) compared to surgery or balloon angioplasty (13 % each). The CCISC reviewed 398 patients ages 4–19 years old undergoing aortic stenting for native or recurrent aortic coarctation and reported an overall complication rate of 12.6 % for this specific age group [21]. The authors concluded that aortic stenting was an effective treatment for coarctation, but it remained technically challenging with a high complication rate. Technical complications decreased over the course of the study and were attributed, in part, to improved catheter and stent technology.

There are several small series and case reports of successful endovascular stent repair of pediatric traumatic aortic injuries [19, 22–24]. These patients are typically older children or adolescents with significant extracardiac injuries or physiological compromise felt to create prohibitive risk for open repair (e.g., bilateral pulmonary contusion, traumatic brain injury with intracranial hemorrhage, abdominal or pelvic injuries at risk for hemorrhage). These studies note size-specific issues related to available grafts for use in children and vascular access for stent graft deployment; if the femoral vessels are too small to accommodate the sheath or stent, operative approaches to the iliac artery or infrarenal aorta may be required.

Perioperative use of unfractionated heparin in children undergoing endovascular stent placement is recommended; therefore, the risk of bleeding from associated injuries with systemic antithrombotic therapy must be weighed against the potential for thromboembolism. Complications of aortic stenting for pediatric aortic injury should mirror the adult experience, including technical complications related to stent deployment or migration, injury to the aorta, and both neurological and peripheral vascular complications from ischemia and thromboembolism. In selected children with significant extrathoracic injuries, endovascular stent repair may temporize an immediately life-threatening injury and defer direct operative aortic reconstruction until other injuries have resolved. It remains important to note that endovascular stent repair has not been widely used in children with aortic injury, and the immediate and long-term efficacy of this approach remains unclear.

In summary, pediatric traumatic aortic rupture is an uncommon but significant, immediately life-threatening injury typically diagnosed using CT angiography. Initial management should be directed at control of heart rate and blood pressure if practical while simultaneously identifying all other associated injuries. Management options require individualization based upon the child's size, associated injuries, and institutional experience. The degree and location of injury, as well as the caliber of the aorta and access vessels, require careful assessment when deciding the method of aortic repair. As experience increases with pediatric endovascular stent grafts, this approach may offer an effective treatment in selected children with aortic injury. The immediate and long-term efficacy of endovascular stenting for pediatric aortic injury remains to be determined.

26.4.2 Extremity Injuries

The upper and lower extremities are the first and third most common sites of pediatric vascular injury, respectively [2, 6]. Penetrating injuries from gunshot wounds, glass, lawn mower blades, or boat propeller blades are common causes of extremity vascular injury in children. Blunt vascular injuries are typically from motor vehicle crashes, falls, or pedestrians struck by vehicles, and these are often associated with fractures. Historically, more than half of pediatric extremity vascular injuries were from glass; in more recent series, gunshot wounds are accounting for an equivalent proportion [6, 25]. Blunt upper extremity injury associated with open or closed supracondylar fracture accounts for a consistent 35–40 % of all reported pediatric vascular injuries. Management of extremity vascular injury in children offers both diagnostic and treatment challenges due to the small caliber of the vessels, the greater effect of arterial spasm, and considerations for further limb growth. Arterial vasospasm may be pronounced and prolonged in children and adolescents in response to both blunt and proximal penetrating injuries. Early consultation and prompt transfer to a regional trauma center with expertise in pediatric vascular and microvascular reconstruction is highly desirable if there is a threatened extremity from vascular injury that exceeds local capacity for treatment or intervention. In the absence of a mangled extremity, limb amputation for traumatic extremity arterial insufficiency is extremely infrequent in the neonatal and pediatric population.

26.4.3 Neonatal and Infant Femoral Artery Injury

In infants and very young children of preschool age (less than 2–3 years old), diagnosis of extremity vascular injury is complicated by the difficulty in precise evaluation of motor and sensory function during preverbal stages of development. Fortunately, vascular injury is less frequent in this age group. Newborn infants have been observed to have a slightly lower normal mean ABI of 0.88; the ABI should normally increase to greater than 0.9 at 1 year of age [26]. Therefore, a threshold ABI of less than 0.9 remains clinically useful in determining the need for confirmatory diagnostic testing for vascular injury with neonates a notable exception. Much of the published experience reflects management of iatrogenic femoral arterial injuries following percutaneous catheterization for diagnostic and/or therapeutic procedures such as cardiac catheterization and arterial line monitoring. These femoral arterial injuries are anatomically focal and there are usually no other associated traumatic injuries. However, there may be significant congenital cardiovascular disease requiring comprehensive management. In this age group, there is consensus that arterial injuries presenting with hemorrhage, arteriovenous fistula, or pseudoaneurysm require repair.

Historically, neonates and infants with an acutely ischemic lower extremity were also explored. Lin and colleagues from Emory University [27] reported a case series of 34 children with iatrogenic femoral arterial injury due to catheterization. Fourteen children had acute leg ischemia associated with a focal femoral artery injury treated by thrombectomy and either primary closure or saphenous vein patch angioplasty. All postoperative morbidity, mortality, and failure to regain palpable pedal pulses were in children less than or equal to 2 years of age, suggesting this younger group was particularly vulnerable. Lazarides et al. reviewed twelve published case series from 1981 to 2006 that provided detailed descriptions of arterial injuries in children [28]. Thirty-one operations were performed for acutely ischemic, threatened extremities in 28 children less than 2.5 years old. Less than half of the extremities regained palpable pulses with a mortality of 25 % and limb-length discrepancy of 15 %. In the setting of an acutely ischemic, threatened extremity, surgical management and outcome in this age group clearly remains challenging.

Clinically distinguishing the viability of an ischemic distal extremity in a neonate or infant can be difficult. This is an age group characterized by extraordinarily small target vessels with profound arterial vasospasm in response to mechanical injury or cold temperature. Unremitting vasospasm can contribute to thrombus propagation into the iliac artery and aorta. Initial management should be aimed at maintaining normal hemodynamics, removal of any arterial or venous catheters present in the affected limb, and warming the distal extremity. In general, symptoms of arterial vasospasm in a neonate should reverse within 3–6 h. The most appropriate early intervention for threatened or nonthreatened limb ischemia associated with femoral arterial thrombosis is prompt initiation of antithrombotic therapy. There must be no clinical contraindications to anticoagulation, and assessment of limb viability should be performed frequently.

Signs of a viable extremity include the presence of a proximal palpable pulse, distal Doppler signals, capillary refill, and absent skin mottling [28]. For this age group, the presence of these signs may help to predict successful nonoperative management of arterial extremity ischemia using systemic anticoagulation with heparin and/or thrombolytic therapy [28, 29]. In infants, systemic anticoagulation and/or thrombolytic therapy may prevent thrombus propagation and increase the probability of vessel patency with healing. There is age-dependent distribution, binding, and clearance of antithrombotic agents, and it is helpful to have guidance from an experienced pediatric hematologist. Evidence-based guidelines for antithrombotic therapy in neonates and infants from the American College of Chest Physicians (ACCP) recommend the use of unfractionated heparin at a loading dose of 75 units/kg intravenously over 10 min, followed by an initial maintenance dose of 28 units/kg/h for infants less than 1 year old and 20 units/kg/h for older children [30]. Titration of heparin dosing should be performed to obtain an activated partial thromboplastin time (aPTT) of 60–85 s or an anti-Xa level of 0.35–0.70. In the absence of contraindications, ACCP clinical guidelines recommend that infants with limb- or organ-threatening femoral artery thrombosis unresponsive to unfractionated heparin should be treated with thrombolytic therapy; if there is contraindication to thrombolytic therapy, surgical intervention is recommended in this setting [30]. This management approach is relatively unique for iatrogenic vascular injuries in this fragile age group with diminutive arterial vessel caliber.

26.4.4 Childhood and Adolescent Extremity Injury

The management of vascular injuries in older children and adolescents follows contemporary adult practice. To account for future somatic growth, most surgeons utilize primary repair when possible and vein patch angioplasty or reversed vein grafts for reconstruction of more complex arterial injuries. Vein grafts are typically harvested from an uninjured limb to prevent iatrogenic disruption of venous drainage from the injured extremity. In the setting of pediatric vascular injury, there are no compelling, evidence-based data regarding the use of interrupted versus continuous suture repair or the use of permanent versus absorbable suture in vascular reconstruction. Therefore, the surgeon should use the techniques that are most familiar to him/her in this setting. Pediatric trauma centers have immediate access to surgeons capable of providing emergent exploration and control of life-threatening hemorrhage; these institutions should also have immediate access to pediatric interventional radiology and surgical specialists in both vascular and microvascular reconstruction.

If immediate vascular repair or reconstruction is not possible during primary exploration for hemorrhage, a temporary shunt may be used as a bridge for maintaining distal perfusion. Successful use of temporary vascular shunts has been reported in civilian and military settings as an adjunct to damage control and as means of injury management prior to transportation for definitive care [31, 32]. There is extremely limited published experience using temporary shunts in children. For smaller children, temporary vascular shunts will require the use of smaller diameter neonatal or pediatric cardiopulmonary bypass cannula, neonatal chest tubes, or pediatric feeding tubes. General technical caveats include loupe magnification and/or the use of an operating microscope, establishing and maintaining normothermia, liberal use of papaverine or topical lidocaine to reverse vasospasm, and generous spatulation of vessels undergoing primary repair using 6–0, 7–0, or 8–0 monofilament sutures [33].

Similar to adults, primary venous reconstruction is desirable when feasible. The use of prosthetic grafts should be limited to the adult-sized adolescent unless autologous grafts are unavailable or impractical. Fasciotomies of the distal extremity compartments should be considered and promptly performed in all children requiring vascular reconstruction with prolonged limb ischemia. Finally, actual blood loss due to vascular injury and its repair may be grossly underestimated in children, and access to massive transfusion capability along with vigilant perioperative monitoring is essential.

Supracondylar fractures of the humerus are an important and relatively common pediatric injury pattern associated with traumatic arterial insufficiency (Fig. 26.1). Failure to promptly recognize brachial artery injury in a child can lead to the development of Volkmann ischemic flexion contracture of the wrist. Children presenting with supracondylar fractures associated

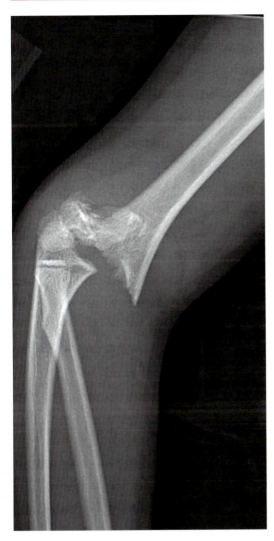

Fig. 26.1 Supracondylar fractures of the humerus are an important and relatively common pediatric injury pattern associated with traumatic arterial insufficiency

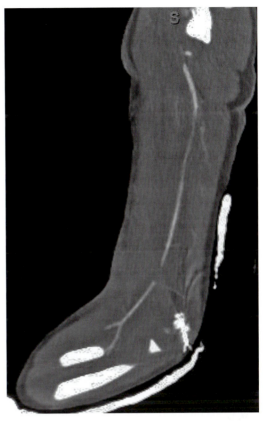

Fig. 26.2 Following reduction, persistent arterial insufficiency determined by either lack of palpable radial pulse, diminished Doppler signals, or decreased flow on Doppler ultrasonography mandates urgent diagnosis and management; some surgeons advocate immediate exploration in this setting, while others will pursue demonstration of brachial artery injury by either duplex or triplex ultrasonography or CT angiography prior to exploration

with a pulseless distal extremity should undergo immediate closed reduction and percutaneous pinning of the fracture. Following reduction, persistent arterial insufficiency determined by either lack of palpable radial pulse, diminished Doppler signals, or decreased flow on Doppler ultrasonography mandates urgent diagnosis and management; some surgeons advocate immediate exploration in this setting, while others will pursue demonstration of brachial artery injury by either duplex or triplex ultrasonography or CT angiography prior to exploration (Fig. 26.2). A

retrospective review of 59 consecutive children with type III supracondylar humeral fractures at Children's Hospital of Boston found evidence of brachial artery injury in 11 (18.6 %) [33]. At exploration, three of these children were found to have brachial artery in spasm. As many of these children are under 10 years of age, the brachial artery is diminutive, and successful repair may require microsurgical techniques [34, 35].

One of the clinically relevant issues with pediatric extremity vascular injury is limb-length discrepancy as a result of chronic arterial insufficiency during growth. Long-term follow-up in pediatric patients undergoing operative repair of extremity arterial injury demonstrates ipsilateral limb shortening in 33–50 % despite rapid development of collateral circulation [36, 37]. Even in the setting of a viable extremity, an aggressive approach at treating arterial insufficiency in a growing child may be important to prevent limb-length discrepancy. Routine follow-up is essential to evaluate for claudication, gait disturbance due to limb-length discrepancy, and changes in ABI. This is also a setting where duplex ultrasonography may have an important diagnostic role in children. Limb-length discrepancy requires extremity plain x-ray films and measurement of bone length, as external measurements are less accurate. Symptomatic arterial insufficiency following pediatric vascular injury requires further diagnostic investigation and intervention. Most surgeons agree that revascularization is indicated for symptomatic extremity arterial insufficiency in a growing child or adolescent. However, the effect of revascularization for chronic extremity arterial insufficiency on reversing limb-length discrepancy remains less clear. In addition, it remains difficult to discern the effect of associated traumatic soft tissue injury, fracture, and nerve injury on limb growth trajectory in children requiring extremity vascular repair.

In summary, pediatric extremity vascular injury is complicated by the small caliber of the injured vessels and the propensity for vasospasm. Management principles are guided by clinical determination of ongoing hemorrhage, hemodynamic status, and limb viability. The ABI remains useful in assessing distal lower limb perfusion in neonates, infants, and children. Selected cases of neonatal and pediatric iatrogenic femoral arterial injury may be successfully managed by antithrombotic therapy. Operative management of childhood and adolescent vascular injuries follows established principles for adult vascular trauma. The use of temporary vascular shunting in children requires access to smaller diameter, size-specific shunts and may be a useful adjunct during damage control. Chronic extremity arterial insufficiency in growing children may result in limb-length discrepancy, highlighting the need for close follow-up.

References

1. Anderson SA, Day M, Chen MK, Huber T, Lottenberg LL, Kays DW, Beierle EA. Traumatic aortic injuries in the pediatric population. J Pediatr Surg. 2008;43(6):1077–81. PMID: 18558186.
2. Barmparas G, Inaba K, Talving P, David JS, Lam L, Plurad D, Green D, Demetriades D. Pediatric vs adult vascular trauma: a National Trauma Databank review. J Pediatr Surg. 2010;45(7):1404–12. PMID: 20638516.
3. Allison ND, Anderson CM, Shah SK, Lally KP, Hayes-Jordan A, Tsao KJ, Andrassy RJ, Cox Jr CS. Outcomes of truncal vascular injuries in children. J Pediatr Surg. 2009;44(10):1958–64. PMID: 19853755.
4. Tepas JJ, Walsh DS. Vascular injury. In: Coran AG, Caldamore AA, Adzick NS, Krummel TM, Laberge JM, Shamberger RC, editors. Pediatric surgery. 7th ed. Philadelphia: Elsevier/Saunders; 2012. p. 361–7.
5. Corneille MG, Gallup TM, Villa C, Richa JM, Wolf SE, Myers JG, Dent DL, Stewart RM. Pediatric vascular injuries: acute management and early outcomes. J Trauma. 2011;70(4):823–8. PMID: 21610390.
6. Klinkner DB, Arca MJ, Lewis BD, Oldham KT, Sato TT. Pediatric vascular injuries: patterns of injury, morbidity, and mortality. J Pediatr Surg. 2007;42(1):178–82. PMID: 17208561.
7. Peclet MH, Newman KD, Eichelberger MR, Gotschall CS, Guzzetta PC, Anderson KD, Garcia VF, Randolph JG, Bowman LM. Patterns of injury in children. J Pediatr Surg. 1990;25(1):85–90. PMID: 2299550.
8. Shah SR, Wearden PD, Gaines BA. Pediatric peripheral vascular injuries: a review of our experience. J Surg Res. 2009;153(1):162–6. PMID: 18541266.
9. Harris LM, Hordines J. Major vascular injuries in the pediatric population. Ann Vasc Surg. 2003;17(3):266–9. PMID: 12704551.
10. Lew SM, Frumiento C, Wald SL. Pediatric blunt carotid injury: a review of the National Pediatric Trauma Registry. Pediatr Neurosurg. 1999;30(5):239–44. PMID: 10461070.
11. Maturen KE, Adusumilli S, Blane CE, Arbabi S, Williams DM, Fitzgerald JT, Vine AA. Contrast-enhanced CT accurately detects hemorrhage in torso trauma: direct comparison with angiography. J Trauma. 2007;62(3):740–5. PMID: 17414357.
12. Inaba K, Potzman J, Munera F, McKenney M, Munoz R, Rivas L, Dunham M, DuBose J. Multi-slice CT angiography for arterial evaluation in the injured lower extremity. J Trauma. 2006;60(3):502–6. PMID: 16531846.
13. Uyeda JW, Anderson SW, Sakai O, Soto JA. CT angiography in trauma. Radiol Clin North Am. 2010;48(2):423–38. PMID: 20609881.
14. Hogan AR, Lineen EB, Perez EA, Neville HL, Thompson WR, Sola JE. Value of computed tomographic angiography in neck and extremity pediatric vascular trauma. J Pediatr Surg. 2009;44(6):1236–41. PMID: 19524747.

15. Chan FP, Rubin GD. MDCT angiography of pediatric vascular diseases of the abdomen, pelvis, and extremities. Pediatr Radiol. 2005;35(1):40–53. PMID: 15692842.

16. Eddy AC, Rusch VW, Fligner CL, Reay DT, Rice CL. The epidemiology of traumatic rupture of the thoracic aorta in children: a 13-year review. J Trauma. 1990;30(8):989–91. PMID: 2388309.

17. Eddy AC, Misbach GA, Luna GK. Traumatic rupture of the thoracic aorta in the pediatric patient. Pediatr Emerg Care. 1989;5(4):228–30. PMID:2602195.

18. Shkrum MJ, McClafferty KJ, Green RN, Nowak ES, Young JG. Mechanisms of aortic injury in fatalities occurring in motor vehicle collisions. J Forensic Sci. 1999;44(1):44–56. PMID: 9987869.

19. Karmy-Jones R, Hoffer E, Meissner M, Bloch RD. Management of traumatic rupture of the thoracic aorta in pediatric patients. Ann Thorac Surg. 2003;75(5):1513–7. PMID: 12735571.

20. Forbes TJ, Kim DW, Du W, Turner DR, Holzer R, Amin Z, Hijazi Z, Ghasemi A, Rome JJ, Nykanen D, Zahn E, Cowley C, Hoyer M, Waight D, Gruenstein D, Javois A, Foerster S, Kreutzer J, Sullivan N, Khan A, Owada C, Hagler D, Lim S, Canter J, Zellers T, CCISC Investigators. Comparison of surgical, stent, and balloon angioplasty treatment of native coarctation of the aorta: an observational study by the CCISC (Congenital Cardiovascular Interventional Study Consortium). J Am Coll Cardiol. 2011;58(25):2664–74.

21. Forbes TJ, Garekar S, Amin Z, Zahn EM, Nykanen D, Moore P, Qureshi SA, Cheatham JP, Ebeid MR, Hijazi ZM, Sandhu S, Hagler DJ, Sievert H, Fagan TE, Ringewald J, Du W, Tang L, Wax DF, Rhodes J, Johnston TA, Jones TK, Turner DR, Pedra CA, Hellenbrand WE, Congenital Cardiovascular Interventional Study Consortium (CCISC). Procedural results and acute complications in stenting native and recurrent coarctation of the aorta in patients over 4 years of age: a multi-institutional study. Catheter Cardiovasc Interv. 2007;70(2):276–85.

22. Milas ZL, Milner R, Chaikoff E, Wulkan M, Ricketts R. Endograft stenting in the adolescent population for traumatic aortic injuries. J Pediatr Surg. 2006;41(5):e27–30. PMID: 16677872.

23. Gunabushanam V, Mishra N, Calderin J, Glick R, Rosca M, Krishnasastry K. Endovascular stenting of blunt thoracic aortic injury in an 11-year-old. J Pediatr Surg. 2010;45(3):E15–8. PMID: 20223302.

24. Goldstein BH, Hirsch R, Zussman ME, Vincent JA, Torres AJ, Coulson J, Ringel RE, Beekman 3rd RH. Percutaneous balloon-expandable covered stent implantation for treatment of traumatic aortic injury in children and adolescents. Am J Cardiol. 2012;110(10):1541–5. PMID: 22853985.

25. Evans WE, King DR, Hayes JP. Arterial trauma in children: diagnosis and management. Ann Vasc Surg. 1988;2(3):268–70. PMID: 3191008.

26. Katz S, Globerman A, Avitzour M, Dolfin T. The ankle-brachial index in normal neonates and infants is significantly lower than in older children and adults. J Pediatr Surg. 1997;32(2):269–71. PMID: 9044135.

27. Lin PH, Dodson TF, Bush RL, Weiss VJ, Conklin BS, Chen C, Chaikof EL, Lumsden AB. Surgical intervention for complications caused by femoral artery catheterization in pediatric patients. J Vasc Surg. 2001;34(6):1071–8. PMID: 11743563.

28. Lazarides MK, Georgiadis GS, Papas TT, Gardikis S, Maltezos C. Operative and nonoperative management of children aged 13 years or younger with arterial trauma of the extremities. J Vasc Surg. 2006;43(1):72–6. PMID: 16414390.

29. Ade-Ajayi N, Hall NJ, Liesner R, Kiely EM, Pierro A, Roebuck DJ, Drake DP. Acute neonatal arterial occlusion: is thrombolysis safe and effective? J Pediatr Surg. 2008;43(10):1827–32. PMID: 18926215.

30. Monagle P, Chan AK, Goldenberg NA, Ichord RN, Journeycake JM, Nowak-Göttl U, Vesely SK; American College of Chest Physicians. Antithrombotic therapy in neonates and children: antithrombotic therapy and prevention of thrombosis. 9th ed: American College of Chest Physicians Evidence-Based Clinical Practice Guidelines. Chest. 2012;141(2 Suppl):e737S–801S. PMID: 22315277.

31. Johansen K, Bandyk D, Thiele B, Hansen Jr ST. Temporary intraluminal shunts: resolution of a management dilemma in complex vascular injuries. J Trauma. 1982;22(5):395–402. PMID: 7077701.

32. Borut LT, Acosta CJ, Tadlock LC, Dye JL, Galarneau M, Elshire CD. The use of temporary vascular shunts in military extremity wounds: a preliminary outcome analysis with 2-year follow-up. J Trauma. 2010;69(1):174–8. PMID: 20622589.

33. Campbell CC, Waters PM, Emans JB, Kasser JR, Millis MB. Neurovascular injury and displacement in type III supracondylar humerus fractures. J Pediatr Orthop. 1995;15(1):47–52. PMID: 7883927.

34. Noaman HH. Microsurgical reconstruction of brachial artery injuries in displaced supracondylar fracture humerus in children. Microsurgery. 2006;26(7):498–505. PMID: 17001639.

35. Reigstad O, Thorkildsen R, Grimsgaard C, Reigstad A, Røkkum M. Supracondylar fractures with circulatory failure after reduction, pinning, and entrapment of the brachial artery: excellent results more than 1 year after open exploration and revascularization. J Orthop Trauma. 2011;25(1):26–30. PMID: 21085027.

36. Whitehouse WM, Coran AG, Stanley JC, Kuhns LR, Weintraub WH, Fry WJ. Pediatric vascular trauma. Manifestations, management, and sequelae of extremity arterial injury in patients undergoing surgical treatment. Arch Surg. 1976;111(11):1269–75.

37. Flanigan DP, Keifer TJ, Schuler JJ, Ryan TJ, Castronuovo JJ. Experience with iatrogenic pediatric vascular injuries. Incidence, etiology, management, and results. Ann Surg. 1983;198(4):430–42.

Military Vascular Injuries

27

Charles J. Fox

Contents

27.1   Introduction

Vascular injury in the military has special significance. Combat-related injuries to major vessels present unique technical challenges and result in hemorrhage that is responsible for nearly 80 % of potentially preventable deaths on the battlefield [1]. The most lethal vascular injuries are those to the torso, which includes the chest and abdomen. Torso injury is reportedly the cause of half of all potentially survivable hemorrhagic deaths, followed by extremity vascular injury, which is responsible for one third [2]. The front lines of a battleground are chaotic, located in harsh environments, and vary widely, depending on the goal and scope of military operations. Surgical care may be rendered in tents or buildings of opportunity that lack suitable light and ventilation or in more established and well-equipped forward surgical hospitals. These austere conditions, combined with the technical demands associated with the treatment of vascular injury, necessitate the early and deliberate preparation of military medics and surgeons at all levels of care to ensure the successful management of vascular trauma [3–5].

27.2   Historical Perspective

During World War II, time lags, practical difficulties, and poor physiologic conditions led DeBakey to conclude after an analysis of nearly

C.J. Fox, MD, FACS
Department of Surgery,
Denver Health Medical Center,
University of Colorado School of Medicine,
777 Bannock Street, M.C. 0206,
Denver, CO 80204, USA
e-mail: charles.fox@dhha.org

A. Dua et al. (eds.), *Clinical Review of Vascular Trauma*,
DOI 10.1007/978-3-642-39100-2_27, © Springer-Verlag Berlin Heidelberg 2014

2,500 cases that vessel ligation, while not the "procedure of choice, is one of necessity" [6]. During the Korean War, a surgical research team was established to study this problem in an effort to improve on the management of combat-related vascular injury [7]. Since the spring of 1952, several reports on successful arterial repairs performed under austere conditions without the benefit of proper instruments gained the attention of the Office of the Surgeon General [8–10]. Hughes demonstrated among 269 repairs an impressive reduction in the amputation rate from 36 % in World War II to 13 % during the Korean War. Time lags and ongoing resuscitation needs remained the ultimate "Achilles heel" of successful vascular surgery during the Korean War [7]. Battlefield environments became more favorable for difficult vascular reconstructions during the Vietnam War. Forward surgical positioning to minimize ischemic time, along with modern resuscitation practices, permitted the widespread application and success of arterial reconstruction. The management of complex injuries such as those involving the popliteal artery and vein, or large cavitary wounds that threaten graft viability, and those associated with severe open contaminated fractures became the focus of attention during this era [11]. The Vietnam Vascular Registry under the leadership of Normal Rich details a careful analysis with completed follow-up of over 1,000 cases and now serves as a reference standard for the application of vascular surgery during the modern conflicts of the twenty-first century [12].

27.3   Recent Advances

With more than 8,000 deaths and approximately 50,000 combat-related injuries in over a decade of modern warfare, the global war on terror (GWOT) has proved to be a formidable and sustained military campaign. During this conflict, advances in many forms have allowed for a concerted effort to reduce deaths from potentially survivable vascular injuries and improve the quality of functional extremity salvage (i.e., saving life and limb) [13–16].

At the beginning of the GWOT, the Department of Defense implemented a testing, training, and fielding program for battlefield tourniquets [17–19]. Effectiveness of early tourniquet application observed in Iraq and Afghanistan has led to doctrinal changes that have produced a surge of patients with vascular injuries who, in the past, would not have reached a field hospital alive [20]. Although current military endeavors regarding the appropriateness of tourniquet use began with trepidation, the forward deployment of surgical capabilities has limited tourniquet duration, thus increasing effectiveness, reducing complications, and ultimately improving survival [21–24]. The development of the Joint Theater Trauma System has also improved surgical care and reduced mortality by implementing clinical practice guidelines and performing outcomes research emerging from the Joint Theater Trauma System, the GWOT Vascular Initiative, and the Walter Reed Vascular Registry.

Other modern advances include the routine use of personal protective gear, the deployment of level II facilities at more forward locations, and the selective application of surgical adjuncts (e.g., temporary vascular shunts, fasciotomies) [25, 26]. Management of complex soft tissue wounds associated with vascular injury with negative-pressure wound therapy and the performance of tibia-level reconstruction for selected injury have also advanced the practice of limb salvage on the modern battlefield [27, 28]. Finally, this is the first conflict whereby endovascular technologies that have been used to diagnose and treat certain types of vascular, pelvic, and solid organ war-related injuries have become more widespread and generally accepted as a mainstay of surgical care [28–32].

27.4   Incidence and Distribution

During the Vietnam War, vascular injuries accounted for 2–3 % of battle-related injuries [12]. However, reports during the current war have demonstrated that the contemporary rate of vascular injury has increased from 9 to 12 % of battle-related injuries, adjusting the rate of vascular injury to five times that reported in prior conflicts [33]. The increased incidence of vascular injury may have several explanations, but certainly protective armor, tourniquets, and an overall increased diagnosing and recording of such injuries have been major factors.

Lower extremity vascular injuries occur at approximately two times the rate of upper extremity injuries, reflecting the relative length of axial vessels and the exposed position of the lower extremity away from protective body armor. The anatomic distribution of arterial and venous injuries is roughly the same. In the lower extremity, the superficial femoral artery is most commonly injured closely followed by the popliteal and tibial arteries (Table 27.1). Injuries to the proximal common femoral and profunda femoris arteries are less common because of

Table 27.1 Distribution and management of 497 patients with 523 vascular injuries using DCR

Location/vascular Injury	Suture	Patch	End-end	Prosthetic	SV interposition	SV bypass	Ligation	Thrombectomy	Total
Abdomen									
Splenic			1				2		3
Renal							1		1
Iliac	1		1	5			2		9
Hypogastric	1						1		2
Neck									
Carotid	2		4		2				8
Chest									
Aorta	1								1
Innominate			2						2
Upper extremity									
Subclavian	1		1	2	2		1		7
Axillary	1	1		1	4	2			9
Brachial	6	1	6	1	48	6	1	2	71
Ulnar	6	1	1	1	1	2	13		25
Radial		1	1		4		18		24
Lower extremity									
Common femoral	4		1	2	6	3	2	1	19
Superficial femoral	4	6	8	2	39	6	3	2	70
Popliteal			5		35	10	4	5	59
Tibial	6	1	5		9	2	28	1	52
Venous									
Saphenous							8		8
Radial							1		1
Brachial					2		9		11
Basilic							7		7
Cephalic	2						5		7
Jugular	1		1				5		7
Subclavian							2		2
Axillary	2						5		7
Hepatic	1						1		2
Splenic							2		2
Hypogastric							1		1
Iliac	3		1				11		15
Femoral	1		2		5		7		15
Superficial femoral	7	1	6	1	6		18	1	40
Tibial	1						13		14
Popliteal	1	1	3		4		13		22
Total	**52**	**13**	**49**	**15**	**167**	**31**	**184**	**12**	**523**

Adapted from Dua et al. [13]

Suture primary repair, *End-End* end-end anastomosis, *SV* saphenous vein

Table 27.2 Distribution and management of 111 US casualties with 113 extremity vascular injuries

Artery	Primary repair	SVG	Prosthetic	Repairs	# Patent	Amputation	Survival	Follow-up[b]
Iliac	1	1	1	3	3 (100 %)		3 (100 %)	347 days (29–1,079)
Femoral	10	20	3	33	29 (87.9 %)	4 (12.1 %)	33 (100 %)	
Popliteal	1	22		23[a]	16 (69.6 %)	7 (30.4 %)	22 (100 %)	
Tibial	9	4		13	11 (84.6 %)	2 (15.4 %)	13 (100 %)	
Brachial	4	28	1	33[a]	30 (90.9 %)	2 (6.7 %)	31 (96.9 %)	
Ulnar	1	3		4	3 (75 %)	1 (25 %)	4 (100 %)	
Radial	2	2		4	4 (100 %)		4 (100 %)	
Total	**28**	**80**	**5**	**113**	**96 (84.9 %)**	**16 (14.2 %)**	**110 (99.1 %)**	

Adapted from Dua et al. [13]

SVG saphenous vein graft

[a]1 Bilateral repair

[b]Mean (range)

their proximity to the protective structures of the torso and their lethality when they do occur. In a detailed analysis of penetrating femoropopliteal injuries during modern warfare, Woodward and colleagues showed that nearly 50 % of lower extremity vascular injuries had a combined arterial and venous component [34]. Because nearly all vascular injuries in wartime are caused by blast or high-velocity weaponry, approximately one third of those with vascular injuries have associated orthopedic injuries and up to 20 % have partial- or full-thickness burns; the same percentage has an additional head or torso injury [35]. All these associated injuries impact the decision making related to the triage and ultimate treatment of vascular injury.

Penetrating mechanisms of injury are by far the most common, with explosive devices and gunshot wounds responsible for nearly all vascular injuries during wartime [6, 7, 12, 25]. In OIF, improvised explosive devices were the cause of vascular injury in 55 % of patients, and gunshot wounds accounted for 39 % of injuries [25, 36, 37]. In one study of these penetrating injuries, 110/111 US casualties survived the immediate repair of an extremity arterial injury. This subgroup had a mean graft patency rate of 84.9 % at 347 days (range 29–1,079 days) and a primary amputation rate of 14.2 % (16/113) after surgical treatment in the US military hospitals of Iraq and Afghanistan. This outcome is especially important given their initial physiologic derangements and may have strong implications for uti-lizing fresh blood products in equal ratios when arterial reconstruction is attempted over a primary amputation (Table 27.2) [13].

27.5 Clinical Presentation

The presentation of vascular injury can be divided into two familiar categories: patients presenting with hard signs of vascular injury and those presenting with soft signs. Approximately half of wartime vascular injuries manifest hard signs, including hemorrhage from a penetrating wound or bleeding into a closed space as evidenced by an expanding hematoma, most commonly in an extremity or the neck. About 30 % of extremity vascular injuries present with an associated fracture or dislocation. Extremity ischemia is another hard sign of vascular injury commonly encountered. Careful physical examination, including use of a stethoscope, may detect the hard sign of a palpable thrill or audible bruit associated with a traumatic arteriovenous fistula. Frequently, these injuries are associated with hemorrhagic shock, with reports of significant blood loss at the scene of the injury or during evacuation. Hemorrhage from a torso vascular injury may present as hemoperitoneum or hemothorax discovered at the time of chest tube placement, thoracotomy, or laparotomy. Alternatively, in patients who are hemodynamically stable and able to undergo contrast angiographic computed tomography, vascular injury may be diagnosed by the presence of blood in the abdomen or chest or an abnormality of a large vessel (e.g., pseudoaneurysm, extravasation).

27.6 Assessment Pearls and Lessons

A concentrated effort has recently focused on reducing potentially survivable deaths from vascular injury and hemorrhagic shock. The effectiveness of early tourniquet application observed in Iraq and Afghanistan has led to doctrinal changes that have produced a surge of patients presenting with vascular injuries that in past conflicts would never have reached a field hospital alive. Optimal management requires proper planning and recognition of the essential priorities necessary to prevent immediate hemorrhagic death (Fig. 27.1). Blast-associated injury involves fractures, thermal injury, and embedded fragments over a majority of the body surface. Following immediate airway control, attention is directed at controlling hemorrhage and obtaining vascular access. External bleeding can often be hidden by warming blankets or military gear as wounded casualties usually arrive in full body armor and may have field tourniquets applied to one or more limbs. Direct pressure is the most effective way to control hemorrhage.

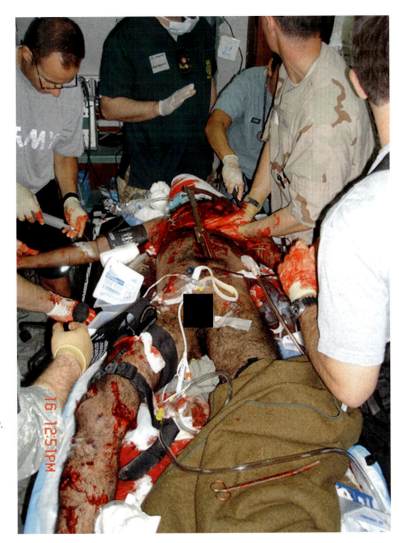

Fig. 27.1 Military trauma results in massive tissue destruction and arterial injury. Aggressive damage control resuscitation is essential for successful limb salvage efforts in combat casualties with vascular trauma with other associated life-threatening injuries (Adapted from Fox et al. [5])

A volume-depleted patient may not always manifest active arterial bleeding at the time of admission. Prehospital tourniquets should nonetheless be inspected and readjusted or replaced once the resuscitation restores adequate peripheral perfusion. For active arterial bleeding, the narrow prehospital tourniquets are commonly exchanged for the much wider EMT pneumatic type (Delfi Medical, Vancouver, Canada) and the wound is best explored in the operating room. Intravenous access may be hindered by shock, and immediate intraosseous access into the tibia or the adult sternum is easy and rapid. Initial laboratory studies will depict the degree of physiologic distress that is used to guide the resuscitation and early operative planning.

Damage control resuscitation, a strategy of liberal blood product administration, minimal crystalloid use, and selective use of recombinant factor VIIa, should begin early in the emergency room and continue intraoperatively. Hemostatic agents or plasma should be used when necessary. The goal is to achieve hemostasis, restore normal physiology, and potentially complete a vascular reconstruction prior to arrival to the intensive care unit. If the graft is done correctly, it should not fail due to correction of coagulopathy and lack of heparin administration. Blood products should be transfused within minutes of arrival with an emergency release of four units of type O packed red blood cells (PRBCs) and four units of thawed AB plasma sent on demand from the blood bank. The blood products are best transfused through a Belmont rapid infuser system (Belmont Instrument Corporation, Billerica, MA) that is reserved in the admitting area. The mean 24-h transfusion requirements are summarized for nearly 500 combat casualties with vascular injury (Table 27.3). Unstable patients with a truncal injury or those with more than one mangled extremity are considered "in extremis" and should trigger a massive transfusion protocol. This involves a standardized release and transfusion of PRBCs, thawed plasma, cryoprecipitate, and platelets. The use of FWB is safe and can be very effective in remote locations where supply is limited or in patients that require a massive transfusion [38].

Table 27.3 Summary of mean 24-h transfusion requirements after damage control resuscitation in 497 casualties

Blood component	Mean (SD)	Range
Packed RBCs	15 ± 13 units	1–70
FFP	14 ± 13 units	1–72
Cryoprecipitate	13 ± 15 units	1–49
Platelets	8 ± 6 units	1–36
Total components	42 ± 39 units	2–236
Total crystalloid	5.8 ± 4.5 l	1–28
Whole blood	6 units	3–10
rFVIIa (1 dose 90–120 g/kg)	2.1 doses	2–6
Massive transfusion (>10 units/24 h)	34 % of study group	

Adapted from Dua et al. [13]
FFP fresh frozen plasma or thawed plasma, *RBC* red blood cells, *DCR* damage control resuscitation, *rFVIIa* recombinant factor VIIa

Active bleeding should be managed by surgical exploration. Progressive ischemic burden can result in ultimate graft failure and subsequent limb loss, and therefore, early recognition is crucial for success. A pattern of soft tissue wounds and fractures is often a very reliable clue that a vascular injury exists. The pulse exam is confirmed with Doppler signals when tourniquets are safely loosened. Recognition and controlling hemorrhage is a key component of the initial assessment and subsequent decision making. These assessments are best done as a team to facilitate operative planning. Angiographic (computed tomographic or catheter based) assessments are useful for cervical and truncal vascular injury or when endovascular interventions are being considered.

27.7 Management Pearls and Lessons

A dedicated two-team approach is recommended for the surgical management of military vascular injuries. For extremity injury this practice reduces ischemic time as the primary team may be preoccupied with thoracotomy, or laparotomy to control hemorrhage, or other damage control maneuvers. A second team can apply external fixation, perform fasciotomies, begin a peripheral vascular exposure, or harvest vein from a noninjured or amputated extremity. It is important to take appropriate time to harvest the vein so as to avoid injury to the conduit which could lead to decreased graft patency. Similarly, care should be taken not to injure the saphenous vein when performing a fasciotomy. Prep, drape, and position the patient to enable unimpeded access to another body cavity or limb in the event of unexpected deterioration or need for additional vein harvesting.

Hemorrhage control is best accomplished away from an expanding hematoma. Careful dissection proximal and distal to the site of injury is generally preferable to dissection and digital occlusion within the hematoma. Communication with the anesthesia team is critical to ensure proper resuscitation and "keeping up" with operative blood loss. Balloon occlusion is often helpful for heavily calcified noncompressible vessels.

For proximal axillo-subclavian wounds, sternotomy or left anterior thoracotomy and clamping of the subclavian artery eliminate the error of uncontrolled dissection through an expanding hematoma of the chest. Alternatively, an endovascular approach, via the common femoral artery, can be used for fluoroscopic-guided intra-arterial balloon control of proximal subclavian vessels. For open control, approach distal axillary and proximal brachial arterial injuries with infraclavicular incisions, and extend across the deltopectoral region into the upper arm as needed. The medial approach is preferred for femoropopliteal injuries. The approach in relation to the knee joint is directed by the level of the wound; however, total division of muscular attachments at the knee is sometimes required to control hemorrhage of transected arteries and veins. You may find that the transected vessel end can be difficult to identify in the destroyed tissue. Although often thrombosed at the time, these vessels must be found and ligated because they will rebleed later after the patient is resuscitated. Retrograde advancement of a Fogarty catheter from an uninjured distal site can also be used to locate the transected artery in a horrific wound that is no longer bleeding. When making a decision to

amputate or salvage an extremity, you should consider the patients' condition, extent of injury, and your willingness to commit the patient to the necessary definitive orthopedic care and physical rehabilitation. No one situation or scoring system can replace the surgical judgment developed by an experience team.

An autologous repair is preferred. For small wounds with preserved muscle, an end-to-end anastomosis or a short reversed saphenous vein interposition graft is the best option. For larger wounds, a long graft well tunneled away from the zone of injury is always preferable to an exposed graft regardless of the composition. Vein grafts are prone to rupture at the anastomosis if they are placed into a dirty contaminated wound. A lengthy and meticulous debridement at the outset is not necessary as these wounds look much better in a few days after subsequent washouts and vacuum dressings. However, debridement of any obviously devitalized tissue is an essential early step of this operation. The saphenous vein is the preferred conduit for military vascular injuries. In the author's experience, prosthetic grafts placed in larger vessels with good muscle coverage have been used successfully. While prosthetic grafts for "clean" subclavian and carotid wounds can yield excellent results, the inferior long-term patency of prosthetic materials and the potential for infection in war wounds have restricted its widespread use in combat-related extremity wounds [39].

Ballistic trauma can transmit kinetic energy and result in intimal injury well beyond the transected arterial segment. Therefore, vascular debridement should be focused on the quality of the luminal surface and strength of the arterial inflow relative to the patients' hemodynamics. In military trauma, lack of adequate lighting, fine surgical instruments, desired monofilament sutures, and loupe magnification may disadvantage the careful tissue handling that is crucial to a successful vascular operation. In overcoming these expected obstacles, a four-quadrant, heel-to-toe anastomosis that is well spatulated is the easiest method to teach and perform in difficult situations. Small Heifetz clips or Bulldog clamps can also minimize the chance of a clamp injury.

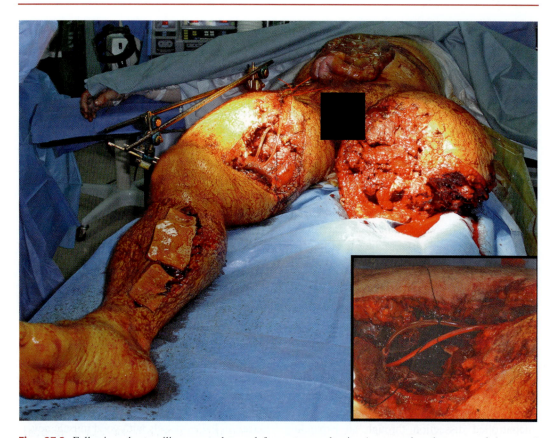

Fig. 27.2 Following hasty iliac control, a left transfemoral amputation, right leg fasciotomy with external fixation, and shunting of the superficial femoral artery and vein were performed for bilateral fragmentation wounds. Insert depicts the use of temporary shunting as a damage control adjunct for delayed repair of the artery and vein. A reversed saphenous graft harvested from the contralateral amputated leg was used to reconstruct the injured femoral artery and vein. At 1-year follow-up, the patient had a viable right lower extremity. He required 194 units of various blood products in the first 24 h (Adapted from Fox et al. [5])

Special precautions are worthwhile and should in particular include routine flushing of the graft and native artery with heparinized saline to dislodge fibrin strands and platelet debris.

The challenges of managing upper extremity injuries should not be underestimated, and they can often require massive transfusions, from ongoing blood loss and resuscitation requirements. The arm swelling and wound expansion that can result highlights the importance of a wide tunnel for a saphenous vein graft. There has been a sustained interest in repair of venous injuries to avoid the potential for early limb loss from venous hypertension or long-term disability from chronic edema. With combined injuries, arterial repair should precede venous repair to minimize further ischemic burden, unless the vein repair requires very little effort. Alternatively, temporary shunting of the artery during venous repair allows for reestablishment of venous outflow prior to definitive arterial injury repair or replacement.

The temporary use of shunts for military trauma is a very effective damage control technique to allow for delayed reconstruction. The value of temporary shunting should be compared with the consequences of simple ligation. For example, ligation of the brachial artery after confirming distal signals and palmar blood flow allows for elective delayed reconstruction if indicated. Surgeons at smaller remote facilities may prefer shunting when rapid evacuation to places capable of matching transfusion requirements or performing emergent complex vascular repairs is necessary (Fig. 27.2).

and the vascular shunt was removed and vascular reconstruction performed [20, 21]. This same sequence may also be effective in the civilian setting where temporary vascular shunts should be considered by less experienced surgeons or those at more rural hospitals. In these instances, a vascular shunt should be placed and secured upon exploration of the vascular injury and the patient evacuated to a larger hospital with expertise in vascular reconstruction.

The third indication for a temporary vascular shunt is in the setting of a patient with extremity vascular injury and other life-threatening injuries and/or severely compromised physiology. In these instances, the vascular shunt is applicable as part of an overall damage control resuscitation strategy allowing for extremity perfusion and reduction of ischemic burden while the patient is resuscitated or other life-threatening injuries are managed. Depending upon the injury scenario, the temporary vascular shunt may be placed prior to or concomitant with laparotomy, thoracotomy, craniotomy, or other procedure. The shunt may remain in place for 12–24 h while the patient is resuscitated and vascular repair can be considered. In rare multiple casualty scenarios which outstrip operating capacity, vascular shunts have been used as an expeditious way to restore extremity perfusion and clear an operating table. In such cases the patient is monitored in the intensive care unit until additional operating room space becomes available and the shunt can be removed in favor of vascular reconstruction.

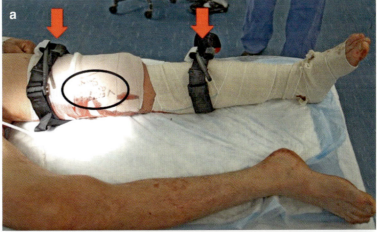

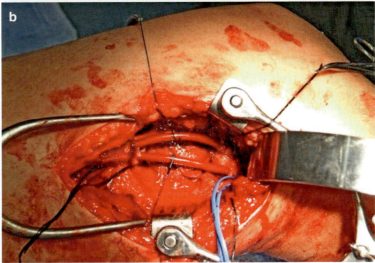

Fig. 28.2 (**a**) After sustaining a penetrating injury to the left thigh, a patient was initially treated with arterial and venous shunting as indicated on the dressing (*circled*). Additionally, tourniquets (*arrows*) were loosely applied and available in the case of shunt dislodgement. (**b**) Operative exposure of the same patient demonstrating in-line vascular shunts in the femoral artery and vein secured with silk sutures and a silastic loop

Finally, vascular shunts are indicated in scenarios of mangled extremity with ischemia or in cases of an extremity amputation in which reimplantation is attempted. As stated previously, vascular injury exploration and shunt placement should take priority in these scenarios to reduce the neuromuscular ischemic time. Once vascular flow is reestablished, then the associated extremity fracture or amputation can be carefully stabilized. In these and other scenarios, vascular shunts are often useful in the extremity vein as well as the artery.

28.4 Timing: When to Apply and for How Long

Shunts should be considered at the time of vascular injury exploration. Once in place shunts have remained patent without systemic anticoagulation for as long as 52 h. However, experience shows that most shunts are in place for 4–6 h and that the risk of shunt-related complications such as thrombosis or thromboemboli increases after 12 h [22]. Shunts which are used in larger vessels (axillary-brachial and femoral-popliteal) have a greater patency than those placed in small, distal vessels (forearm and tibial). In most instances patency of large proximal vascular shunts is maintained without systemic anticoagulation, which is often contraindicated in trauma. Even in cases where anticoagulation is not possible, local and regional heparinized saline (1,000–10,000 units/l) should be used to reduce platelet aggregation and thrombus formation at the time of shunt placement. It is the authors' observation that a low level of systemic anticoagulation is necessary to maintain patency in a shunt used in small, distal arteries. Experience from the war in Iraq showed that despite a higher rate of thrombosis, use of shunts in distal arteries did not detract from overall limb salvage.

28.5 Technical Considerations

Use of a temporary shunt begins with exposure and control of the vascular injury. In the extremity this may be facilitated with the use of tourniquets in order to temporarily control hemorrhage. If there is no bleeding from a wound, the tourniquet may not be necessary and control can be gained by operative exposure at or just proximal to the site of injury. Control of mesenteric vascular injuries can usually be obtained at or just proximal to the site of hemorrhage although control of the aorta above the celiac artery may be necessary. Once broad control of bleeding and the injury site is obtained, the exact site of the disrupted vessel(s) should be exposed. Dissection of the proximal and distal aspects of the injured vessel(s) is performed, and these segments are gently encircled with silastic vessel loops. One can next determine the extent of the injury which may range from a contusion with varying degrees of occlusion to transection of the vessel. At this stage in the operation, the surgeon must determine his or her mode of management: ligation, placement of a shunt, or vascular reconstruction. As previously noted, this decision depends on several factors including anatomic location of the vascular injury, physiological status of the patient, the experience of the surgeon, and the capacity of the medical facility in which the operation is taking place.

Before placing the vascular shunt, the open edges of the injured segment must be exposed and flow established using a combination of Fogarty thromboembolectomy catheters and flushes of heparinized saline. These steps establish proper inflow and outflow of the injured segment, and failure to do so equates to placing the shunt in an occluded vascular segment with no perfusion. At the least, the proximal inflow vessel must be opened, allowing brisk bleeding and flushing of platelet aggregate or thrombus. Regional heparinized saline should also be flushed in the injured vascular segment including the inflow and outflow using a soft plastic catheter or a metallic infusion instrument such as a St. Mark's injection tip. If there are no serious concomitant injuries, systemic anticoagulation should considered at this point as well.

Once the edges of the vascular segment have been debrided such that there is space to place the shunt, the distal end should be inserted and allowed to bleed in a retrograde fashion (i.e., "back bleed"). When grasping the shunt for positioning and insertion, it is important not to grasp too aggressively or to crimp the shunt. While most shunts are robust and resist impingement on their inner lumen, some have a wire lining which can be deformed with too aggressive of handling. Crushing or crimping of the internal lumen will result in restriction of flow and early thrombosis or occlusion. The depth of insertion will depend upon the length of the shunt as well as the length of the vascular defect.

Once the distal end of the shunt is placed, the proximal aspect of the vascular injury should be allowed to flush (i.e., "fore bleeding"), clearing any elements of platelet debris or thrombus. The proximal end of the shunt is then placed into this segment and perfusion established. Gentle release and then retraction of the silastic vessel loops at the proximal and distal aspects of the vascular injury are helpful in placement and securing of the device. If the vessel has contracted and the lumen significantly reduced in size, insertion can be facilitated by use of a small right-angled dissecting device inserted into this lumen and opened to spread or gently dilate the intended insertion site. Although the shunt should not be inserted any deeper than is necessary to secure it into a true luminal position, the important point is to make this step as easy and fluid as possible. Because the short, in-line shunts are not designed to loop, they often require deeper insertion in order to easily position the opposite end. In contrast, the longer, looped shunts tend to be more flexible and accommodating of very minimal insertion depth. Once the shunt is in the desired location and flow confirmed with continuous wave Doppler, it can be secured using silk ties around the edges of the vessel in which it is inserted.

28.6 Types of Shunts

Shunts used for vascular injury today were originally designed to provide cerebral perfusion during carotid endarterectomy and include (among others) the Sundt©, Javid©, Pruitt-Inahara©, and Argyle©. These devices have varying inner diameters ranging from 1.9 to 5.7 mm and fall into two categories including the short "in-line" and the long "external" or "looped" shunts (Table 28.1). The Sundt© shunt (Fig. 28.3) is a silicone elastomer reinforced with a spiral stainless steel wire within the wall to prevent kinking. The Sundt© has atraumatic bulb-tipped insertion ends and comes in a short (10 cm) in-line and a long (30 cm) external or looped design. The Javid© (Fig. 28.4) is a long, external shunt composed of a polished polymer and tapered ends to allow atraumatic insertion. The Pruitt-Inahara© (Fig. 28.5) is a long, external shunt made out of polyvinyl chloride and secured inside the vessel lumen by inflatable balloons on the proximal and distal ends. The Pruitt-Inahara© also has a side port that may be used for transducing blood pressure or infusing therapeutics. The Argyle© (Figs. 28.6 and 28.7) is a polyvinyl chloride in-line shunt available in 15 or 28 cm lengths. Each container of Argyle© shunts contains 8, 10, 12, and 14 Fr diameters. These shunts have all performed equally well with regard to insertion and patency in the military and civilian settings over the past decade. The choice of shunt may be left to the surgeon, but any of these commercially manufactured devices are preferred over improvised devices such as chest tubes, nasogastric tubes, or even intravenous tubing [23].

Table 28.1 Summary of commonly available temporary vascular shunts

Shunt model	Manufacturer	Style	Proximal diameter	Distal diameter	Length (cm)
Sundt©	Integra LifeSciences	In-line or looped	2.1–3.1 mm[a] 3.9–5 mm	1.3–2.2 mm[a] 2.7–4 mm	10, 30
Javid©	Bard Peripheral Vascular	Looped	17 Fr	10 Fr	27.5
Pruitt-Inahara©	LeMaitre Vascular	Looped	8–10 Fr	8–10 Fr	31
Argyle©	Bard Peripheral Vascular	In-line	8–14 Fr	8–14 Fr	15, 28

Fr French scale
[a]Denotes inner diameter, all other diameters reflect outer diameters

Fig. 28.3 The Sundt©
vascular shunt
(Integra LifeSciences) is a
silicone elastomer tube
reinforced with a spiral
stainless steel wire within the
wall to prevent kinking. The
ends are bulb tipped and
designed to be atraumatic to
ease insertion. It is available
as a short (**a**), 10 cm, in-line
and a long (**b**), 30 cm,
external or looped design.
Proximal internal luminal
diameters range from 2.1 to
3.1 mm with distal internal
diameters of 1.3–2.2 mm.
An optional 1 cm portion of
non-reinforcement (*arrow*) is
available to permit clamping
of the shunt

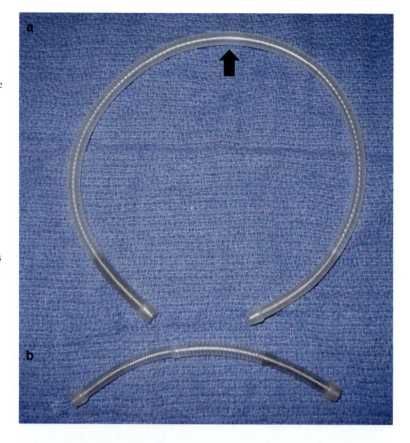

Fig. 28.4 The Javid©
(Bard Peripheral Vascular)
is a long (27.5 cm), external
or looped shunt composed
of a polished polymer and
tapered ends to allow
atraumatic insertion. The
external diameter tapers from
17 Fr at the proximal end to
10 Fr at the distal end

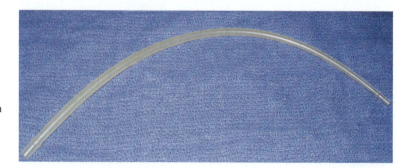

28.7 Vascular Shunting of Visceral Vascular Injury

Operative steps performed as part of damage control surgery have led to improved survival of patients sustaining severe abdominal trauma including mesenteric vascular injury. Although less common than extremity vascular injury, mesenteric injuries may also be amenable to the use of temporary shunts as part of this damage control approach. The rationale behind using these adjuncts in the abdomen is similar to that in the extremity as are the basic steps to vascular injury control, preparation, and shunt insertion. The same types of shunts used in the extremity vessels may be used in the mesentery, and like the extremity, low levels of anticoagulation should be considered if not contraindicated because of associated injury.

Fig. 28.5 The Pruitt-Inahara©
(LeMaitre Vascular) is a long
(31 cm), external shunt made
out of polyvinyl chloride and
secured inside the vessel
lumen by inflatable balloons
(*black arrows*) on the
proximal and distal ends.
The Pruitt-Inahara© also has a
side port (*red arrow*) that may
be used for transducing blood
pressure or infusing
therapeutics

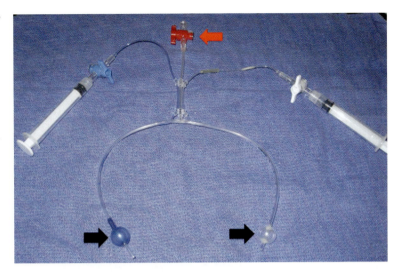

Fig. 28.6 The Argyle©
(Bard Peripheral Vascular)
is a 10 cm (**a**) or 28 cm (**b**),
polyvinyl chloride, in-line
shunt available in 8, 10, 12,
and 14 Fr diameters. A linear
radiopaque line (*arrow*) is
embedded within the wall of
the shunt to aid in
visualization on radiographs

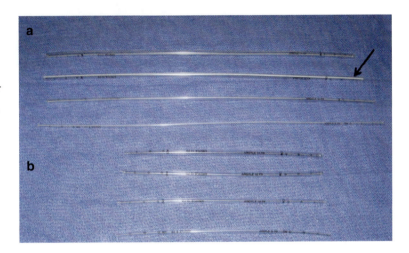

At least one recent translational large animal study has confirmed the feasibility and effectiveness of mesenteric artery shunting, and clinical case reports of this maneuver exist in the literature. Reilly and colleagues [12] described use of a vascular shunt to maintain midgut perfusion through a superior mesenteric artery injury in a patient having sustained a gunshot to the abdomen. In this case the shunt was placed as a temporizing measure to perfuse the intestine while the patient's coagulopathy and physiological derangements were corrected. With expanded use of damage control surgery and an increasing acceptance of temporary shunts for use in the setting of extremity vascular injury, it is likely that these adjuncts will continue to be an effective tool in select cases of mesenteric vascular trauma.

28.8 Shunt-Related Complications

The most common shunt-related complications are thrombosis and distal embolization. Thrombosis or occlusion is the more common of these complications and occurs more frequently when shunts have been placed in small, distal extremity vessels such as the tibial or forearm arteries [18, 24]. Shunt thrombosis is also prone to occur if one has not adequately cleared preexisting clot from

Fig. 28.7 Operative exposure demonstrating an injury to the left iliac artery with an Argyle© vascular shunt secured with silk sutures and vessel loops

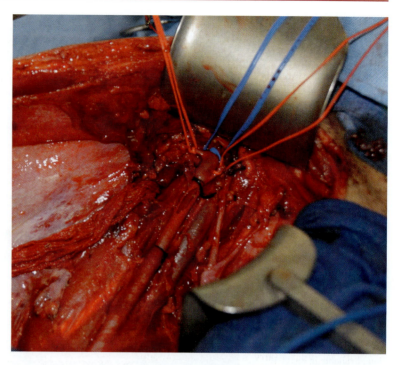

the inflow and outflow vessels or if the shunt's internal lumen has been crimped by aggressive handling. Finally the risk of occlusion is directly related to dwell time and increases significantly beyond 8–12 h. While research has shown shunts to remain patent in animal models for as long as 24 h without systemic anticoagulation, it is the authors' experience that dwell times greater than 8–12 h are associated with high rates of thrombosis. In scenarios requiring extreme shunting or dwell times of greater than 12 h, one should attempt to provide low levels of systemic anticoagulation to reduce these risks.

Interestingly when shunts do occlude, they appear to do so without distal embolization. While this observation is not uniform, it is rare that temporary vascular shunts lead to clinically significant distal thromboembolism. As an example the higher rate of thrombosis in small or distal arteries during the Iraq experience did not negatively impact the ability to complete vascular reconstruction or to salvage the limb. In most cases of thrombosis, the shunt is simply removed, thrombectomy performed, and vascular reconstruction accomplished as would have been required at the time of initial exploration.

Although a potentially serious complication, dislodgement of the temporary vascular shunt is extremely rare in the military or civilian experience. Even with the military's extensive medical evacuation experience, shunts appear to be stable once secured with appropriate maneuvers. Rare cases of dislodgment have been due to inadequate securing of the devise or the shunt having become entangled in the wound closure or dressing material. Because this complication could result in significant and even life-threatening hemorrhage, the military recommends placing a loose tourniquet on the extremity proximal to the shunt location in case it were to become dislodged.

The effect of shunts on the endothelium of the native vessel at the time of insertion and perfusion is an area of investigation. Ding et al. [25] studied the effects of shunts in a porcine model of superior mesenteric artery injury and found that irreversible damage occurred to the endothelium in contact with the device starting at 9 h of dwell time. These findings support efforts to minimize dwell time to only that which is necessary. Furthermore, this study suggests that once a shunt is removed, that an amount of vessel which has been in contact with the shunt should be debrided prior to vascular reconstruction. Importantly, emerging outcomes data on wartime extremity vascular injury suggests that there are no mid- or long-term sequelae of shunt use. Gifford and colleagues have reported that after 24 months of follow-up, those patients who had shunts used in the management of their injury had better freedom from amputation than those that did not [26]. This observation was especially pronounced in those with high mangled extremity severity scores and suggests these devices do not lead to clinically significant myointimal hyperplasia or stenosis.

28.9 Summary and Future Directions

Recognition of the need to improve quality and not just statistical limb salvage following extremity vascular injury has led to a broader acceptance and use of temporary vascular shunts. Specifically the burden of injury from the war and resulting translational research has shown benefit from more expedited reperfusion of injured limbs with an ischemic component. As such the future of this adjunct appears to be bright and will likely include the development of trauma-specific vascular injury shunts able to be recognized and used routinely by general and acute care surgeons for both extremity and mesenteric injuries. Shunts of the future may have larger internal diameters better suited to perfuse a limb and include infusion ports to allow for delivery of therapeutics able to mitigate ischemic injury [27]. Trauma-specific shunts with a side-port lumen may also allow for performance of arteriography and infusion of an anticoagulant to prevent shunt thrombosis or thromboembolism. In this context scenarios of extended shunt dwell times could be envisioned, allowing for stabilization of contaminated soft tissue wounds prior to shunt removal and vascular reconstruction. Just as temporary intraluminal devices for vascular trauma evolved a century ago, it is quite likely that innovation in their design, delivery, and clinical use will continue to expand in near and midterm.

References

1. Tien HC, Spencer F, Tremblay LN, Rizoli SB, Brenneman FD. Preventable deaths from hemorrhage at a level I Canadian trauma center. J Trauma. 2007;62(1):142–6.
2. Teixeira PGR, Inaba K, Hadjizacharia P, et al. Preventable or potentially preventable mortality at a mature trauma center. J Trauma. 2007;63(6):1338–46.
3. Eastridge BJ, Mabry RL, Seguin PG, Cantrell JA, Tops TL, Uribe PS, et al. Death on the battlefield (2001–2011): implications for the future of combat casualty care. J Trauma. 2012;73(6 Suppl 5):S431–7.
4. Kelly JF, Ritenour AE, McLaughlin DF, Bagg KA, Apodaca AN, Mallak CT, et al. Injury severity and causes of death from Operation Iraqi Freedom and Operation Enduring Freedom: 2003–2004 versus 2006. J Trauma. 2008;64(2):S21–6.
5. Tuffier T. French surgery in 1915. Br J Surg. 1917;4:420–32.
6. Bowlby A. The development of British surgery at the front. BMJ. 1917;1:705–21.
7. Blakemore AH, Lord JW. A nonsuture method of blood vessel anastomosis. Ann Surg. 1945;121(4):435–52.
8. DeBakey ME, Simeon FA. Battle injuries of the arteries in World War II. Ann Surg. 1946;123(4):534–79.
9. Spencer FC. Historical vignette: the introduction of arterial repair into the US Marine Corps, US Naval Hospital in July-August 1952. J Trauma. 2006;60(4):906–9.
10. Eger M, Golcman L, Goldstein A, Hirsch M. The use of a temporary shunt in the management of arterial vascular injuries. Surg Gynecol Obstet. 1971;132(1):67–70.
11. Rasmussen TE, Clouse WD, Jenkins DH, Peck MA, Eliason JL, Smith DL. Echelons of care and the management of wartime vascular injury: a report from the 332nd EMDG/Air Force Theater Hospital, Balad Air Base, Iraq. Perspect Vasc Surg Endovasc Ther. 2006;18(2):91–9.
12. Reilly P, Rotondo M, Carpenter JP, Sherr SA, Schwab CW. Temporary vascular continuity during damage control: intraluminal shunting for proximal superior mesenteric artery injury. J Trauma. 1995;39(4):757–60.
13. Feliciano DV. Management of peripheral arterial injury. Curr Opin Crit Care. 2010;16(6):602–8.
14. Malan E, Tattoni G. Physio- and anatomo-pathology of acute ischemia of the extremities. J Cardiovasc Surg. 1963;4:212–25.
15. Subramanian A, Vercruysse G, Dente C, Wyrzykowski A, King E, Feliciano DV. A decade's experience with temporary intravascular shunts at a civilian level I trauma center. J Trauma. 2008;65(2):316–24.
16. Burkhardt GE, Spencer JR, Gifford SM, Propper B, Jones L, Sumner N, et al. A large animal survival model (Sus scrofa) of extremity ischemia/reperfusion and neuromuscular outcomes assessment: a pilot study. J Trauma. 2010;69(1):S146–53.

17. Gifford SM, Eliason JL, Clouse WD, Spencer JR, Burkhardt GE, Propper BW, et al. Early versus delayed restoration of flow with temporary vascular shunt reduces circulating markers of injury in a porcine model. J Trauma. 2009;67(2):259–65.

18. Rasmussen TE, Clouse WD, Jenkins DH, Peck MA, Eliason JL, Smith DL. The use of temporary vascular shunts as a damage control adjunct in the management of wartime vascular injury. J Trauma. 2006;61(1):8–12.

19. Peck MA, Clouse WD, Cox MW, Bowser AN, Eliason JL, Jenkins DH, et al. The complete management of extremity vascular injury in a local population: a wartime report from the 332nd Expeditionary Medical Group/Air Force Theater Hospital, Balad Air Base, Iraq. J Vasc Surg. 2007;45(6):1197–204.

20. Chambers LW, Green DJ, Sample K, Gillingham BL, Rhee P, Brown C, et al. Tactical surgical intervention with temporary shunting of peripheral vascular trauma sustained during Operation Iraqi Freedom: one unit's experience. J Trauma. 2006;61(4):824–30.

21. Taller J, Kamdar JP, Greene JA, Morgan RA, Blankenship CL, Dabrowski P, et al. Temporary vascular shunts as initial treatment of proximal extremity vascular injuries during combat operations: the new standard of care at Echelon II facilities? J Trauma. 2008;65(3):595–603.

22. Granchi T, Schmittling Z, Vasquez J, Schreiber M, Wall M. Prolonged use of intraluminal arterial shunts without systemic anticoagulation. Am J Surg. 2000;180(6):493–6.

23. Sriussadaporn S, Pak-art R. Temporary intravascular shunt in complex extremity. J Trauma. 2000;52(6):1129–33.

24. Dawson DL, Putnam AT, Light JT, Ihnat DM, Kissinger DP, Rasmussen TE, et al. Temporary arterial shunts to maintain limb perfusion after arterial injury: an animal study. J Trauma. 1999;47(1):64–71.

25. Ding W, Ji W, Wu X, Li N, Li J. Prolonged indwelling time of temporary vascular shunts is associated with increased endothelial injury in the porcine mesenteric artery. J Trauma. 2011;70(6):1464–70.

26. Gifford SM, Aidinian G, Clouse WD, Fox CJ, Porras CA, Jones WT, et al. Effect of temporary shunting on extremity vascular injury: an outcome analysis from the Global War on Terror vascular injury initiative. J Vasc Surg. 2009;50(3):549–55.

27. Simon F, Giudici R, Duy CN, Schelzig H, Oter S, Gröger M, et al. Hemodynamic and metabolic effects of hydrogen sulfide during porcine ischemia/reperfusion injury. Shock. 2008;30(4):359–64.

Index

A. Dua et al. (eds.), *Clinical Review of Vascular Trauma*,
DOI 10.1007/978-3-642-39100-2, © Springer-Verlag Berlin Heidelberg 2014

Printing and Binding: Stürtz GmbH, Würzburg